S. Niwa J.P. Paul S. Yamamoto (Eds.)

# Total Knee Replacement

Proceeding of the International Symposium
on Total Knee Replacement,
May 19–20, 1987, Nagoya, Japan

With 199 Figures

Springer-Verlag
Tokyo Berlin Heidelberg New York London Paris

SHIGEO NIWA, M.D.
Professor
Department of Orthopedics
Aichi Medical University
Aichi, 480–11 Japan

JOHN P. PAUL, B.Sc. Ph.D.
Professor
Bioengineering Unit
University of Strathclyde
Glasgow G4 ONW
Scotland, UK

SUMIKI YAMAMOTO, M.D.
Head
Centre for Rheumatic Disease
Matsuyama Red Cross Hospital
Matsuyama
Ehime, 790 Japan

**ISBN-13: 978-4-431-68077-2** **e-ISBN-13: 978-4-431-68075-8**
**DOI: 10.1007/ 978-4-431-68075-8**


**Softcover reprint of the hardcover 1st edition 1988**



Typesetting: Asco Trade Typesetting, Hong Kong

# Preface

Back in September of 1974, I acquired much valuable information while attending the International Conference on Total Knee Replacement in London, which was organized by The Medical Engineering Working Party and the Tribology Group of the Institution of Mechanical Engineers, and the British Orthopaedic Association. I was greatly inspired by the conference, and it formed the beginning of my studies on total knee replacement. The co-editors of this proceedings, Prof. J. Paul and Dr. S. Yamamoto, are both acquaintances made originally at that conference.

The International Symposium on Total Knee Replacement held in Nagoya, Japan, on 18–19 May 1987 was attended by many participants, including Prof. Walker, who had presented his studies earlier in London. During the past decade and a half, remarkable technical progress has been made in total knee prostheses. In this symposium, cemented total knee replacement (TKR), noncemented TKR, design considerations of total knee prostheses, problems concerning the patello-femoral joint, and the newly developed total knee prosthesis were the main topics discussed.

I believe that much new information, including that about the challenges which still remain, along with a fresh view towards continuing studies, are presented here for the reader.

I would like to express my sincere gratitude to the support of the Knee Joint Research Society in Japan and to the participants in the symposium for their great help in publishing this book.

Shigeo Niwa

# Contents

# Key Note Lecture

# Computer Graphics Design of Total Knee Replacement

P.S. WALKER[1]

**Summary.** While many existing designs of total knee are derivative, relying for the most part on features which are present in other existing designs, rigorous application of the engineering design method can theoretically result in an improved end result. There should be more innovative features due to the attention paid to the creative phase. The device should be safer and more successful due to the methodical approach to anaylsis, testing, and optimization. The surgical application should be more reproducible and accurate due to the iterative approach to design and instrumentation. Finally, the design should highlight those areas which are in need of further research for future breakthroughs. In brief, the design method involves the following steps: (a) Define the objectives, (b) list the criteria, (c) divide the criteria into musts (absolutes) and wants (relative), (d) give the wants a score, (e) formulate solutions (creative phase), (f) eliminate solutions not satisfying musts, (g) score remaining solutions, (h) select best one to three solutions for further study; (i) carry out testing, analysis, and optimization as needed, (j) make final decision.

Starting with the objective of designing a condylar replacement knee with maximum versatility and simplicity, we have used existing knowledge and new research to produce a design where each feature is optimized as much as possible.

The shape of the femoral component was derived by sectioning a large number of knees and obtaining the average condylar geometry. The tibial profile shape was similarly determined.

The tibial bearing surface was generated by moving the femoral component in a multitude of positions to produce a surface giving required motion and laxity, and stability suitable for cruciate retention or sacrifice.

The patellar flange and component is an often neglected aspect, which was designed by producing partially conforming surfaces, allowing normal variation of motion in all degrees of freedom without excess conformity, which can lead to loosening. The tibial fixation pegs/posts/blades for both press-fit or cemented application were designed after exhaustive testing of pressure distribution in response to offset loading, shear forces, and torques.

The instrumentation was designed with the objectives of maximum simplicity and accuracy.

Based on our experience with this design process and with our previous designs, the areas which are in need of further research are the patellofemoral joint, a new material or materials for the bearing surfaces, and more accurate cuts on the bone.

**Keywords:** Computer graphics—Design—Follow-up—Total knee replacement

## Introduction

Many of the existing designs of total knee are derivative, relying for the most part on features which were already present in other designs. Component geometry has usually been obtained from planar radiographic information or from approximation to a number of anatomical samples. Anthropometric studies, which have been useful for deciding upon the range of sizes, have been restricted to linear measurements. The articulating surfaces have often been simplified for ease of definition and manufacture. The relative geometry between the femoral and tibial surfaces, which determines the range of motion, laxity, and stability, has covered the extremes from complete conformity to complete lack of conformity. For a particular fixation method, such as cement or biological ingrowth, there have been a wide variety of means of anchoring the components to the bone. Despite the extensive knowledge gained from theoretical, experimental, and clinical studies, there is still no clear evidence of the optimum design features, and a variety of design solutions may be valid.

However, with the advances made in computer technology over the past few years, techniques of design which can significantly enhance the design process are now available. Computergraphics is one of these techniques, which is particularly useful to a problem such as implant design because of the importance of geometry and fit. Rather than relying on two-dimensional data for bone geometry, three-dimensional shapes can readily be

[1] Orthopedic Biomechanics Laboratory, Brigham and Women's Hospital, Boston, USA; Institute of Orthopaedics, Royal National Orthopaedic Hospital, Stanmore, UK

described and displayed. Color enhancement, hidden-line removal, solid shading, and displaying from multiple directions, provide almost real-life visualization. Fit of a component onto the bone and the relative motion between two or more components can be seen by superposition. Surfaces can be generated for specific motion patterns using specialized software. Analyses can more readily be carried out, such as motion, contact stresses, and component material stresses. Finally, prototypes as well as final molds and parts can be rapidly produced by transmitting data electronically and using computer-assisted machining (CAM).

Nevertheless, it must be remembered that the computer is a sophisticated tool, and the engineering design process must not be lost sight of. In brief, the design process involves the following main steps:

Definition of objectives
Formulation of solutions
Selection of best one to three solutions for further study
Carrying out testing, analysis, and optimization
Final decision.

Using this method, there should be more innovative features due to the attention paid to the design formulation phase. The device should be safer and more durable due to the methodical approach to analysis, testing, and optimization. The surgical application should be more reproducible and accurate due to the iterative approach to design and instrumentation. Finally, those areas which are in need of further research for future design ideas will be highlighted.

### Major Objective and Criteria

The major objective was to design a condylar replacement knee with maximum versatility, durability, and simplicity, applicable for cement or press-fit, and with or without the cruciate ligaments. The criteria for the different aspects of the design were as follows.

**Femoral component.** The overall profiles and curvatures should be closely anatomical for accurate fit and replication of normal kinematics, cruciate lengths, and quadriceps lever arm. A symmetrical component was desirable, so long as this could be justified geometrically.

**Patellofemoral joint.** The femoral flange should be anatomical to allow retention of the normal patella, and there should be a smooth transition from the flange to the distal condyles. There should be adequate laxity to allow for variations in tracking. Conformity should be sufficient to limit wear and deformation to acceptable limits.

**Tibial surface.** Using the available plastic material, polyethylene, the main criterion was to minimize the contact stresses, consistent with achieving anatomical motion and laxity. At the same time, there should be adequate stability with or without the cruciate ligaments. A further criterion was component interchangeability, to allow, for example, a standard-sized femoral to be used with a large tibial. These various criteria for the tibial surface appear to be conflicting, but as will be seen, a solution was reached without undue compromise.

**Tibial fixation elements (e.g., pegs, posts, keels).** These should enable the component to be used with cement or press-fit, with compromise of neither. For cemented application, there should be retardation of interface breakdown. For press-fit, the fixation elements should maximally resist offset loading (e.g., varus), shear, and torque.

**Instrumentation.** This should be simple enough to avoid logistical errors or uncertainty in use. The number of parts should be minimized for ease of inventory control in the operating room. Accuracy of cuts should be within 2° with prevention of extreme errors of more than about 4°.

## Existing Knowledge

### Evolution of Designs

To formulate a new design, a useful first stage is to identify the strong and weak points of the present designs. This will be done in the present article with a brief review and a report of our own institutional data on retrieved total knees and clinical follow-ups. Metal-plastic total knee replacement (TKR) was first introduced in the late 1960s. Among the first designs were the Polycentric, the Freeman-Swanson, the Geomedic, and the DuoCondylar [61]. During the 1970s, many other designs were introduced, some being adaptions to address the problems with the early designs, and others with new concepts. During that decade, clinical problems were reported due to inadequate instrumentation, inaccurate component alignment, poor cement technique, excessive device constraint, absence of patellofemoral replacement, and lack of ligament balancing. However, reviews published in the early 1980s suggested that for some designs at least problems occurred in only a few percent of cases at up to 10 years follow-up [13, 16, 29, 58].

## Analysis of 90 Retrieved Metal-Plastic TKRs

Previous retrieval studies have shown that the wear was potentially more serious than in total hips due to the high stresses on the plastic surface. The present study was particularly valuable in that a large number of implants was studied over long follow-up times. The series consisted of 90 TKRs removed from patients at the Brigham and Women's Hospital [33]. The plastic in all cases was ultra-high-molecular weight polyethylene. The implant time ranged from 3 months to 10 years with a mean of 5.6 years. Twenty TKRs were in place for more than 8 years, and only five for less than 2 years. The cases were all condylar replacements, with a variety of femoral-tibial geometries. Most of the designs were Unicondylar, Duocondylar, and Duopatella, but the Marmor, Geomedic, and a variety of others were also included.

The reason for removal in over a third of the cases was loosening of the tibial components, while the next most frequent category was pain in the patellofemoral joint, usually in designs without a flange. Pain for other reasons, instability, sepsis, and component breakage, made up the remainder. In analyzing the wear, it must be recognized that fragmented cement particles in loose components could have an effect.

The plastic components were examined using low-power microscopy. Thin sections of plastic from each component were cut with a scalpel and examined under transmitted light microscopy. Small cubes were cut from 20 components and studied with scanning electron microscopy. Similar blocks of plastic from 21 components were used for molecular weight analysis, using high-temperature gel-permeation chromatography (Jordi Associates, Millis, MA, USA).

Embedded acrylic cement particles were seen in 43% of components, while craters where cement had been present were seen in 74% of components. The plastic was often severely abraded in the vicinity. Deformation or cold flow occurred in most components. It was seen on the main bearing area, near the edges due to subluxation, and on the tibial eminence due to digging in of the metal femoral component in internal-external rotation. Abrasion, seen as scratches, grooves, and stretching of multiple fibers of plastic on the surface, also occurred on most components.

An important type of surface breakdown, delamination, occurred on over a third of components. This was seen as subsurface cracking, raised flakes of material, multiple cracks and fragmentation, and surface cavities (Fig. 1). The subsurface cracks were usually parallel to the surface and were at least 100 $\mu m$ in width. Sections of unused plastic often showed many small cavities or discontinuities. In some cases, fine lines could be seen in a network. This pattern became accentuated in used implants, and in some of the longer-term cases almost complete breakdown of the material could be seen. Since the material is compression-molded by fusion of small granules, it is believed that the fine lines represent granule

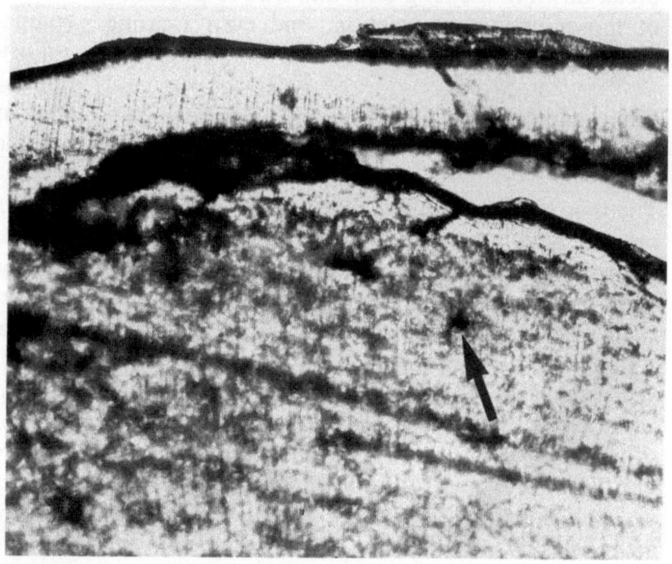

**Fig. 1.** A section through the polyethylene surface showing delamination wear, probably caused by excessive subsurface stresses. Note the intergranular cracking and defects (*arrow*)

boundaries and that high stresses and inadequate fusion led to the breakdown.

It has been found in laboratory wear tests that wear increases with high-contact stress and low molecular weight [49]. In our group of samples, there was a wide variety of molecular weight. The high-molecular weight fraction ranged from 723 000 to 4 670 000. The low-molecular weight fraction values were from 46 000 to 654 000. The overall wear per year correlated with best ambulatory status, while for similar components from one manufacturer there was a linear relation between overall wear and years of follow-up. There was also a relation between wear per year and molecular weight. Particularly striking were compressive-molded flat Marmor components, which would show high-contact stresses. These components had high molecular weight and showed minimal wear at 8–10 years follow-up.

The most striking finding from this wear study was the overall severity, far greater than has been reported for total hips. In many cases, much of the wear was due to abrasion from bone or cement, which is avoidable by attention to surgical technique. However, at the metal-plastic contact points, the stresses have been measured and calculated to be higher than the compressive strength of the plastic. The stresses are higher the less the conformity, with the highest von Mises stresses being subsurface. With repetitive loading, this will lead to fatigue failure, seen as cracks, eventually liberating particles from the surface. The initiation of the cracks will be enhanced by small fusion defects in the plastic, while low molecular weight will lead to more extensive and rapid crack propogation. It appeared that the plastic surface could severely break down in the long term and lead to problems of loosening, tissue reaction, and even wearing through the plastic completely.

## Clinical Follow-up of 1069 Kinematic Condylar Knees

The first 1069 consecutive cases in 798 patients of primary Kinematic Condylar TKR (Fig. 2) carried out by nine staff orthopedists at the Brigham and Women's Hospital were reviewed [17, 59].

The follow-up times were: 0–1 years, 386 cases; 1–2 years, 191 cases; 2–3 years, 113 cases; 3–4 years, 67 cases; 4–5 years, 43 cases; 5–6 years, 20 cases; 6–7 years, 2 cases. There was an age range of 12–90 years, with an average age of 67 years and 77% of the cases were female. There were 47.7% osteoarthritis (OA), 46.8% rheumatoid arthritis (RA), and 2.4% juvenile rheumatoid arthritis (JRA). For 667 cases, there was a complete clinical history, with a minimum of 1 year follow-up. There were 836 cases available for the radiographic alignment study; in 616 cases, a minimum of 6 months' follow-up was available for the radiographic interface study.

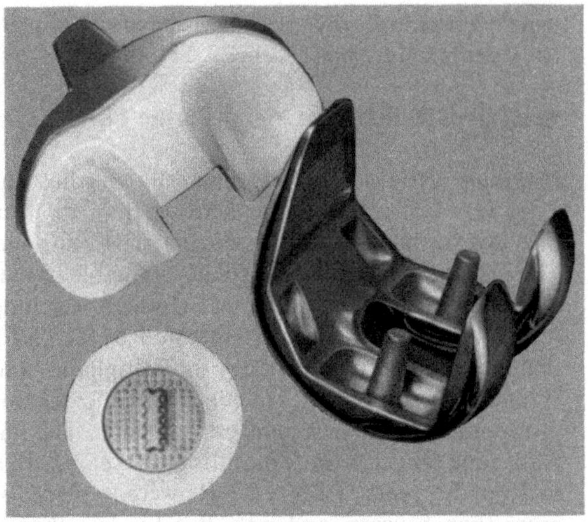

**Fig. 2.** The Kinematic Condylar Total Knee Replacement with a metal-backed tibial component

The most recent radiographs were measured for component and leg alignments by digitizing points on the bones and components into a computer. The cement-bone interface was studied for radiolucent lines (RLL) in seven tibial zones (anteroposterior view) and five femoral zones mediolateral (view). The total RLL score was calculated as the sum of the RLL thicknesses (to the nearest millimeter) measured in each zone. Thus, a uniform 1-mm RLL all round the tibial component would have a score of 7.

Postoperatively, 93% of the patients had no or minimal pain on all activities; 82% could negotiate stairs normally, and the others had to lead with the other leg. The range of motion averaged 2.5°–107°.

The aseptic revisions were as follows: loose femoral component, no cases; loose tibial component, one; skin necrosis (patellectomy to close), one; patella button loose, six; patella subluxing, five; patella transverse fracture, two; patella painful, one; and patella dislocation, one. These total 17 of 667 cases (2.5%). Other complications were: deep sepsis (nine retained, one exchanged), 11 cases; transient problems (skin, hematoma, etc. no additional surgery), 29 cases

It was notable that all of the patellar loosenings occurred in rheumatoid patients, implicating poor bone quality or valgus alignment as possible causes.

From the radiographic alignment data, the mean and standard deviations (means ± SD) of various angles were calculated. In the frontal view, the tibial component was aligned in 2° of varus, SD 2.7°. The femoral component was at 6.5° of valgus, SD 3.8°. In the sagittal view, the tibial component was sloped back 3° ± 4.7°. The femoral was flexed 4° ± 6°.

The incidence of interface radiolucency on the femoral and tibial components was 14% and 30%, respectively. The RLLs on the tibial component occurred primarily at the extreme medial or lateral zones, the inner zones having less than half the incidence (Fig. 3). RLL around the peg occurred in only a few cases. There was a slight trend for the incidence of RLL to increase with time, but these were mainly small RLLs at the sides. The scores for the femoral components were mainly 1, indicating a 1-mm RLL in only one zone, usually the posterior or anterior flange, where it is difficult to achieve good cement pressurization and where high stresses and micromotion occur.

The data on the 21 cases with RLL scores greater or equal to 4 were particularly interesting. Of these 21 cases, there were 12 cases of cement filling wedge-shaped defect or thick cement layer, seven cases of both medial and lateral RLL where the cause was not evident, and two cases with varus or valgus deformity.

It was evident that the wedge-shaped defects were the most common situation when radiolucent lines occurred (Fig. 4). This can be addressed using metal wedges and longer stems [9]. Loosening of major components was not a problem, though longer-term loosening is still a possibility. The patella was the main problem with loosening probably due to poor bone and high valgus and subluxation due to a variety of factors.

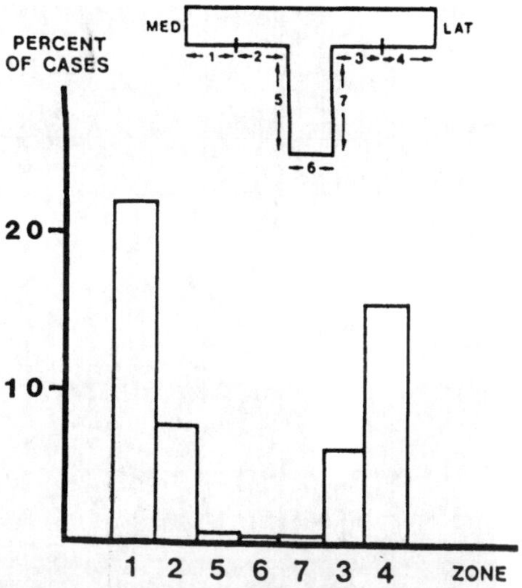


**Fig. 3.** The incidence of radiolucency in each zone at the tibial component-bone interface for 616 cases of Kinematic Condylar with 0.5–7 years follow-up

## Summary of Current Status

A study of the causes of failure in the retrieval study indicated that some of the main causes of component loosening (mostly tibial) were inadequate coverage, insufficiently rigid plastic unicondylar components, poor cement technique, and misalignment. Disregarding the avoidable wear due to direct bone or cement abrasion, it appeared that the stresses on the plastic surface are excessive [5], leading to a delamination type of wear which could result in serious long-term problems. Apart from alternative design configurations such as sliding meniscus bearings [23], the femoral-tibial surfaces should be as conforming as possible, consistent with adequate motion and laxity and sufficiently low interface shear stresses. When using metal trays, the use of thin (e.g., 6-mm) components has to be ruled out, especially with heavy patients or those with long life expectancy.

Loosening of metal femoral components has been only a minor problem. Experiments and analyses of various types of design of tibial component have led to the conclusion that single-piece metal-backed components with a central peg provide a reasonably normal stress distribution at the interface and in the bone [6, 35, 43, 46, 60, 62]. The relatively low loosening rate of central peg designs, a few percent over a period of 5–10 years, has been already mentioned. Attention to achieving good cement penetration at surgery is likely to be a factor [31]. The slow progression of the RLL is also encouraging, even though there is a theoretical basis for expecting steady propagation with time [55]. A central peg will extend the fixation life if the radiolucent line extends completely across the upper surface. Nonetheless it is likely that radiographic views underestimate the extent of fibrous tissue at the bone-cement interface, based on data on component-bone deformations [24, 52].

Many of the tibial loosenings and radiolucencies reported in the literature can be ascribed to misalignment [4, 12]. In our Kinematic follow-ups, even though the average alignments were ideal, the standard deviations of 3°–4° were excessive. This has since been improved to 2°–3° using an intramedullary (IM) guide system, a finding reported

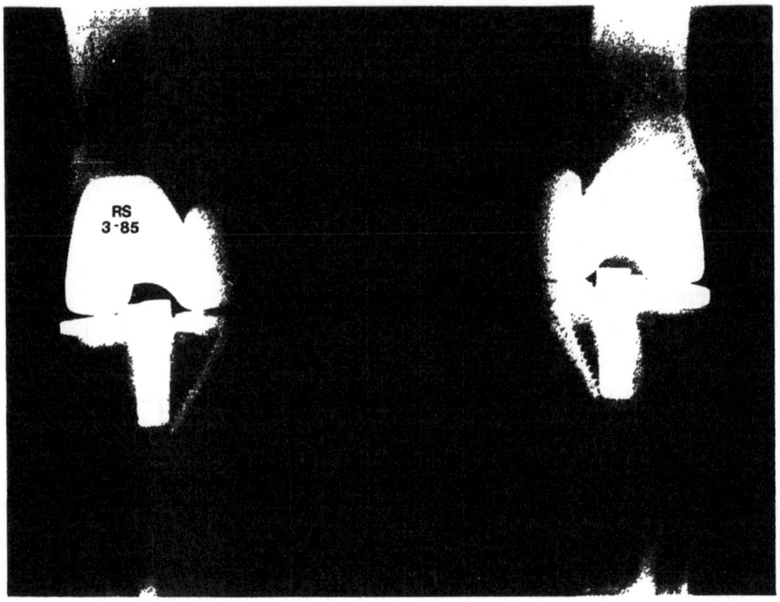


**Fig. 4.** A typical example of radiolucency beneath a wedge of cement used to fill a bone deficiency

by others [34]. Thus, there would appear to be a strong case for the use of an IM guide, especially for the femur.

By far the biggest single problem in our series was at the patellofemoral joint. Others have reported a similar experience [10, 11, 20, 29, 40, 57]. The problems have included clicking and catching, subluxation, dislocation, loosening, bone fractures, and mechanical failure. In the last category, wearing through of the plastic to the metal backing or dissociation of the plastic from the metal has presented a serious metal-on-metal wear problem.

In conclusion, although many of the early problems have been solved or reduced in significance, several important problems remain.

## Femoral Surface Design

Previous studies have determined the overall dimensions of the knee [39] or details of the sagittal profiles of the femoral condyles, modeling them by circular arcs or spirals [44, 53, 54]. Other features such as the shape and angle of the patellar groove have been studied [19]. Three-dimensional considerations have been relatively recent, using polynomials [65], geometrical analogs [64], or triangular surface plates [15].

For our study, points around serial sections were stored in a computer data file to provide a surface description. Twenty-three knees were used. To define a reproducible axis system, radius gages in a jig were used to determine the centers of the posterior condyles, and a metal rod was drilled through to define a transverse axis. The second axis passed through the center of the rod and was parallel to the femoral long axis. The third axis was mutually perpendicular. The knee (including the tibia) was embedded in foam and 24 uniform sagittal slices were cut, exposing 25 sections. The sections were digitized into a computer and the coordinates scaled linearly to magnify or reduce the femur to a standard medial-lateral width of 80 mm. To produce an "average knee," the profiles of all 23 knees for the same section number were superimposed on the computer screen. An interactive profile averaging technique [51] was used to determine the average profile. The averages for all 25 sections were so obtained and reconstructed in the computer (Fig. 5). Graphical programs enabled the visualization at any viewing angle, while solid modeling (using MOVIE.BYU) enabled better visualization at the oblique angles.

For the purposes of femoral component design, a piecewise mathematical analog was constructed. The posterior condyles were modeled as spherical, the distal condyles as toroidal, and the patellar groove as conical with a toroidal base and sides. This parametrized model accurately modeled the surfaces. The asymmetry of the anatomical femoral condyles was found to be primarily due to rounding off and chamfering of corners, rather than asymmetry of the bearing surfaces. The profiles of the lateral and medial condyles and the base of the patellar groove essentially lay on three parallel planes.

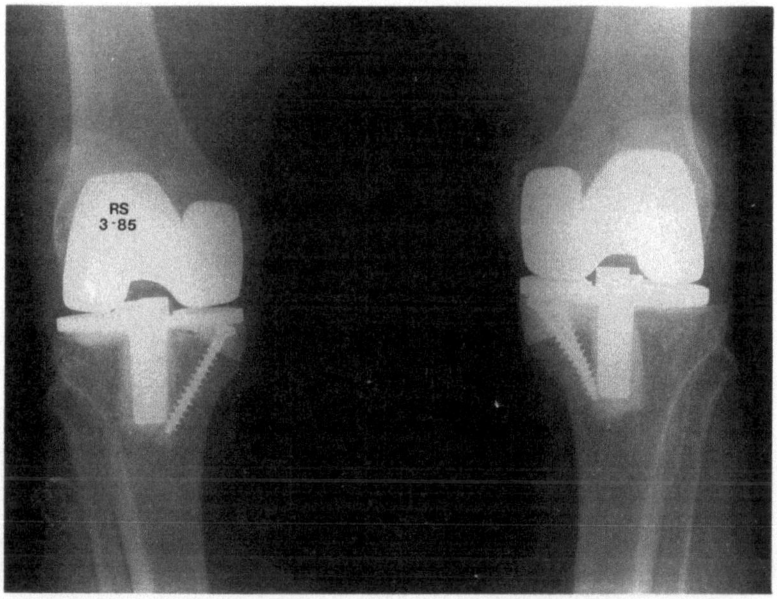

Fig. 5. Computer graphics displays of the average knee

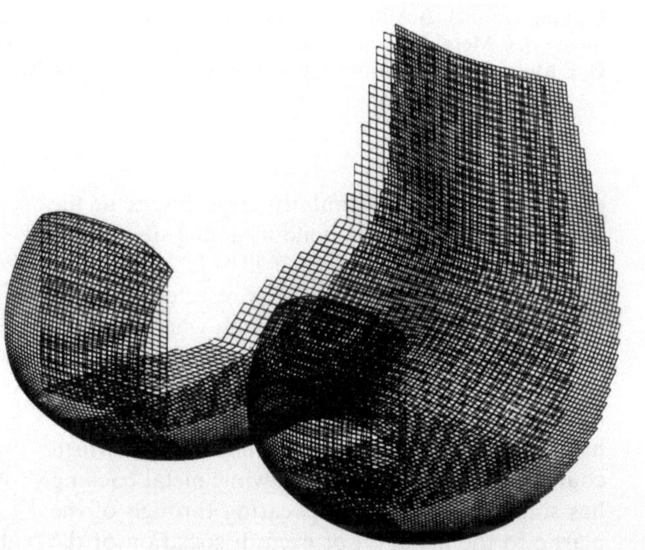

Fig. 6. The femoral component, described by a modified mathematical analog of the anatomical surfaces

The radius of the femoral condyles in the frontal plane was 20 mm. However, for the femoral component design, this was increased to 30 mm to facilitate medial-lateral laxity and reduce the contact stresses. Provision of normal medial-lateral laxity was necessary in our design to facilitate femoral-tibial component interchangeability. A benefit of the 30 mm radius was a perfect and continuous transition from the patellar flange to the distal condyles. The femoral component surface is shown in Fig. 6.

## Patellofemoral Joint

Correct biomechanics of the patellofemoral joint is crucial to the function of the knee. Even if the patella itself appears to be functioning correctly, a disadvantageous lever arm, with the resulting quadriceps inefficiency, has been implicated in impaired ability to ascend and descend stairs [3]. In a number of follow-up studies of TKR, cited earlier, failure of this joint is more common than problems with the femoral and tibial components combined. This is perhaps not surprising considering that the forces on the small patellar bone can reach up to about six times body weight at varying locations

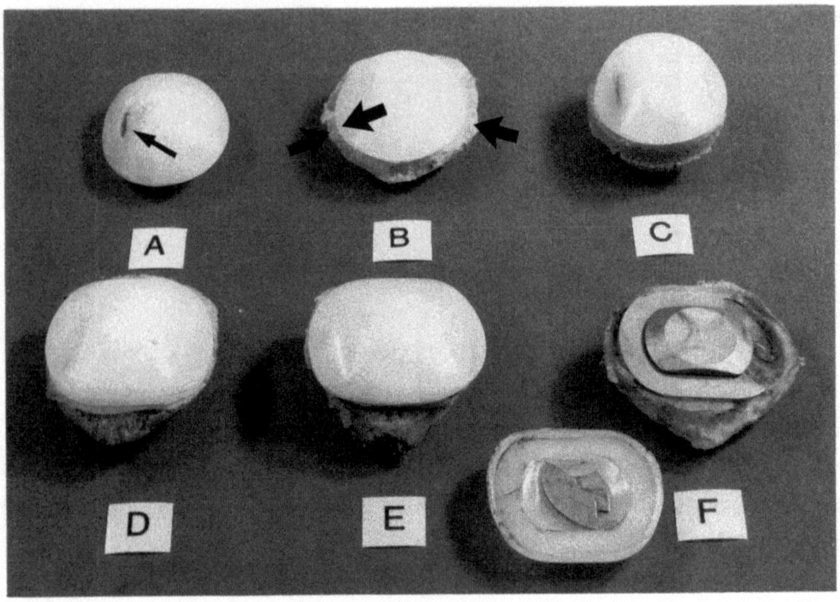


**Fig. 7.** Experimental wear patterns of different patellar designs. **A** Removed from a patient. Note the exposed metal backing (*arrow*). **B** All-plastic dome. This is deformed elliptically, and shows bone deformation under the contacts (*arrows*). **C** Metal-backed dome, worn through to the metal. **D** Conforming design with less wear and deformation than **B**. **E** Metal-backed conforming; almost worn to metal. **F** Metal-backed, showing fracture and plastic dissociation

on the surface, with similarly large forces in the quadriceps and patellar tendon acting at varying directions to the patella itself [2, 14, 26, 45]. Almost half of the patellar bone is resected to insert the patellar resurfacing component, which leads to elevated stresses within the bone and on the bone surface [22, 38]. Construction of patellar replacements has presented a dilemma. All-plastic designs have been susceptible to deformation [25], which could contribute to loosening, while metal backing has sometimes resulted in wearing through of the plastic to the metal [7] or even dissociation of the plastic and metal, leading to serious metal-on-metal wear.

In an effort to address some of these problems, additional studies were carried out.

## Wear and Deformation

To study wear and deformation (Hsu and Walker, unpublished data), a cyclic-motion test machine was constructed. The femoral component was mounted on a shaft which oscillated through an angle of 45°. The patellar button was mounted on real or artificial bone and attached to the end of a pneumatic load cylinder. The patella was loaded onto the patellar flange with a force of 1500 N (twice body weight), while the femoral component oscillation corresponded to a flexion range of 55°–100°. Distilled water was used as lubricant. The tests were run for 500 000 cycles or until failure. The contact areas were measured at regular intervals using Fujifilm. Various designs of the patellar component were tested against a Kinematic Condylar femoral component: an all-plastic dome-shaped patella, a plastic dome-shaped patella with metal-backing, an all-plastic conforming patella (conforming in skyline view only), and a plastic conforming patella with metal-backing. Figure 7 shows some of the results.

In all cases, the contact occurred initially as two small patches each about 20 mm$^2$ in area on the lateral and medial sides. This area increased rapidly at first but then slowed down considerably once the contact area had doubled.

With the all-plastic dome, the plastic became elliptical, being squeezed in form the sides, consistent with clinical observations [25]. The bone beneath the contact areas suffered some compression failure. With the metal-backed dome, the wear progressed through to the metalbacking, replicating the condition observed in a few clinical cases [7].

The all-plastic conforming patellas showed reduced deformation of the plastic and underlying bone compared with the dome-shaped patella due

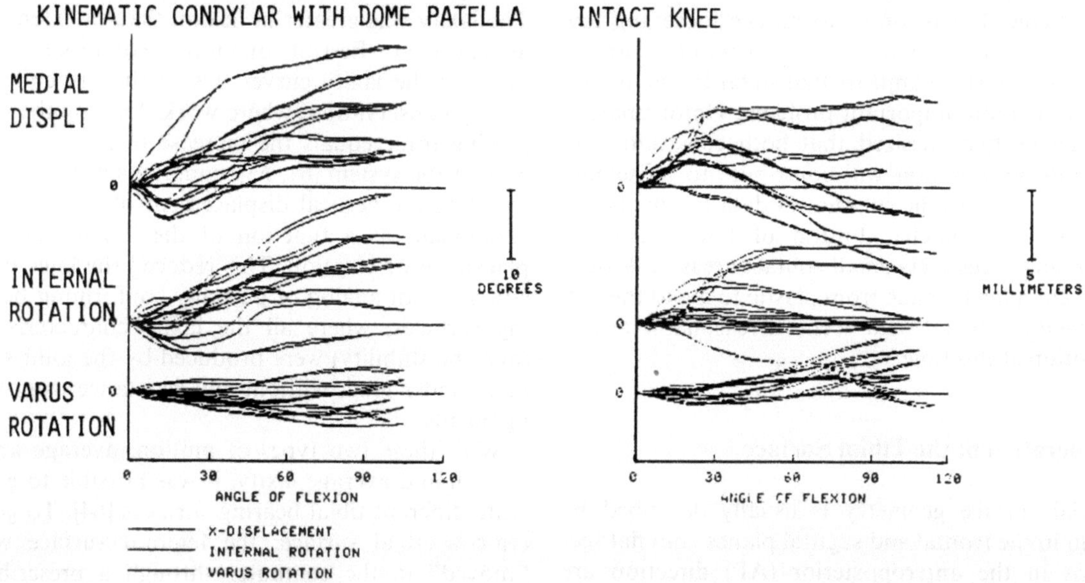


**Fig. 8.** Tracking of the normal patella relative to the femur. The graphs show medial-lateral motion, internal-external rotation, and varus-valgus rotation. Variations between knees and for each particular knee can be seen

to the increased thickness of plastic beneath the contact areas. The increased plastic thickness above the metal backing also resulted in a much greater time before wearing through to the metal. However, compared with the all-plastic patella, the plastic thickness was reduced to make room for the metal, and it was only a matter of time before wearing through took place.

### Motion and Tracking

The second study [30] used a dynamic test machine [47, 50] to measure the 3D motion of the patella relative to the femur before and after prosthetic replacement. Eight fresh specimens were mounted in the machine to a defined axis system. The source and sensor of a Polyhemus 3-Space Tracker were attached to the femur and patella, respectively. As the knee was dynamically flexed and extended using force in the quadriceps, the 3D patellofemoral motion was recorded. The motion was first recorded for the intact knee. Then, a Kinematic Condylar Total Knee, preserving the posterior cruciate, was inserted using standing instrumentation. Motion was recorded with the natural patella. Motion was next recorded with an unconstrained dome patella inserted. To test a more conforming patellar replacement, the original PCA patella was tested with the standard Porous Coated Anatomic (PCA) total knee.

The motions which were the most relevant are shown in Fig. 8. The eight intact knees showed different motions. However, there was one common feature in all but one, a lateral to medial displacement of 3–6 mm in the initial stage of flexion accompanied by an internal rotation of up to 10°. This behavior was due to the patella being initially tilted over to the lateral side in extension, caused by the Q-angle, a relatively small quadriceps force, and a shallow patellar groove. In the flexion range of 30°–110°, the medial displacement and internal rotation remained relatively constant or changed only gradually. Varus rotation linearly increased to as much as 10° during flexion.

After prosthetic replacement with the natural patella and the dome patella, the motion was again variable from knee to knee, but the ranges were very similar to those for the intact knee. The initial range of flexion was seen to be important. It appeared necessary for the femoral flange to be sufficiently wide and deep superiorly in order to capture the patella and ensure that it tracked correctly without subluxation. The motion for the constrained PCA patella was again variable from knee to knee but the ranges of the motion parameters were reduced by about a half due to the constraint. This would impose shear forces and torques on the patella, possibly leading to loosening (the current PCA patella is less constrained).

Thus, the two above studies seem to suggest conflicting design criteria. In order to reduce deformation and wear, greater conformity is an advantage, but in order to reduce loosening low conformity is likely to be better. From the various clinical reports, it appears that so far loosening has been the more important problem. Unfortunately, it can be hypothesized that both constraint and overall deformation will contribute to loosening, and there is insufficient clinical data on this point. However, a patellar button of low constraint, avoiding excessively small contact areas in flexion, and completely made from plastic to avoid the risk of metal-to-metal wear seems a reasonable design solution at this time.

## Generation of the Tibial Surface

Tibial surface geometry is usually described by radii in the frontal and sagittal planes, and flat sections in the anteroposterior (AP) direction are frequently used. The result is a variety of laxity and stability patterns [56] some of which are unphysiological. The concept used here for generating the tibial surface was to describe the required motion, laxity, and stability mathematically, and then to move the femoral component in multiple positions in space so as to generate the tibial surface as the 3D envelope of the femoral surface.

Anatomical knee motion can be described by three rotations and three displacements. While there is no single motion path, but rather a dependence on the activity and the muscle actions, certain characteristics seem to be common. Flexion-extension is the dominant motion, but internal-external rotation and AP translation of the femur on the tibia have been found to be significant. Based on test rig experiments [8, 32, 47] and as recently shown in living subjects, the rotation is 15°–20° and occurs primarily in the 0°–30° flexion range. The AP translation is about 8 mm, occurring steadily throughout flexion. Based on our test rig simulations of knee flexion-extension under quadriceps action [47], the motion parameters were described by polynomial equations as a function of flexion angle.

Another important consideration of joint motion is laxity, which is the motion induced at a fixed angle of flexion when a force or torque is applied. A common example is the AP motion measured in a "drawer" or Lachman test. From an extensive study of knee laxity in AP, medial-lateral (ML) internal-external rotation, and varus-valgus rotation with the knee under compressive load, it was noted, as in several similar studies, that the laxity was greatest about the neutral point, but at the extremes the stiffness increased rapidly [37]. The laxity was greater in flexion than in extension as expected. Best-fit quadratic equations were fitted to the laxity curves. Using the principle of energy conservation, where work done by the displacing force equals the increase in potential energy of the system [61, 63], equations were written to relate the vertical displacement of the femoral component as a function of the horizontal displacement or rotation. This reduced the knee prosthesis to an analog of partially conforming bearing surfaces, where all the laxity characteristics (and the stability) were produced by the joint surfaces under load, without any assistance from the ligaments.

With these two types of motion, average knee motion and average laxity, it was possible to generate different tibial bearing surfaces [64]. To generate a tibial surface, the femoral surface was "moved" in the computer through a prescribed path of motion in multiple discrete steps. A horizontal gridwork of nodes was defined on the tibial surface. The lowest y-values at each node from the multiple femoral positions were collected to define the tibial surface. The tibial surface which was generated depended upon the type of motion. For example, average knee motion gave a concave medial surface but a lateral surface flat in the AP direction, reflecting the AP translation of the lateral femoral condyle. The maximally conforming surface was for a fixed axis femoral motion. The least conforming surface was flat, representing infinite laxity.

After surface generation, the femur was then placed through its original motion path. The contact points were determined and the local radii of curvature along the AP and ML axes were calculated. Using elasticity theory for double elliptical contacts [48], the contact areas and maximum compressive stresses were calculated ($E_{plastic} = 600$ MPa).

The most conforming surface, for fixed axis femoral motion, gave low contact stresses in extension and somewhat higher contact stresses in flexion when the posterior femoral condyles of smaller sagittal radius came into contact (Fig. 9). At the other extreme, for the totally unconstrained flat tibial surface, the stresses were five times higher in extension and two times higher in flexion. Average knee motion gave stresses between the two values, somewhat higher on the lateral side than on the medial. For average laxity, the maximum stresses in flexion were only 25% higher than for the fixed axis surface. In extension, the laxity stresses were higher than for average knee motion, because ML laxity was included.

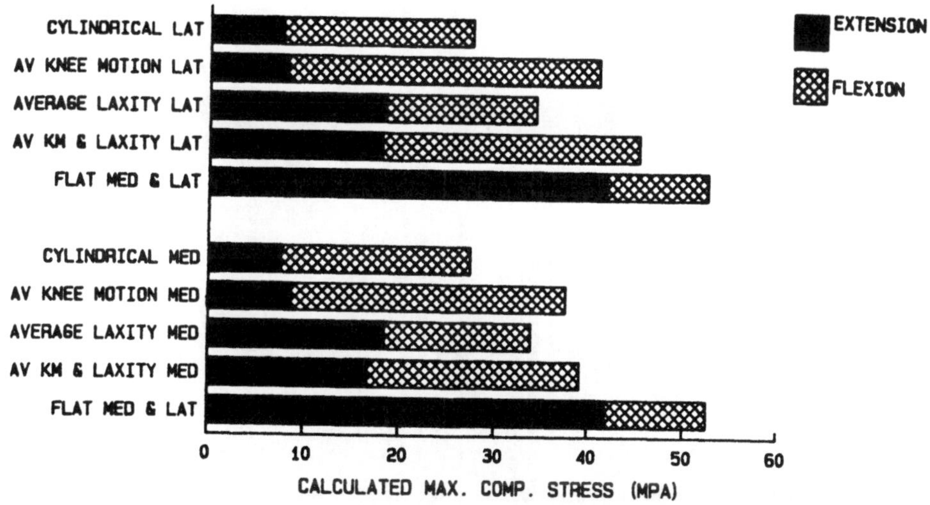


**Fig. 9.** The femoral-tibial contact stresses in extension and flexion for different types of generated tibial surfaces for a force of 1000 N on each condyle

**Fig. 10.** A tibial surface, generated using laxity criteria, for total knee replacement. This can be used with or without cruciate ligaments

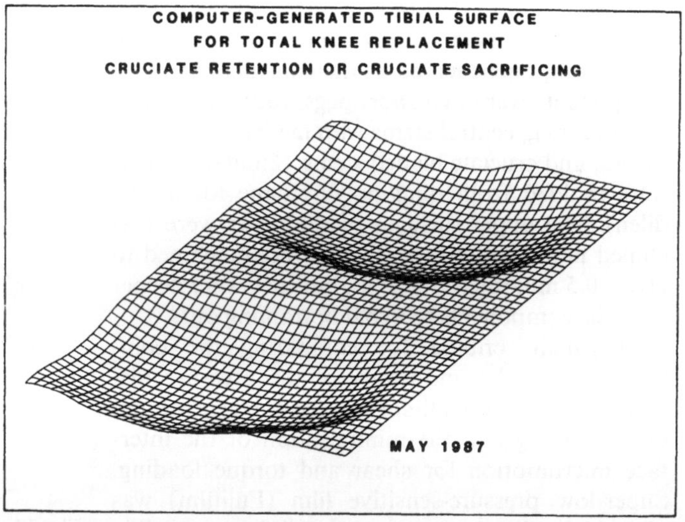


However, the laxity surface was considered the best overall solution, in that it provided maximum stresses only slightly higher than ideal and accommodated adequate laxity, especially in rotation and in the AP direction. An example of a generated tibial surface which could be applied to a TKR is shown in Fig. 10. This surface was based on allowing $\pm 15°$ of internal-external rotational laxity and a total of 4 mm of AP drawer. In addition, $\pm 3$ mm of ML laxity was included to allow interchangeability of femoral and tibial sizes. The stability provided by this surface would enable it to be used with or without the cruciate ligaments. With the cruciates preserved, the ligaments and joint surface would theoretically contribute equally to the stability.

## Tibial Fixation Design

In the review of the current status reported above, loosening of the femoral and tibial components was not seen to be a serious problem in follow-ups of up to 10 years. Nonetheless, the incidence of radiolucency and its progress over time suggests that additional loosening may emerge in the 10- to 20-year follow-up period. Knees which are misaligned at surgery or where the bone stock is deficient are at higher risk and particularly need optimum fixation. Another consideration in our case was that the fixation was required to be applicable to both cement and press-fit, without compromise to either. For the tibial component in particular, this places new requirements on the design of the

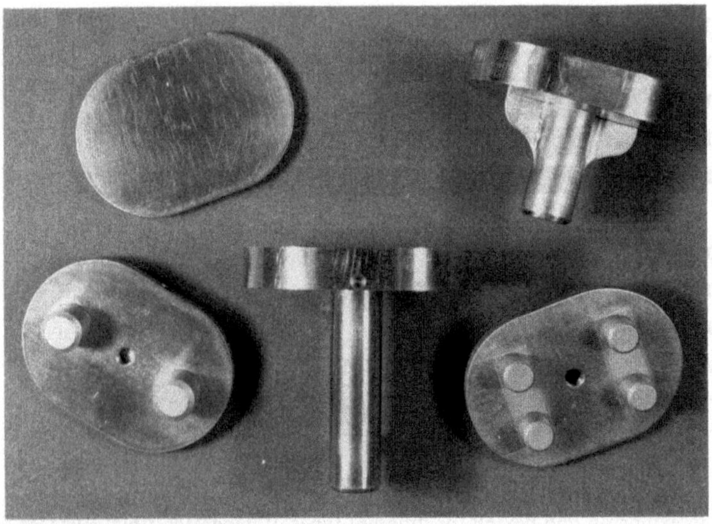

**Fig. 11.** Different possible tibial component design with various fixation elements

fixation elements, such as pegs, posts, and keels.

In order to test the press-fit configurations, which is the most demanding, various possible designs of component were machined (Fig. 11) [66]. A flat component served as the control. The other components were two short pegs, four short pegs, a central peg, central stems with medial and lateral blades, and cruciate bladed stems. Simulated tibias were molded from rigid polyurethane foam (Pedilen). The upper surfaces of the tibias were machined flat. The holes and slots were machined to give a 0.5 mm interference fit, but they were deeper than the components to avoid bottoming out.

The main criteria for comparing the components was the uniformity of the pressure distribution on the tibial surface for the central and offset loading and the minimization of the interface micromotion for shear and torque loading. Super-low pressure-sensitive film (Fujifilm) was placed between the component and the upper tibia surface and a load applied in a test rig, producing a pressure pattern image on the Fujifilm. The control pattern was for a vertical force applied at the center of the component. Offset loading was simulated by loading at 25% from one side (varus or valgus) and 25% from the front or back (anterior or posterior). Shear loading was simulated by anterior-to-posterior loading and by torque loading. All loading conditions for all components were repeated on four separate tibias. Cadaveric tibias were also used for confirmation of results.

To quantify the pressure patterns, video images were input to a VAX computer and analyzed using a Gould DeAnza image processor. For central and offset loading, the load distribution over four regions of the surface was measured. For shear loading, the micromotion was seen as increased density due to small elongations of the contact points. Examples of pressure patterns are shown in Fig. 12.

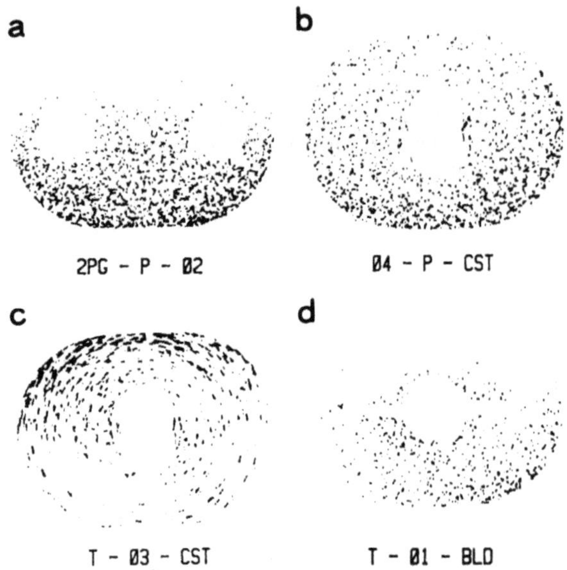


**Fig. 12a–d.** Typical pressure patterns at the component-bone interface. Pressure patterns at the component-tibia interface. **a** Posterior loading, two-peg design. **b** Posterior loading, central stem design (note the more uniform pressure distribution). **c** Torque, central stem design. **d** Torque, central stem and blades (note the reduction in micromotion)

For central loading, the pressure distribution was uniform. The exception to this was the cruciate-bladed design which showed uneven and nonreproducible pressure patterns. This was due to the difficulty of accurate manufacture and of precisely cutting slots in the bone, even under ideal

**Fig. 13.** A graph showing a measure of the resistance of components to shear loading. A low value indicated low interface micromotion. The superiority of the central peg with blade and four-peg components is seen

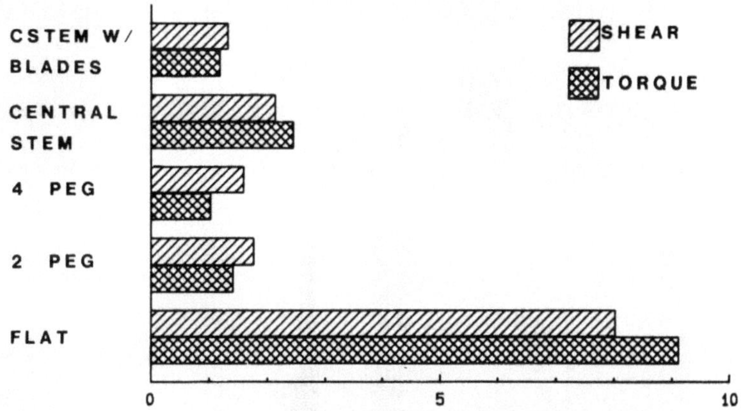


laboratory conditions. This component was eliminated from further tests.

Under offset loading, the pressure distribution was clearly biased. For the flat component, elevated pressures were seen under the loaded area, with low or zero pressure seen at the opposite side of the component. However, the type of fixation modified this pattern. The two pegs gave only slight modification, but the four pegs improved the distribution further. The most improvement was given by the central peg component and the central peg plus blades component. In varus loading for example, the peak pressure was reduced by 24% compared with the flat plate, due to the moment carried by the central peg. The relative comparison between components was similar for all the offset loading conditions.

In shear loading, based on the minimization of shearing motion at the interface, the flat plate was naturally the poorest. The best performance was by the components with a large surface area at maximum radius, namely the four peg and the central peg with blades (Fig. 13).

Overall, the best performance in these press-fit experiments was shown by the central stem with side blades. For practical application to both cement and press-fit, the design was modified slightly. The central stem was smaller in diameter than previous pegs (e.g., Total Condylar) to reduce the total size of the cavity occupied by the peg plus the cement. The blades were enlarged at the medial and lateral sides forming keels and reduced in height toward the central stem. This put the maximum metal at the largest radius, avoided structural compromise of the bone, and cutting too much into the cement mantle, as is the case with the large blades. In addition, the keels were swept back to bring the ends of the keels into the center of the lateral and medial plateaus, in hard bone beneath the main loaded regions [28]. For cemented application, drilling holes at the ends of the keels is an advantage for cement integrity, load transfer, and retarding radiolucency from moving in from the sides. A further benefit is that extension stems can be readily added to the central stem. The final component is shown in Fig. 14.

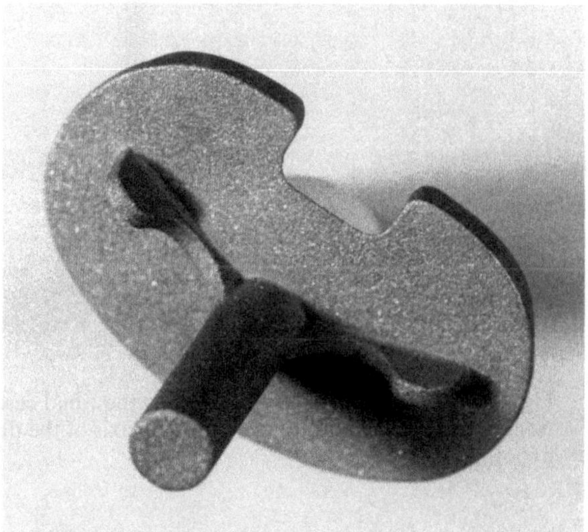

**Fig. 14.** Final design of tibial component for cemented or press-fit application

## Instrumentation and Technique

The goal is to place the tibial component at 90° to the long axis in both planes and to place the femoral component at 5°–7° of valgus with respect to its long axis and perpendicular in the sagittal plane. This is closely equivalent to restoring the normal mechanical axis [42]. The 2°–3° of varus tilt of the upper tibia [27] is not included; the back-

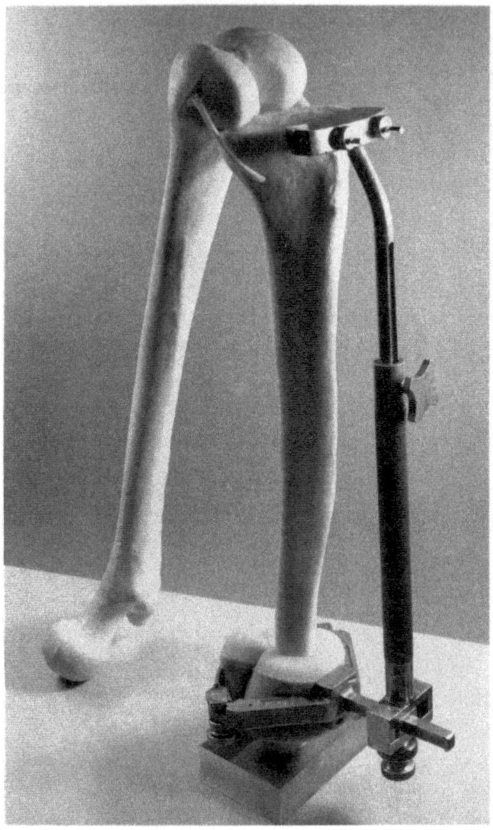

**Fig. 15.** The upper tibial cutter enables the tibial resection to be made perpendicular to the long axis of the tibia in both planes

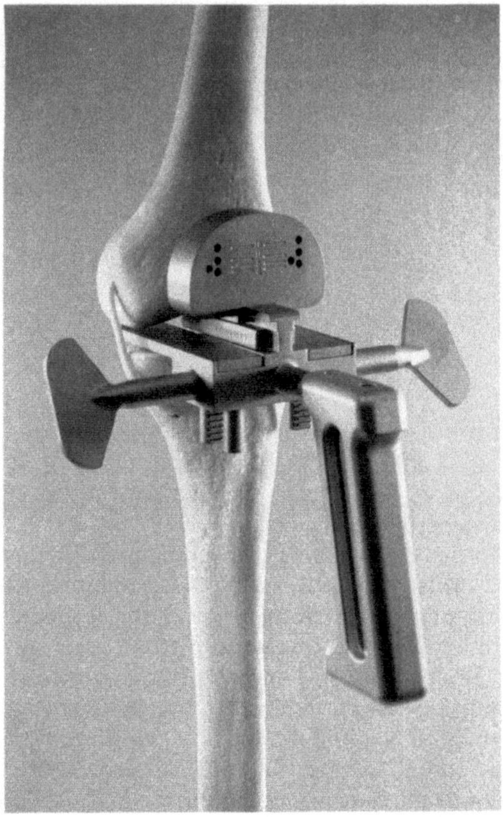

**Fig. 16.** The Gobot distractor which is keyed to the femur at the correct degree of valgus with the intramedullary tuning fork

ward slope is also not included but is accounted for in the design of the plastic tibial surface. The proximal tibial cutting guide (Fig. 15) is placed on the anterior tibia, with two short pins to fix the cutting surface. The long rod should bisect the malleoli distally and be parallel to the long axis of the tibia in the sagittal plane. The sagittal plane adjustment is made with a distal thumb screw. The upper tibia is cut using an oscillating saw.

The anterior prominences are cut from the distal femur for better seating of the distal femoral cutting block to be used later. A starter hole is drilled in line with the medullary canal and the right or left alignment fork, 5° or 7°, is introduced into the medullary canal (Fig. 16). The femoral distractor is slid onto the alignment fork and the leg is extended. The distractor is now keyed to the correct valgus in the frontal plane, and perpendicular in the sagittal plane.

The lateral and medial arms of the distractor are screwed up to the distal femoral condyles. If the lateral and medial ligaments are imbalanced, appropriate soft tissue releases are performed at this time. The tibial component thickness markings are read off. The drill guide is slid up to the anterior femur and two 3-mm pins are tapped through the holes corresponding to the selected tibial thickness.

The drill guide and distractors are removed, leaving the pins in place. The knee is flexed to 90° and the cutting block is placed on the pins. Using an oscillating saw, the distal femoral condyles are resected. The cut should be perpendicular to the long axis of the femur in the sagittal plane and at the correct valgus angle.

With the knee still at 90° of flexion, the distractor is inserted so that it rests flat on the cut proximal tibia. It is distracted to the same amount as in extension or slightly less if a more lax posterior cruciate ligament is preferred. The drill guide is located against the distal femoral surface and two 3-mm pins are tapped in. The distractor is removed and the cutting block is placed on the pins. With the cutting block in place, the posterior condyles, the anterior femur, and the chamfer are cut. The size of the femoral component is based upon the correct anterior cut. Notching or excessive anterior resection of the femur should be avoided. The interchangeability in our system allows for one size difference up or down between femoral and tibial components, without compromise to motion and tracking.

A tibial template is used to cut a central hole with the bone punched downward to act as a plug. Guillotine blades cut the bone for the tibial component keel. If cement is to be used, additional holes are drilled at the locations of the keels on the lateral and medial sides. If patellar resurfacing is to be performed, this is carried out next using various guides.

Tracking of the patellofemoral articulation should be stable during flexion and extension of the joint with the trial components prior to capsular closure.

With all trial components inserted, the stability, range of motion, and tracking are checked. The uncemented components should lie flat on the bony cuts without excessive toggle during flexion/extension of the knee. A final check of overall valgus knee alignment is made at this time.

For cemented application, all bony surfaces are cleaned using pulsatile lavage, dried thoroughly, and packed with sponges during mixing of the cement. The cement is applied in a soft state and pressed into the bony interstices with a tibial pressurizer [31]. The components are placed, starting with the tibial side, then the femoral side, and then the patellar component. The leg is extended and held for a few moments, then flexed again. Excess cement which is extruded is removed and then the leg is held in extension until the cement is hardened. After curing of the cement, all excess is removed. Range of motion, stability, ligament tension, and patellar tracking are again checked.

As noted earlier, when femoral component alignment relied on an external guide rod, although the average alignment was close to ideal, the standard deviation was 4° in the frontal plane and 6° in the sagittal plane with extreme errors of up to 10°. This meant that many cases were unacceptable and became liable to loosening problems. With the intramedullary guide system, the standard deviation was reduced to 2.5° in both planes, an acceptable result.

## Interface

The important topic will only be covered briefly. The evidence to date seems to indicate that with conventional condylar replacements with metal backing and central peg, using current cementing techniques and accurate instrumentation, there will be only a few percent fixation problems at up to 10 years follow-up. It may be that failures will emerge after that time but the indications are that this is unlikely to be at a rapid rate. The results to date with biological ingrowth [27] have been mixed, although the knees have generally functioned as well as cemented knees even if fibrous tissue rather than bone ingrowth has occurred. There are indications for cement-free implants, including patients with long life expectancy, active individuals, postsepsis, where bone grafting is required, and revisions [17]. Our approach has been to reexamine press-fit, where smooth or slightly roughened metal is interfaced directly with the bone. This type of interface has a long and successful history in McKeever and MacIntosh arthroplasty. In an experimental series of 17 patients using a Kinematic Condylar adapted for press-fit, the results were at least as good as in cemented knees in both the recovery phase and follow-up to 2 years [18]. These results have now been maintained up to 4 years. In press-fit interfaces, both radiographically and from reported histological studies of various implants, a layer of fibrous tissue forms adjacent to the metal with a new subchondral-like plate beneath. This amounts to a compliant interface with a strong bone layer, which could be extremely stable in the long term. To enhance the press-fit interface, a further layer of compliant material such as a velour could be added to the implant. This initially produces more uniform stresses on the bone surface [21], protecting the trabecular bone from fatigue failure [41], and will stimulate more rapid fibrous tissue formation.

## Final Design System

The methods for the design of a new total knee system have been described. Computer-graphics were used extensively because of the importance of morphology and fit and as an aid to analysis. The design process was implemented as an orderly and methodical approach to design in an attempt to optimize the final knee system. The major objectives of the system were defined as versatility, durability, and simplicity. Criteria were then specified for each of the components and the instrumentation.

The first stage was to identify the problem areas and deficiencies of the present designs. These included loosening and subluxation of the patellar component, excessive stresses and wear of the tibial plastic, loosening of the tibial component, undefined motion, laxity and stability characteristics, and inaccuracies of instrumentation. Each of these problem areas was addressed by experiments and theoretical analyses in an effort to achieve improved design features.

The final total knee system includes a combination of modular femoral, tibial, and accessory components to deal with a wide variety of pathological conditions.

The femoral component is manufactured in five sizes and two styles, a condylar and a stabilizer with an intercondylar box. The component is anatomically shaped to the degree necessary. The patellar flange is broad and deep for controlled tracking without subluxation and there is adequate laxity in the groove for the plastic patellar button. The symmetrical femoral shape is consistent with the anatomy and reduces the required inventory. The central peg enables extension stems to be added, while build-ups can be added to one or both condyles to compensate for bone loss.

The tibial tray, also in five sizes and symmetrical, includes a number of new features. There is a short central stem, proven to be effective for cement fixation, augmented by two swept-back keels for rotation and shear control in the press-fit mode. Extension stems can be added while wedges can be attached for bony defects. The plastic bearing components snap securely into the tray, with the choice of the condylar or stabilizer designs. The condylar bearing surface is computer generated to accommodate a full range of motion and laxity, with a very smooth action, while minimizing the contact stresses. The condylar surfaces are sufficiently stable to be used with or without cruciates. ML laxity allows femoral tibial size interchangeability. To maximize wear life, there are two pockets in the metal tray beneath the centers of the lateral and medial contact regions.

The instrumentation has the minimum number of parts, such that it is simple to use but provides accurate results. The femoral cuts are based on an intramedullary guide for alignment to within about 2° and a distractor to enable appropriate bony cuts and ligament tensions to be made. Special jigs and guides enable the tibial stem and blades to be cut perpendicular to the bone surface.

Surgical experience and clinical follow-ups will reveal whether the intended practical and functional advantages are realized.

**Acknowledgments.** The Design group for the Computer Knee was P.S. Walker, F.C. Ewald, C.B. Sledge, R.A. Zimmermam, and M.P. Poggie. This work is a composite of a number of separate studies carried out in the Orthopaedic Biomechanics Laboratories at the Brigham and Women's Hospital, Boston, MA, USA and the Veteran's Administration Medical Center, West Roxbury, MA, USA, teaching affiliates of Harvard Medical School. Significant contributions were made by students from Massachusetts Institute of Technology, and fellows from University of Tokyo Medical Center, Peking Union Medical College Hospital, 6th People's Hospital, Beijing, and University of Tsukuba, Japan. The particular contributors are referenced in the text.

The author thanks Ann Carpenedo and Kathy Tamilio for preparation of the text and illustrations.

Thanks are due to the Veterans Administration Rehabilitation Research and Development, the National Institutes of Health, and Howmedica, division of Pfizer Inc. for funding and support of much of this work.

## References

1. Ahmed AM, Burke DL, Hyder A (1987) Force analysis of the patellar mechanism. J Ortho Res 5: 69
2. Ahmed AM, Burke DL, Yu A (1983) In-vitro measurement of static pressure distribution in synovial joints: II. Retropatellar surface. J Biomechanical Engineering 105: 226
3. Andriacchi T, Stanwyck TS, Galante JO (1986) Knee biomechanics and total knee replacement. J Arthroplasty 1: 211
4. Bargren JH, Blaha J, Freeman MAR (1983) Alignment in total knee arthroplasty. Clinical Orthopaedics 173: 178
5. Bartel DL, Bicknel VL, Wright TM (1986) The effect of conformity, thickness and material on stresses in UHMWPE components for total joint replacement. J Bone Jt Surg 68-A: 1041
6. Bartel DL, Burstein AH, Santavicca EA Insall IN (1982) Performance of the tibial component in total knee replacement. J Bone Jt Surg 64-A: 1026
7. Bayley JC (1988) Patellar component failure following total knee replacement. In: Proc. The Knee Society, Atlanta
8. Blankevoort L, Huiskes R, deLange A (1984) An in vitro study of the passive kinematic behaviour of the human knee joint. Advances in Engineering, Winter Annual Meeting of the American Society of Mechanical Engineers, Bioengineering Division, New Orleans
9. Brooks PJ, Walker PS, Scott RD (1984) Tibial component fixation in deficient bone stock. Clin Orthop 184: 302
10. Clayton ML, Thirupath R (1982) Patellar complications after total condylar arthroplasty. Clin Orthop 170: 152
11. Conway WF, Gilula LA, Serot DI (1986) Breakage of the patellar component of a kinematic total knee arthroplasty. Orthopaedics 9: 532–534
12. Cornell CN, Ranawat CS, Burstein AH (1986) A clinical and radiographic analysis of loosening of

total knee arthroplasty components using a bilateral model. J Arthroplasty 1: 157
13. Eftekhar NS (1983) Total knee replacement. Results with the intramedullary adjustable total knee prosthesis. J Bone Jt Surg 65-A: 293
14. Ellis MI, Seedhom BB, Amis AA, Dowson D, Wright (1979) Forces in the knee joint whilst rising from normal and motorised chairs. Engineering in Medicine 8: 33
15. Essinger JR, Leyvraz PF, Heegard JH, Force analysis program: a 3-D knee model for prosthesis design testing. Proceedings of Orthopedic Research Society, San Francisco, p 290
16. Ewald FC, Jacobs MA, Miegel RE, Walker PS, Poss R, Sledge CB (1984) Kinematic total knee replacement. J Bone Jt Surg 66-A: 1032
17. Ewald FC, Walker PS, Hsu HP, Uematsu O, Kelley KM (1986) Is total knee replacement better than total hip replacement? Proceedings of American Academy of Orthopedic Surgeons, New Orleans, p 102
18. Ewald FC, Walker PS, Poss R, Miegel RE, Reilly DT, Thomas WH, Sledge CB (1986) Uncemented press-fit total knee replacement. Proceedings 2nd Scientific Meeting of the Knee Society, University Park Press, Baltimore
19. Ficat RP, Hungerford DS (1977) Disorders of the patello-femoral joint. Williams and Wilkins, Baltimore
20. Figgie HE, Goldberg VM, Heiple KG, Moller HS, Gordon NH (1986) The influence of tibial-patellofemoral location on function of the knee in patients with the posterior stabilized condylar knee prosthesis. J Bone Jt Surg 68-A: 1035
21. Garg A, Walker PS (1986) The effect of the interface on the bone stresses beneath tibial components. J Biomechanics 19: 957
22. Goldstein SA, Coale E, Weiss APC, Grossnickle M, Meller B, Matthews LS (1986) Patellar surface strain. J Orthop Res 4: 372
23. Goodfellow JW, Tibrewal SB, Sharman KP (1987) Unicompartmental Oxford meniscal Knee arthroplasty. J Arthroplasty 2: 1
24. Green DL, Bahniuk E, Liebelt RA, Fender E, Mirkov P (1983) Biplanar radiographic measurements of reversible displacement and migration of total joint replacements. J Bone Jt Surg 65-A: 1134
25. Hood RW, Wright TM, Burstein AH, Insall JN (1981) Retrieval analysis of 20 polyethylene patella buttons. Proceedings of Orthopedic Research Society, Las Vegas, p 210
26. Huberti HH, Hayes WC (1984) Patello-femoral contact pressures. J Bone Jt Surg 66-A: 715
27. Hungerford DS, Krackow KA, Kenna RV (1985) Alignment in total knee arthroplasty. The Knee Papers of the 1st Scientific Meeting of the Knee Society University Park Press, Baltimore, chap 2
28. Hvid I, Hansen SL (1985) Trabecular bone strength patterns at the proximal tibial epiphysis. J Orthop Res 3: 464
29. Insall JN, Binazzi R, Soudry M, Mestriner LA (1985) Total knee arthroplasty. Clinical Orthop 13: 192
30. Kaltwasser P, Uematsu O, Walker PS (1987) The patello-femoral joint in total knee replacement. Proceedings of Orthopedic Research Society, San Francisco, p 292
31. Kim YH, Walker PS, Deland JT (1984) A cement impactor for uniform cement penetration in the upper tibia. Clin Orthop 182: 206
32. Kurosawa H, Walker PS, Abe S, Garg A, Hunter T (1985) Geometry and motion of the knee for implant and orthotic design. J Biomechanics 18: 847
33. Landy M, Walker PS (1985) Wear in condylar replacement knees- a 10 year follow-up. Proceedings of Orthopedic Research Society Las Vegas, p 96, (1988) J Arthroplasty (in press)
34. Laskin RS (1986) RMC total knee replacement: a review of 166 cases. J Arthroplasty 1: 11
35. Lewis JL, Askew MJ, Jaycox DP (1982) A comparative evaluation of tibial component designs of total knee prostheses. J Bone Jt Surg 64A: 129
36. Le Fortune LA, Cavanagh PR (1985) The measurement of normal knee joint motion during walking using intracortical pins. In: Whittle M, Harris D (eds) Biomechanic measurements in orthopaedic practice. Clarendon Press, Oxford
37. Markolf KL, Bargar WL, Schoemaker SC, Amstutz HC (1981) The role of the joint load in knee stability. J Bone Jt Surg 60-A: 570–585
38. McLain RF, Bargar WF (1986) The effect of total knee design on patellar strain. J Arthroplasty 1: 91
39. Mensch JS, Amstutz HZ (1975) Knee morphology as a guide to knee replacement. Clin Orthop 112: 231
40. Merkow RL, Soudry M, Insall JN (1985) Patella dislocation following total knee replacement. J Bone Jt Surg 67-A: 1321
41. Miegel RE, Walker PS, Nelson PC, Inadomi J, Needalman L, Maxine M. (1986) A compliant interface for total knee arthroplasty. J Orthop Res 4: 486
42. Moreland JR, Hanker GJ (1985) Lower extremity axial alignment in normal males. The Knee Papers of the 1st Scientific Meeting of the Knee Society. University Park Press, Baltimore, chap 6
43. Murase K, Crowninshield RD, Pedersen DR, Chang TS (1983) An analysis of tibial component design in total knee arthroplasty. J Biomechanics 16: 13–22
44. Rehder U (1983) Morphometrical studies on the symmetry of the human knee joint: Femoral condyles. J Biomechanics 16: 351
45. Reilly DT, Martens M (1972) Experimental analysis of the quadriceps muscle force and patellofemoral joint reaction force for various activities. Acta Orthop Scand 43: 126
46. Reilly D, Walker PS, Ben-Dov M, Ewald FC (1982) Effects of tibial components on load transfer in the upper tibia. Clin Orthop 64A: 129
47. Reuben JD, Rovick JS, Walker PS, Schrager J (1986) Three-dimensional kinematics of normal and cruciate deficient knees-a dynamic in vitro study. Proceedings of Orthopedic Research Society, New Orleans, p. 385
48. Roark RJ, Young C (1975) Formulas for stress and strain. McGraw-Hill, New York

49. Rose RM, Goldfarb HV, Ellis E, Crugnola AM (1983) On the pressure dependence of the wear of UHMWPE. Wear 92: 99
50. Rovick JS, Reuben JD, Robertson DD, Walker PS (1987) Control of knee kinematics by ligaments. Proceedings of Orthopedic Research Society, San Francisco, p 126
51. Rovick JS, Walker PS (1986) Design of an off the shelf knee orthosis using averaging techniques. Proceedings of Rehabilitation Engineering Society of North America Minneapolis, p 107
52. Ryd L, Lindstrand A, Rosenquist R, Selvick G (1986) Tibial component fixation in knee arthroplasty. Clinical Orthopaedics 213: 141
53. Seedhom BB, Longton EB, Wright V, Dowson D (1972) Dimensions of the knee. Annals of Rheumatic Disease 31: 54
54. Shinno N (1961) Statico-dynamic analysis of movement of the knee. Tokushima Experimental Medicine 8: 101
55. Steege JW, Lewis JL, Keer LM, Wixson RL (1987) Crack propagation at the bone-cement interface. Proceedings of Orthopedic Research Society, San Francisco, p 54
56. Thatcher JC, Zhou X-M, Walker PS (1987) Inherent laxity in total knee prostheses. J Arthroplasty 2: 199
57. Thornhill TS, Dalziel RW, Sledge CB (1982) Alternatives to arthrodesis for the failed total knee arthroplasty. Clin Orthop 170: 131
58. Townley CO (1985) Anatomic total knee resurfacing arthroplasty. Clinical Orthop Rel Res 192: 82
59. Uematsu O, Hsu H-P, Kelley KM, Ewald FC, Walker PS (1987) A radiographic study of Kinematic total knee replacement. J Arthroplasty 2: 317
60. Vasu R, Carter DR, Schurman DJ, Beaupre GS (1986) Epiphyseal-based designs for tibial plateau components. J Biomechanics 19: 647
61. Walker PS (1977) Human joints and their artificial replacements. Thomas, Springfield, chap 6
62. Walker PS , Greene D, Reilly D, Thatcher J, Ben-Dov M, Ewald FC (1981) Fixation of tibial components of knee prostheses. J Bone J Surg 63A: 258
63. Walker PS Wang CJ, Masse Y (1974) Joint laxity as a criterion for the design of condylar knee prostheses. Proceedings of conference on total knee replacement. Institution of Mechanical Engineers, London
64. Walker PS, Zhou XM (1987) The dilemma of surface design in total knee replacement. Proceedings Orthopedic Research Society, San Francisco, p 291
65. Wismans J, Veldpaus F, Janssen J, Huson A, Struben P (1980) A three-dimensional mathematical model of the human knee joint. J Biomechanics 13: 677
66. Zimmerman RA, Hsu H-P, St. Ville J, Granholm JW, Walker PS (1987) A method for evaluation of press-fit tibial component designs. Proceedings Orthopedic Research Society, San Francisco, p 294

# *Discussion*

*Hoshino* (Tokyo Medical and Dental University): How do you know if the hole is correct for the nail into the medullary canal?

*Walker* (Harvard Medical School): I'm not sure how it could be wrong. Preoperative planning with assessment of the radiographs is important to ensure that the femur is reasonably normal in terms of its curvature. There is of course an inherent error in drilling a hole into the medullary canal because it can be out by 2° or 3°. It is necessary to rely on some landmarks and if the intermedullary canal in addition to external features are used reasonable security is provided I think.

*Hoshino*: But in most cases the landmark is pathological, it is not normal, and so would you say that a lot depends on the judgment of the surgeon?

*Walker*: Yes of course, each case must be considered separately.

*Ranawat* (Cornell University Medical Collage): Could you comment on the depth of the patellofemoral groove of the femoral component? I think that the shallowness of the anterior bulge of the femoral component to the linear motion of 45°–75° is critical for the longevity of the patellofemoral joint replacement. Did you take this into consideration at all?

*Walker*: I think there are two aspects to this. If the bulge is large, the tension in the patella will be very high and exacerbate fractures, which is what I think you were alluding to. This is also connected to other mechanical aspects such as roll back; if there is excessive roll-back this may also exacerbate high stresses in the patella. The other aspect is the lever arm of the quadriceps; if the lever arm is diminished too much by reducing the height of the flange and the thickness of the patella, higher quadriceps forces are necessary in stair climbing and rising from a chair. I think that approaching the normal anatomy is not a bad idea in terms of correct lever arms and thicknesses.

*Goldie* (Karolinska Institute): Could you comment on how the axis of the stem of the tibial component is placed in relation to the long axis of the tibial shaft? It has been suggested that it should be placed posteriorly, but still giving the tibial plateau as large a coverage as possible of the tibia itself.

*Walker*: It is certainly true that the intermedullary canal is anterior on the tibial surface and that the contact points of load bearing are posterior to the center and, therefore, it would seem that in order to achieve maximum support for the tibia it is necessary to have more posterior rather than anterior support. In designs like the Total Condylar or Kinematic, the peg is fairly large in the anterior-posterior dimension and it probably does achieve enough support in the posterior direction.

However, another aspect is that if that if the stem is to be extended in, for example, revision cases, the existing stem should probably be in line with the canal, so that you can continue with a long intermedullary rod.

*Goldie*: In designing the patellar button or replacement, do you consider that there is very often a patellar misalignment before surgery due to some abnormality?

*Walker*: I think that surgeons are really the experts in that problem of realignment. I would say that undercorrected valgus is probably not very good for the patella, because of large lateral pressures. It is a very complicated system because rotation of the components on the bone has an effect on patellar tracking. Engineers as you know tend to deal with the normal knee.

*Goodfellow* (Oxford University): With regard to preservation of the cruciate mechanism, did you mean preservation of both cruciate ligaments or just that of the posterior ligament?

*Walker*: Just the posterior ligament.

*Goodfellow*: Do you not believe that both cruciate ligaments are important? While the posterior ligament is responsible for the roll-back, the anterior ligament is necessary for the roll-forward.

*Walker*: I think that a great deal can be compensated for by the bearing surfaces. For example, designs that are anteroposteriorly flat and only preserve the posterior cruciate ligament are perhaps not optimum because there is no substitute in those designs for the anterior ligament. I think it is necessary to prevent excessive posterior rollback. So, I think it is possible in the design to compensate for the absence of the anterior ligament, but perhaps the function is superior if it is possible to preserve both ligaments in the knee. In the literature, it can be seen that function is not perfect, for example, there is the inability of patients fo climb up and down stairs correctly, and the absence of the anterior cruciate ligament may well be a factor here.

*Krackow* (John Hopkins University): Some designs now use a tibial plateau which is aligned to be perpendicular when viewed in the sagittal plane. There are other systems which now go up to as much as 10° of posterior slope on the tibial plateau in the sagittal plane. Would you comment on the advisability of sloping the tibia downward?

*Walker*: Following the anatomy, there is no question that the upper tibial surface slopes back 5°–10°. In terms of the bearing surface, of course, this can be compensated for in the design of the plastic surfaces, so that if a perpendicular component is introduced in both planes the bearing surfaces can be absolutely correct. However, the question is—does this impose shearing stresses on the interface? I personally do not think this makes very much difference: The shearing forces go anteriorly and posteriorly and it is hard to see that a small posterior tilt will significantly affect the magnitude of the shearing stresses.

# Special Lecture

# Mechanics of the Knee Joint and Certain Joint Replacements

J.P. Paul[1]

**Summary.** The loads transmitted by the structures at the knee joint during activities of daily living comprise a complex three-dimensional dynamic system. This is true for the normal knee, the knee with pathological changes and a knee with a joint replacement of any kind.

As in all mechanical analyses reasonable assumptions must be made about the relevant activities, the loads developed, the orientation of the structures and the identification of soft tissues carrying load at particular instants of time. The effects of these assumptions are interpreted for the loads in the normal and the prosthetic knee joint.

Straight line level walking is considered to be the activity generating most cycles of fatigue loading or wear of structural components on knee joint prostheses. Other activities such as stair or ramp negotiation, and sitting or standing from sitting generally will have higher values of load which may be responsible for generating the levels of stress corresponding to the failure of fixation. The whole body mechanics of these movements is reviewed and the consequent effects on joint loading predicted for normal and joint replacement patients.

Passive joint movements are considered in respect of loading of ligamentous structures. Attention is given to the differences in ligamentous orientation between the normal knee and the knee with different types of knee joint replacement.

**Keywords:** Knee—Mechanics—Loading—Ligaments—Walking—Running

In 1974 there was strong interest in total knee arthroplasty reflected in the meeting "Total Knee Replacement" at the Institution of Mechanical Engineers, London [12] and the Workshop on Total Knee Arthroplasty, Charlottesville, Virginia [3]. At that time total hip arthroplasty and finger joint arthroplasty were achieving significantly better results than total knee arthroplasty. In the intervening time, knee joint replacement results have significantly improved. This paper reviews the mechanics of the knee in the normal individual with regard to kinematics and load transmission and explores the consequences for implanted joint replacements.

Since the knee is at the centre of the longest limb of the human body and generally has little overlying soft tissue coverage, it might be expected that definitive information would be available on its kinematics and load-bearing characteristics. The knee joint, however, is particularly difficult for analysis in mechanical terms for the following reasons:

- Throughout its range of movement the axes of the tibia and femur are inclined to each other in three-dimensional space
- The articulating surfaces of the tibia and femur comprise asymmetrical shapes of three-dimensional curvature whose characteristics are variable between individuals
- It allows a large amount of angulation about the flexion/extension axis, but the smaller angulations about perpendicular axes are highly significant to the function of the joint
- The angular movements at the joint occur about continuously changing instantaneous axes.

The loading transmitted at the joint can be described as three perpendicular force components together with three components of moment about corresponding reference axes and all of these load actions are significant:

- The knee is controlled in space by a complex system of one- and two-joint muscles, and there is at present no specific way of analysing the loads transmitted by specific muscles
- The kinematics of the joint are controlled by a complex system of ligaments, two of which are inaccessible to external palpation or measurement
- The joint surfaces, the meniscal cartilages and the ligaments deform under load with the consequence that the kinematics of the joint are variable depending on the load being transmitted.

Cadaver tests are frequently reported indicating the structures likely to carry load, the orientation of the structures and the pressures developed at the joint surfaces. Such tests occasionally indicate the load distribution due to straightforward axial

[1] Bioengineering Unit, University of Strathclyde, Glasgow, Scotland

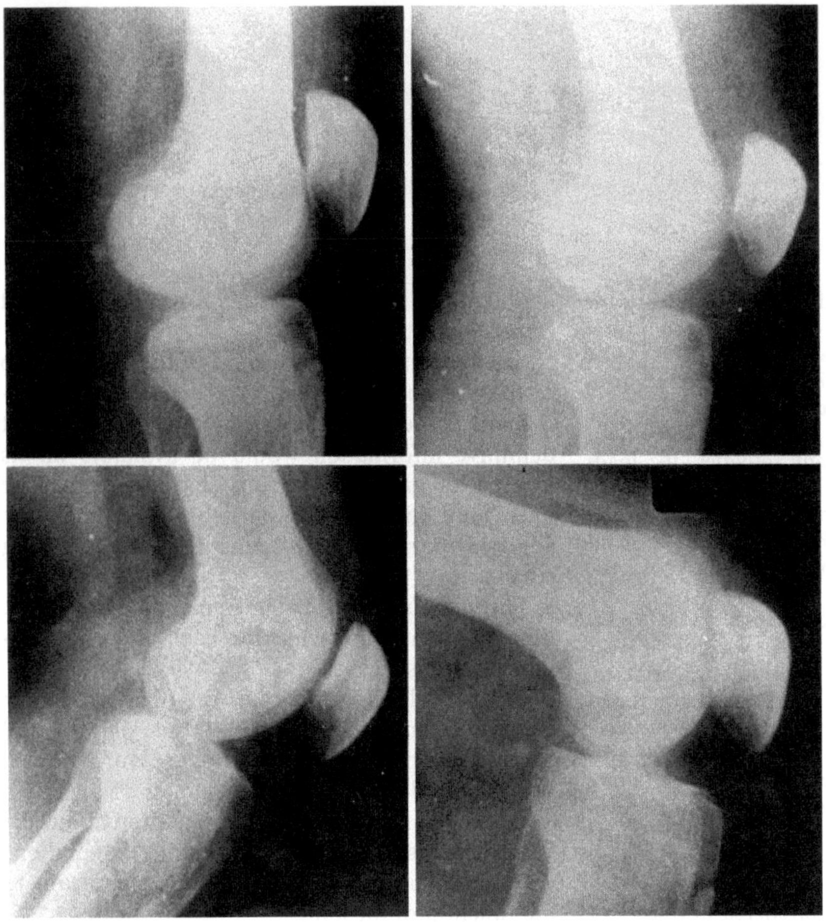

**Fig. 1.** Lateral radiographs of a normal knee at flexion angles of 0°, 15°, 60°, and 90°

compression of the extended leg. The knee, however, is generally subjected to a three-dimensional system of external loads. The transmission of these loads corresponds to tension in appropriate muscles, and unless consideration is given to these force actions, cadaver tests may give rise to highly approximate if not erroneous conclusions.

If the knee is viewed from the lateral direction, X-rays can be taken to show the relative positions of femur and tibia at increasing angles of flexion as shown in Fig. 1. The actual centre of transmission of force between these two bones in the dynamic situation will depend on the characteristics of the lubrication system present, but as a first simplifying assumption it can be taken that the load line passes perpendicular to the common tangent of the surfaces at their point of closest approach as shown radiologically. Figure 1 shows the familiar phenomenon of the translation of the centre of pressure posteriorly on the femoral condyles with increasing flexion angle. As far as the tibia is concerned it will be noted that the centre of pressure appears to be comparatively stationary lying on the line defining the internal margin of the posterior cortex of the tibia. Nisell et al. [18] show the movement of the contact point with knee flexion angle, as presented in Fig. 2. Unfortunately their graph appears to indicate that a substantial amount of hyperextension was present and there are no data covering the range between that position and 30° flexion, which includes the range most utilised during the stance phase of locomotion. Iseki and Tomatsu [13] undertook a similar study in three dimensions with the use of silicone rubber models of the joint space in cadaver tests. Their data show a corresponding progression in the position of the contact point relative to the tibia, although the work cannot be compared directly with that of Nisell et al. since the latter's work was undertaken on living volunteers and measurements were taken while the knee was carrying body weight at different flexion angles. It is an interesting exercise to determine the locus of the instantaneous centre of the knee joint relative either to the tibia or femur, but a number of factors should be borne in mind with regard to this. The

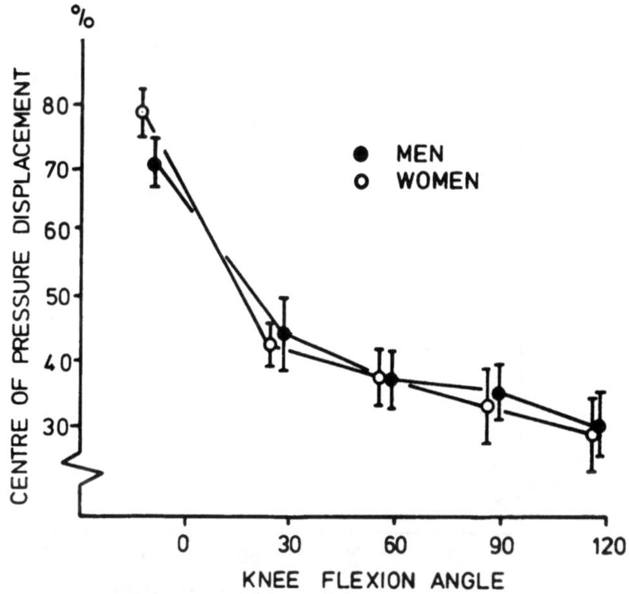


**Fig. 2.** Displacement of the centre of pressure of the knee relative to the tibia at different flexion angles. The ordinate defines the position of the centre of pressure from the posterior margin of the tibial plateau as a percentage of the total antero-posterior dimension. Adapted from Nisell et al. [17]

mathematics of the calculation of the position of an instantaneous centre is very sensitive to small errors in the determination of the position of markers. The precise position of the centre of pressure can be variable depending on the instantaneous deformation of cartilage and ligamentous structures. The locus of the centre of pressure can be erratic and variable in patients with degenerative conditions at the joint. Another fundamental point should be borne in mind that, whereas for a pair of cylindrical surfaces the resultant joint force must intersect the relevant axes of the cylinder regardless of the distribution of the pressure round the circumference, the same does not hold for non-circular bearing surfaces. Therefore in general the resultant knee joint force will not pass through the instantaneous centre of rotation and analyses which assume that the line of the resultant joint force passes through the instantaneous centre are in error.

The loads developed by the application of a flexion or extending moment to the knee may be resisted by the structures indicated on a simplified basis in Fig. 3, and this illustrates the basic problem in any analysis of muscle forces. It is usual to ignore the effect of joint friction in this analysis. The maximum moment transmitted in flexion and extension may be 35 Nm [16, 20]. Such et al. [24] indicate friction couples of typically 5 Nm magnitude due to joint friction and soft tissue resistance. This indicates that no great error results from excluding the effects of friction. Antagonistic muscle

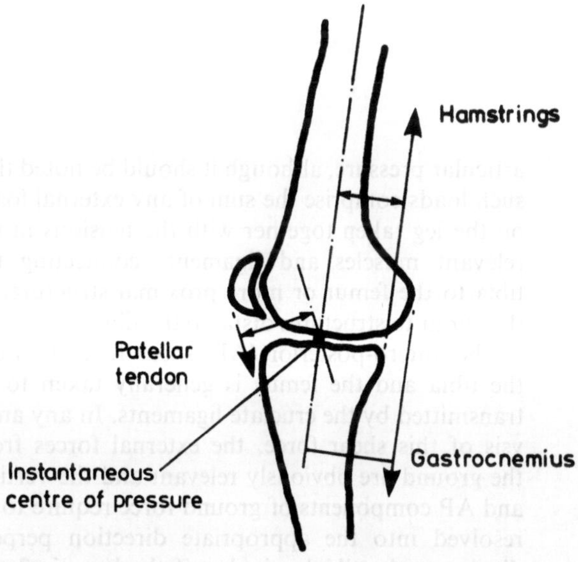


**Fig. 3.** Structures involved in transmitting flexion and extension moments

action may be present and if present no reasonable estimate of muscle force can be made from external observation unless complex schemes of interpretation of EMG signals are utilised as cited by Hof and Van der Berg [10]. Appropriate lever arms can be inferred from cadaveric or X-ray measurements as presented in Fig. 4, which is taken from the work of Nisell et al. [18]. Loads transmitted along the axis of the tibia are obviously transferred from the tibia to the femur by

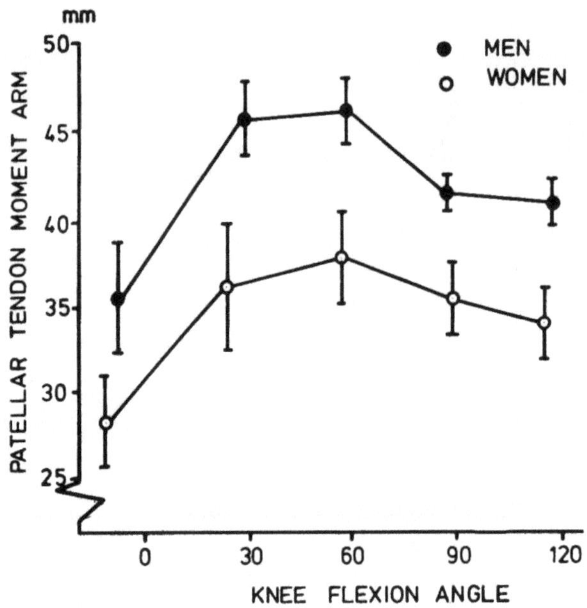


**Fig. 4.** Variation with knee angle of the lever arm of the patellar tendon relative to the tibio-femoral contact point. Adapted from Nisell et al. [17]

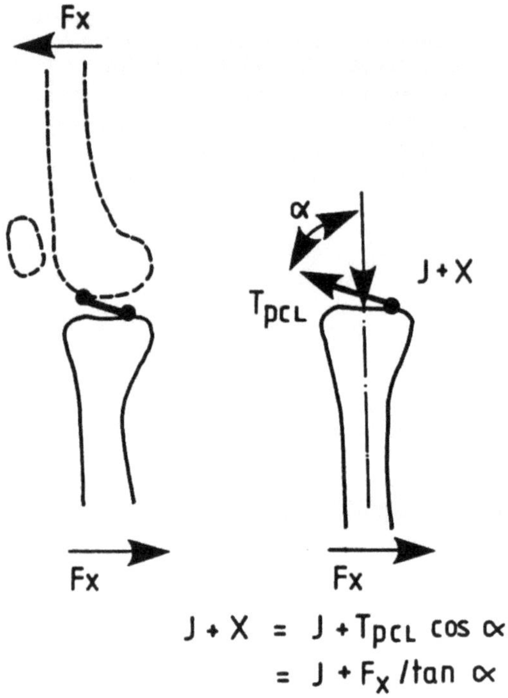


**Fig. 5.** Transmission of antero-posterior shear force by the cruciate ligaments augments the joint force

articular pressure, although it should be noted that such loads comprise the sum of any external loads on the leg taken together with the tensions in the relevant muscles and ligaments connecting the tibia to the femur or more proximal structure, or the femur to structures distal to the tibia.

The antero-posterior (AP) shear force between the tibia and the femur is generally taken to be transmitted by the cruciate ligaments. In any analysis of this shear force, the external forces from the ground are obviously relevant and the vertical and AP components of ground force require to be resolved into the appropriate direction perpendicular to the tibial axis; but if the knee is flexed account must be taken also of the appropriate component of the patellar tendon, hamstrings and gastrocnemius tendon forces. Figure 5 illustrates the effect that since the cruciate ligaments are inclined in space to the axis of the tibia, the application of shear force results in a corresponding increase in the joint force.

In normal walking the knee is subjected to moments tending to adduct the tibia and in some circumstances the loading may be abducting. Since the tibio-femoral joint is essentially bicompartmental, as shown in Fig. 6, small values of moment in association with longitudinal force may be transmitted by a redistribution of the pressure between the two compartments of the joint, as shown in Fig. 7. The concept of transmission of the moment by difference in joint pressure is related in the figure to a linear variation of contact pressure,

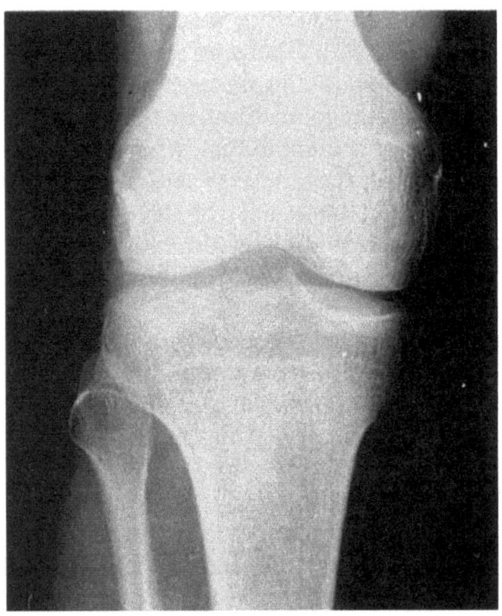

**Fig. 6.** Antero-posterior radiograph of the knee

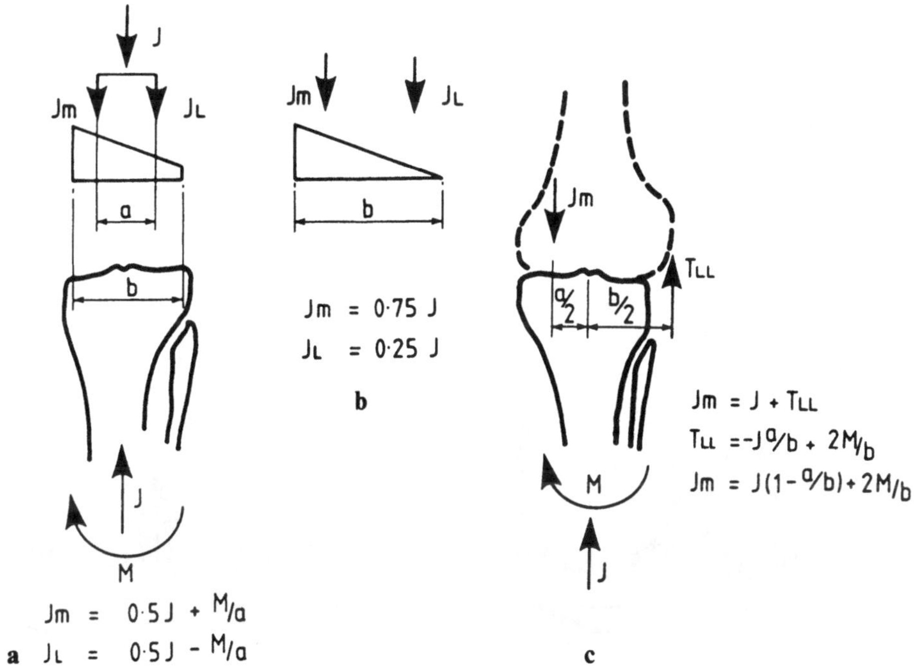


**Fig. 7a–c.** Transmission of adducting moments by the knee. **a** Redistribution of joint pressure under small moments. **b** Limiting condition with pressure tending to zero at lateral margin. **c** Hypothesised loading with larger moments developing tension in lateral structures

which is realistic to a first approximation if the cartilage is assumed to be linearly elastic. If this is not so, the overall sharing of load between the two compartments is still a mechanism for transmission of adducting moment, although the details of the pressure distribution would be different. Two loading situations are shown in Fig. 7a, b; moment increase beyond the limiting conditions shown in Fig. 7b would tend to open the joint surfaces on the lateral side. This would obviously be resisted by the development of tension in the lateral collateral ligament and in the fascia lata; the analysis is not sensitive as to whether one or other of these structures is the principal load-bearing component. An alternative mechanism for transmission of this moment is, however, by difference in tension in the medial and lateral hamstrings or in the medial and lateral heads of the gastrocnemius. Major differences in the EMG patterns of these muscles have not been reported and science has not yet developed far enough to be able to interpret whether in fact this differential tension exists. It is, however, the case that during the stance phase of locomotion, the fascia lata are in tension due to contraction of the tensor fascia lata and gluteus maximus.

Medio-lateral shear forces require to be transmitted by the knee and most analyses assume that this would be transmitted by contact between the tibial eminence and the femoral condyles. However, knees with no reported problems in medio-lateral force transmission can be seen on X-ray to have very little area of possible contact in this region. Due to the medio-lateral distance between the areas of origin and insertion of each of the cruciates, they also have the mechanical capacity to resist medio-lateral relative movement at the knee. Generally the loads transmitted in this direction in normal activity are small and the author is aware of no in-depth analysis of this situation. In trauma due to lateral impact, the major injuries seem to correspond to overloading of the collateral ligaments corresponding to bending in adduction or abduction.

There is still uncertainty about which structures of the knee are involved in a transmission of internal or external rotating moment. Histories of sports injuries point to the cruciate ligaments having an important role in this load transmission and it is interesting to speculate on the precise loading, which may be as illustrated in Fig. 8. There is no clearly defined axis about which rotation of the tibia about its long axis relative to the femur will take place. A reasonable approximation is that it will occur at the centre of the area representing the tibial eminence as seen in the superior view. This

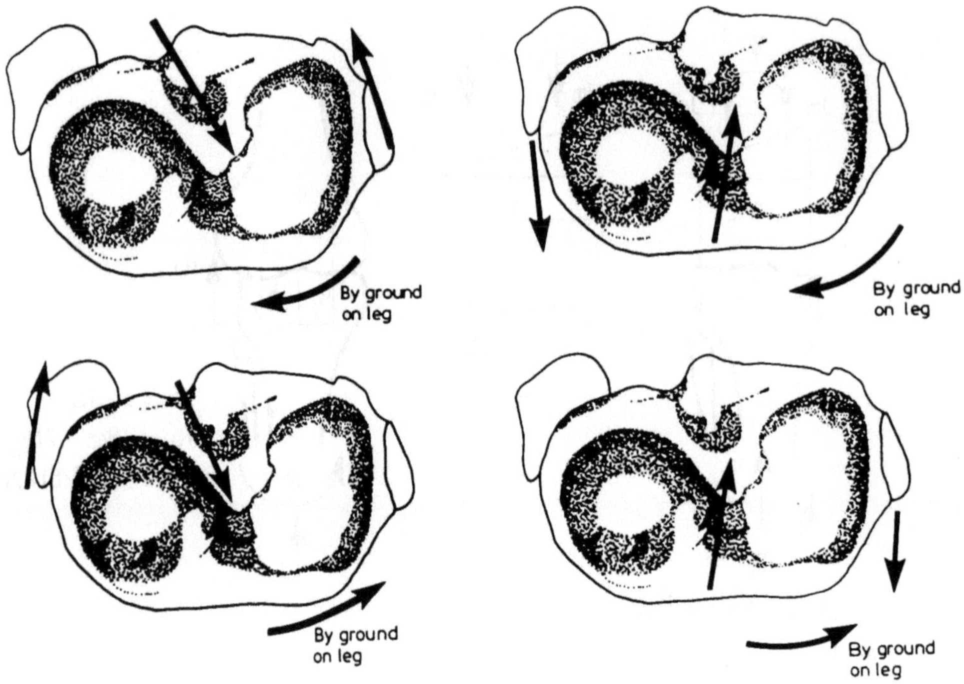


**Fig. 8.** Views of the tibial plateau from above, subject to external moments tending to rotate the tibia clockwise or anticlockwise relative to the femur

implies that the cruciate ligaments will have quite small lever arms relative to this axis as shown in Fig. 8. If the joint is subject to no loading other than torsion, it would appear that tension in one of the cruciates would balance tension in one of the collateral ligaments as shown in the figure, and this implies that those fibres of the collateral ligaments which are most nearly perpendicular to the long axis of the tibia will be more highly loaded. This situation of the knee being subject to torsional load in the absence of other loads is an unlikely abstraction, and certainly during locomotion there will be tension in other structures which could assist in transmission of the torsion.

The above discussion of load transmission specifically by ligaments is based on the concept of the knee subjected to a series of loads in isolation. As has been pointed out in almost all situations there is load transmitted between the tibia and femur at the joint and therefore analysis of the loads tending to produce relative movement at this interface should take account of this. Hsieh and Walker [11], Shoemaker and Markolf [23] and Gollehon et al. [7] have explored the actions of the cruciate and collateral ligaments in load transmission of this type. Shoemaker and Markolf in particular stress the importance of joint load in assessing the function of ligaments. They point out a two fold increase in the stiffness of the knee to AP displacement, corresponding to applied force when the knee is axially loaded, compared with zero load, and a similar phenomenon exists in respect of the torque/rotation relationship when considered in the loaded and unloaded situation. In the tests of Shoemaker and Markolf the joint load applied at maximum was 925 N. Taking a typical value of coefficient of friction for cartilage on cartilage in the presence of synovial fluid of 0.01, this would suggest forces resisting AP displacement of less than 10 N and torques resisting rotation of less than 1 Nm. Both of these figures are small compared with the values applied to the cadaver specimens, and it appears therefore that there must be some load-bearing mechanism additional to the friction, possibly the "ball in saucer" phenomenon, corresponding either to the dish shape of the tibial plateau or to the indentation of the cartilage on the plateau.

Bresler and Frankel [1], Morrison [16] and Paul [21] have shown the moments about reference axes in the knee during straight-line level walking on a smooth surface by young healthy individuals, giving values in flexion and extension in the range 30–50 Nm for flexion and adduction, 10 Nm in torsion. Possibly because of the convenience of analysing this type of gait in the laboratory, these

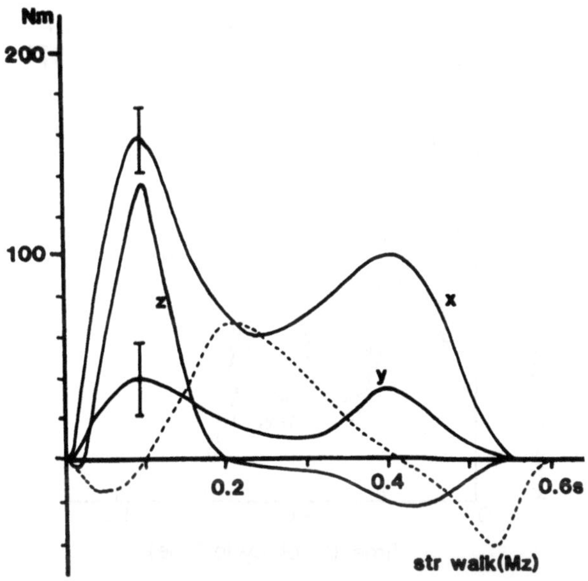


Fig. 9. Variation with time of moments developed about the axes of the knee during a 90° walking turn (*solid lines*). *Positive values* correspond to the external load tending to flex (*z-axis*), adduct (*x-axis*) and inwardly rotate the foot (*y-axis*). The *broken line* corresponds to flexion moments developed in straight-line walking. *Bars* represent ± 1 SD (seven tests)

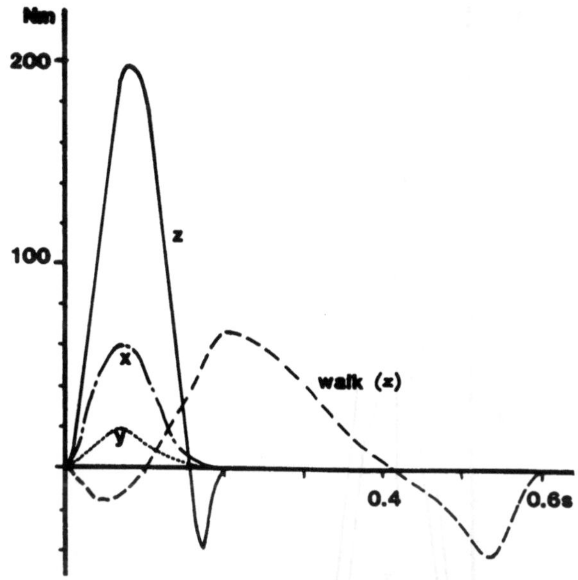


Fig. 10. Variation with time of moments developed about the axes of the knee during straight-line running. *Positive values* correspond to the external load tending to flex (*z-axis*), adduct (*x-axis*) and inwardly rotate the foot (*y-axis*). The *broken line* corresponds to flexion moments developed in straight-line walking

data and the corresponding joint forces are generally utilised in assessments of the required load-bearing capacity of joint replacements. Harrison and Nicol [9] have determined corresponding values in some other activities. Figure 9 illustrates the averages of tests conducted on seven young male volunteers undertaking a right angle turn whilst walking. The moments in this activity are compared with the flexion extension moment for the same individuals in straight-line level walking. It is seen that the flexion, adduction and torsion moments are approximately double the values that are developed in straight-line walking.

Figure 10 shows the corresponding data for test subjects running in a straight line. This activity gives a flexing moment approximately three times the level walking value, while the other two moments are sensibly unaltered. Where a running turn is accomplished, as illustrated in Fig. 11, the flexing and adducting moments are four to five times the level walking values, and the torsion moment up to ten times higher. These latter two activities are unlikely to be accomplished by patients with joint replacements, but the aggravating effect of these activities cannot be ignored. It should be noted that the ground to foot forces in turning whilst walking and straight-line walking are very similar in magnitude; the enhanced moment values correspond to the greater lever arms through which the ground forces act relative to the knee in the configurations adopted.

The forces transmitted between tibia and femur can be calculated in the manner of Morrison [16] or Paul and Poulson [22] and average curves, as shown in Fig. 12, can be produced to show the variation of joint force with time at different walking speeds. It is interesting to note that even at slow walking speeds, the joint force exceeds two times body weight for straight line level walking. In the running turn, values of joint force of up to 13 times body weight have been calculated. It is obvious therefore that design of knee joint replacements should be in accordance with the level walking data obtained and that patients should be strongly advised against undertaking any activities involving a twisting movement while the foot is stationary on the ground and any movement involving a lateral push-off between the foot and the ground.

Patients requiring joint replacement surgery may have a ligamentous structure which closely resembles the normal in strength and stiffness or it may be so lax as to lead to instability of the joint. Generally the surgeon will attempt to retain as much of the ligamentous structure as possible and

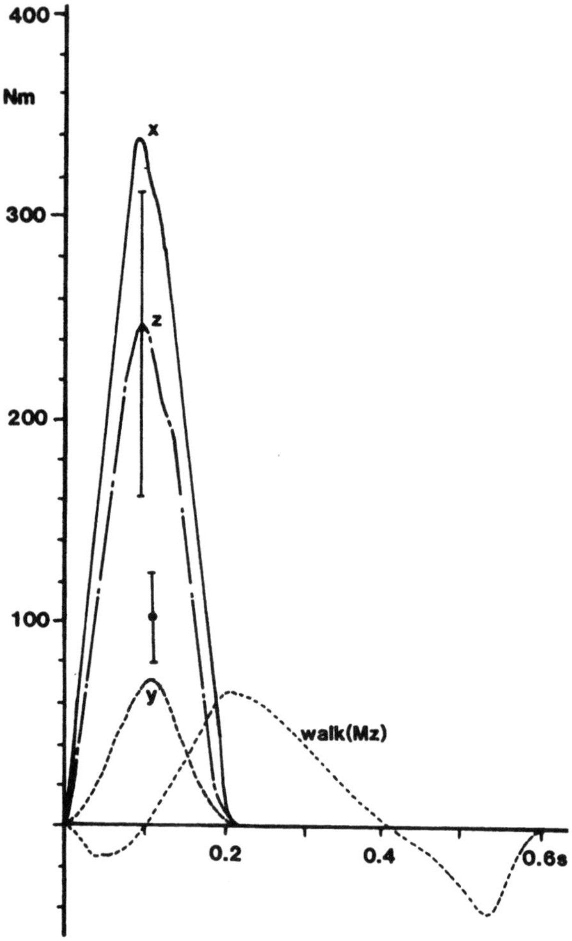


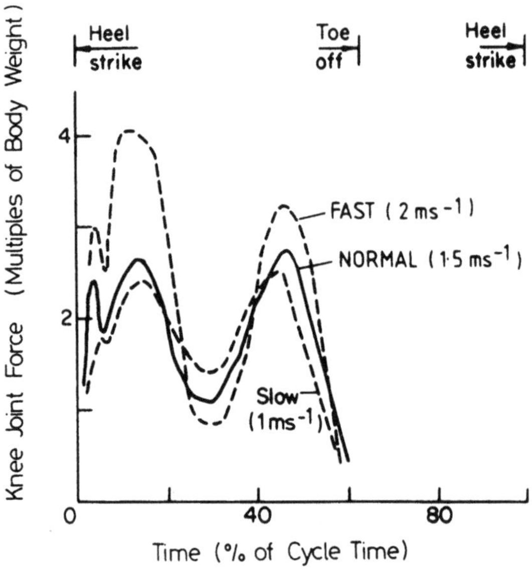


**Fig. 12.** Calculated values of knee joint force variation with normalised time in straight-line level walking at different speeds

◀**Fig. 11.** Variation with time of moments developed about the axes of the knee during a 90° running turn. *Positive values* correspond to the external load tending to flex (*z-axis*), adduct (*x-axis*) and inwardly rotate the foot (*y-axis*). The *broken line* corresponds to flexion moments developed in straight-line walking. *Bars* represent ± 1 SD (seven tests)

lax tissues may be tightened. It is important therefore that following surgery the patient should have a joint system in which the kinematics of the implant match, as far as possible, the constraints of the ligaments. This, however, is difficult, due to the complex curvature of the articulating surfaces. There is considerable uncertainty in the literature however on the constraints applied by the ligaments; these have been explored by several authors [4–6, 25, 26]. Comparisons of their data are shown in Figs. 13–16. It appears from these figures that there is as much evidence of the ligaments tightening in flexion as there is for them slackening, and the question must be posed whether in fact there is any significant tightening of the ligaments in the normal individual since in normal individuals the knee may easily be flexed beyond 120°. The data of Iseki and Tomatsu [12] and Nisell et al. [17] indicate that considerable changes in the axis of the knee are necessary to accommodate the restraints of the ligamentous structure. It is obvious therefore that a fully constrained joint having a single axis of rotation must result in loading the ligamentous structure as it flexes. This corresponds to the well-reported results of patients with knee joint replacement who, in many cases, have difficulty in achieving 90° flexion. A similar situation must occur with any implanted joint where the bearing surfaces are cylindrical since this implies a fixed joint centre. Where the profile of the femoral component makes some attempt to match the condyles of the natural knee, there appears to be a greater chance of success. This success can be achieved more easily if the cruciate ligaments are sacrificed, although the stability of the knee joint in torsional loading may be prejudiced by this, as previously discussed. If the joint replacement and the ligamentous structure are incompatible, the consequences may be: (a) Restriction of flexion angle; (b) loss of accessory rotation of the tibia and the femur accompanying knee flexion; (c) enhancement of loading transmitted at the joint surfaces and consequently at the joint-bone interfaces.

In the design of joint replacements for the knee,

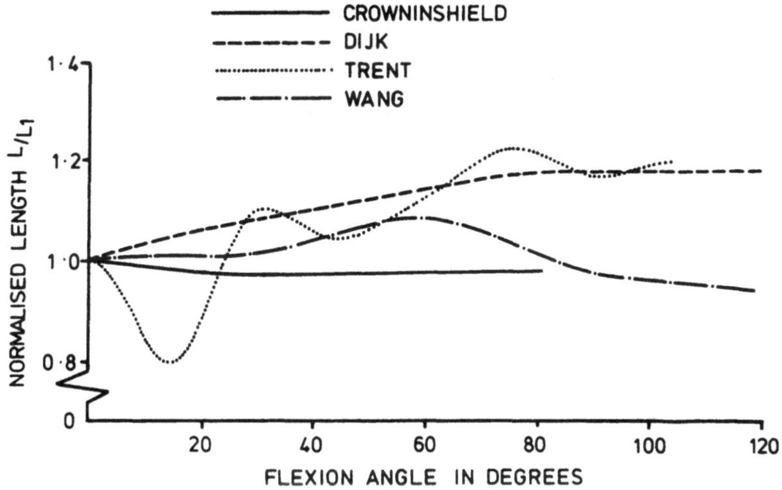


**Fig. 13.** Posterior cruciate ligament, anterior fibres, variation of normalised length with flexion angle. Normalised length is the ratio of measured or calculated length at a specific angle of flexion divided by the length at zero flexion. Calculated data after Crowninshield et al. [4], experimental data after Edwards et al. (1970), Wang et al. [24], Trent et al. [23], and Dijk [5]

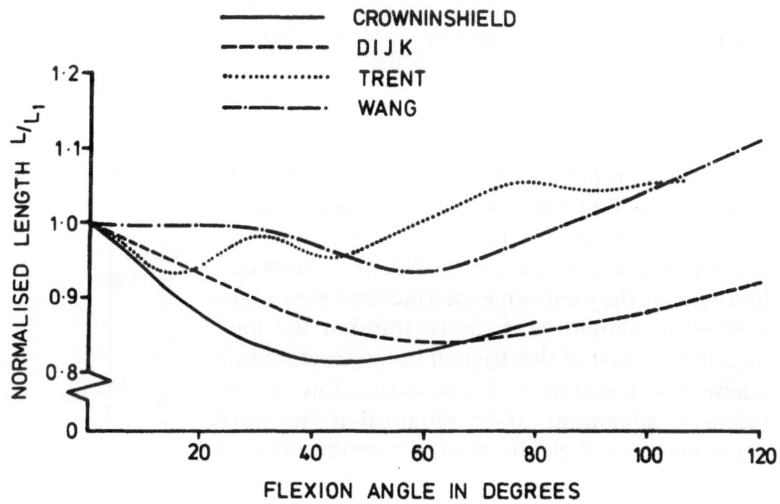


**Fig. 14.** Posterior cruciate ligament, posterior fibres. For explanation see legend to Fig. 13

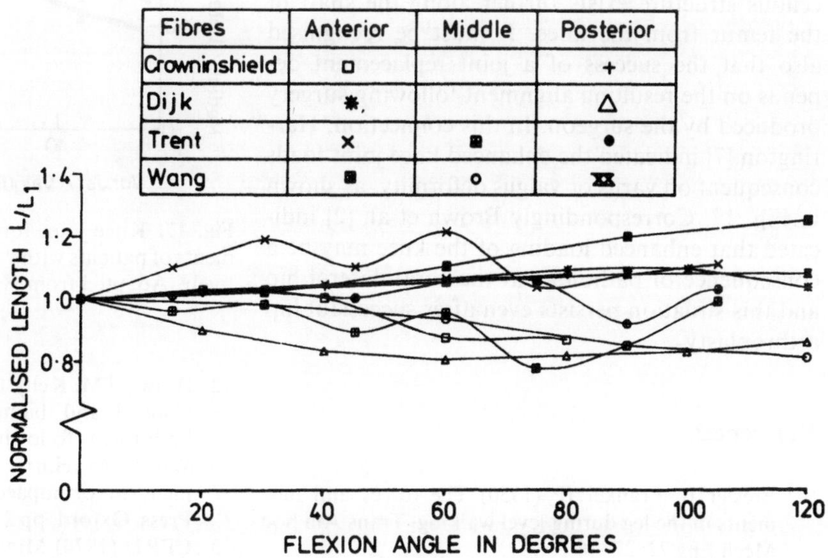


**Fig. 15.** Anterior cruciate ligament. For explanation see legend to Fig. 13

| Fibres | Anterior | Middle | Posterior | Oblique | Deep |
|---|---|---|---|---|---|
| Crowninshield | + | | □ | ✱ | Δ |
| Wang | | × | | | |
| Edwards | ▣(T)●(M)■(B) | | ○(T)××(M)◆(B) | | |

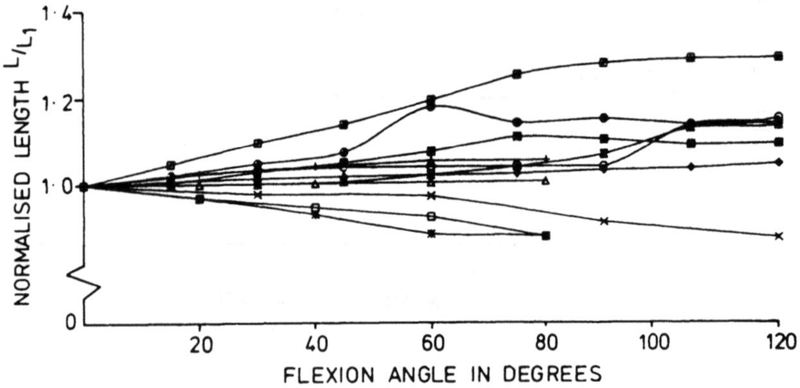


**Fig. 16.** Medial collateral ligament. *T, M, B* top, middle and bottom fibres, respectively. See also legend to Fig. 13

the relative rolling and sliding of the surfaces under load will produce wear, which may generally be taken to be proportional to the magnitude of the joint loading. Failure is equally likely to occur, however, at the joint-bone interface and every possible effort should be made to transmit the joint load to that part of the original bony structure best adapted to transmit it. There is therefore a considerable advantage to be obtained if the tibial component is sufficiently rigid to transmit the joint load to the cortical regions, which are best adapted to transmit it. The problem is not so acute in respect of the femoral condyles since a stronger cancellous structure exists further along the shaft of the femur from the knee. It must be recognised also that the success of a joint replacement depends on the resulting alignment following surgery produced by the surgeon. In this connection, Harrington [7] indicated the enhanced knee joint loads consequent on varus or valgus deformity, as shown in Fig. 17. Correspondingly Brown et al. [2] indicated that enhanced loading of the knee may be a consequence of pathology at the contralateral hip and this situation persists even after successful hip arthroplasty.

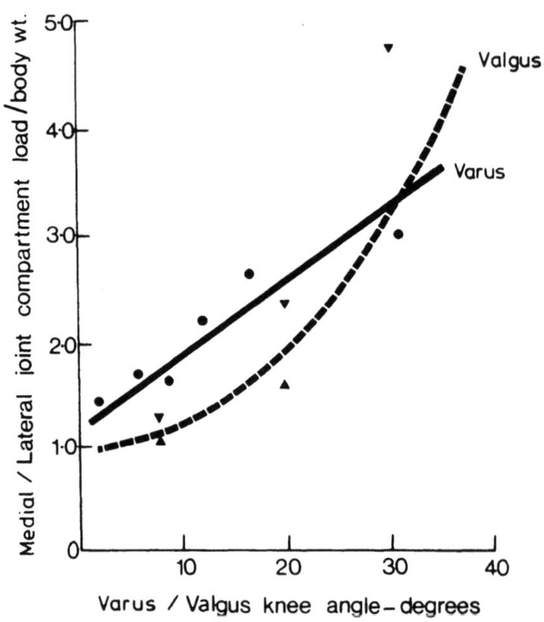


**Fig. 17.** Knee joint force in medial or lateral compartments of patients with varus or valgus deformities, respectively. Adapted from Harrington [7]

## References

1. Bresler B, Frankel JP (1950) The forces and moments in the leg during level walking. Trans Am Soc Mech Eng 72: 27–36
2. Brown TM, Kelly IG, Paul JP, Hamblen DL (1985) Clinical and biomechanical assessment of lower limb forces following joint replacement surgery. In: Whittle M, Harris D (eds) Biomechanical measurement in orthopaedic practice. Oxford University Press, Oxford, pp 224–247
3. CPRD (1974) Minutes of a workshop on total knee

arthroplasty. National Research Council, National Academy of Sciences of USA, Washington DC
4. Crowninshield R, Pope MH, Johnson RJ (1976) An analytical model of the knee. J Biomech 9: 397–405
5. Dijk RV (1983) Behavior of the cruciate ligaments in the human knee joint. Thesis, Catholic University of Nijmegen
6. Edwards RG, Lafferty JF, Lange KD (1970) Ligament strain in human knee joint. J Basic Engineering 131–136
7. Gollehon DL, Torzilli PA, Warren RF (1987) The role of the posterolateral and cruciate ligaments in the stability of the human knee. J Bone Jt Surg 69A: 233–242
8. Harrington IJ (1975) The effect of congenital and pathological conditions on the load transmitted at the knee joint. In: [12] pp 1–7
9. Harrison DW and Nicol AC (1988) Knee joint loads during running and turning activities. In Biomechanics in Sport Inst Mech Eng London pp 13–18
10. Hof AL, Van der Berg J (1981) EMG to force processing. J Biomech 14: 747–792
11. Hsieh H, Walker PS (1976) Stabilizing mechanisms of the loaded and unloaded knee joint. J Bone Jt Surg 58A: 87–93
12. Institution of Mechanical Engineers (1975) Total knee replacement. MEP, London
13. Iseki F, Tomatsu T (1976) The biomechanics of the knee joint with special reference to the contact area. Keio J Med 25: 37–44
14. Louie JK, Mote CD Jr (1987) Contribution of the musculature to rotatory laxity and torsional stiffness at the knee. J Biomech 20: 281–300
15. McLeod PC, Kettelkamp DB, Srinivasaw V, Henderson DL (1975) Measurements of repetitive activities of the knee. J Biomech 8: 369–373
16. Morrison JB (1968) Bioengineering analysis of force actions transmitted by the knee joint. Biomedical Engineering 164–170
17. Nisell R (1985) The biomechanics of the knee. Acta Orthop Scand Suppl 216
18. Nisell R, Nemeth G, Ohlsen H (1986) Joint forces in extension of the knee. Acta Orthop Scand 57: 41–46
19 Otis JC, Gould JD (1986) The effect of external load on torque production by knee extensors. Jnl Bone and Jt Surg 68A, 65–70.
20. Paul JP (1975) Force actions transmitted in the knee of normal subjects and by prosthetic joint replacements. In: [12] pp 126–131
21. Paul JP (1971) Comparison of EMG signals from leg muscles with the corresponding force actions calculated from walkpath measurements, In: Human locomotor engineering. Inst Mech Eng, London pp 16–26
22. Paul JP, Poulson J (1974) The analysis of forces transmitted in the human body. In: Bartolozzi G (ed) Proceedings of 5th Conference on Experimental Stress Analysis, May 1974. CISM, Udine pp 3.34–3.42
23. Shoemaker SC, Markolf KL (1985) Effects of joint load on the stiffness and laxity of ligament—deficient knees. J Bone Jt Surg 67A: 136–146
24. Such CH, Unsworth A, Wright V, Dowson D (1975) Qualitative study of stiffness in the knee joint. Ann Rheum Dis 34[4] 286–291
25. Trent PS, Walker PS, Wolf B (1976) Ligament length patterns, strength, and rotational axes of the knee joint. J Clin Orth 117: 263–270
26. Wang CJ, Walker PS Wolf B (1973) The effect of flexion and rotation on the length patterns of the ligaments on the knee. J Biomech 6: 587–596

## *Discussion*

*Goodfellow* (Oxford University): You said, and I agree, that the lengths of the cruciate ligaments do not alter significantly from full extension to full flexion. Is that not because they do in fact always run through the instant center of that rotational movement? Is the instant center not that point at which they cross, which means that they are able to stay the same length?

*Paul* (University of Strathclyde): Yes, I agree with you, and that makes the data showing a change in length I presented from all these investigators so surprising. On the other hand, it is something of a simplification to talk of the cruciate ligaments as if they were each a single structure: They have discrete areas of origin and insertion, and their fibers are by no means tethered one to the other. In fact, the ligaments are a collection of links rather than a single rigid link.

*Goodfellow*: But the neutral fiber, if there is one in such a bundle, would pass though the instant center?

*Paul*: Yes.

*Goodfellow*: Following on that, you said it was not appropriate to measure the lever arms of the muscles as if they radiated from the instant center. But if you do not measure them from there, I cannot see where you do measure them from.

*Paul*: In the mechanical analysis, one always has more unknowns than one has equations. A common mechanical technique is to use a reference axis though which one of the forces that is unknown can be taken to act. The joint force vector does not necessarily pass through the instantaneous center.

# Original Papers

# Part 1
# Cemented Total Knee Replacement I

# Clinical Results of Kinematic Total Knee Replacement

T. Sasaki[1], K. Yasuda[2], T. Yagi[2], J. Monji[2], Y. Aoki[2], and Y. Tomiyama[2]

**Summary.** The kinematic knee prostheses are intended as a "graduating system" and consist of four different types. We can choose a favorable type of prosthesis at the time of surgery depending on the severity of the pathological condition of the knee joint. We performed 225 kinematic knee replacements and followed up 201 knees (101 rheumatoid, 100 osteoarthritic).

Using Ewald's knee-rating system, the average score for all 201 knees was 86 points with 176 knees (88%) having a good or excellent rating at 2–6 years 8 months postoperatively. The average postoperative range of motion was 100° in rheumatoid arthritis and 109° in osteoarthritis.

Major complications included three loosenings, two fractures, one dislocation of the patella, three ruptures of the extension mechanism, and one impingement due to recurred synovitis.

The results obtained in this study are apparently better than those in previous series using the anametric, total condylar, and GUEPAR types. Our results, using the posterior cruciate retension type, almost correspond to those reported by Ewald.

**Keywords:** Graduating system—Kinematic knee—Complications—Clinical evaluation—Comparison with previous series

## Introduction

We have performed total knee replacement on rheumatoid or osteoarthritic knees in terminal stages since 1973. The type of prosthesis is chosen according to the pathological condition of the knee joints, for example, the severity of deformity and instability and degree of restriction in mobility, so as to use the most suitable prosthesis. We treat our patients on the principle that the preserved function of the living body should be utilized as much as possible in total knee replacement. The kinematic knee system was developed by Walker et al. in 1978 from conventional prostheses. According to the severity of pathological changes of the knee joint and the condition of the ligament, an optimal type can be selected from four types of prosthesis during the operation (recently, six types of prosthesis have become available). Total knee replacement using the kinematic knee system may be said to be, in fact, the selection of prostheses by a "graduating system."

Until 1979 we chose prostheses from the anametric, total condylar, and GUEPAR types. However, we have used the kinematic knee system since 1980. Regarding clinical results of the use of the kinematic knee system, relatively few papers have been published [2]. In particular, the results obtained in a relatively large series of Japanese patients have never been reported to our knowledge. The aim of the present paper is to review the results obtained in our patients who have undergone total knee replacement using the kinematic knee system and compare them with those of previous series.

## Materials and Methods

Two hundred and twenty-five consecutive total knee replacements using the kinematic knee system in 174 patients were performed between June 1980 and April 1985 by one of four staff surgeons at our institutions. Seven patients (nine knees) died prior to this report and 11 patients (five knees) have been lost to follow-up. The remaining 156 patients (201 knees) were available for clinical and radiographic evaluation. The average age of patients was 63 years (range, 23–83 years); there were 124 knees in women and 32 in men. The diagnosis was rheumatoid arthritis in 101 knees and osteoarthritis in 100 knees. Ten of 201 knees were revision operations of other prostheses. The operative techniques and postoperative rehabilitation have been previously published [4].

[1] Hokkaido Prefectural Rehabilitation Center for Crippled Children, Sapporo Unit, Affiliated with the Sapporo Medical College, Sapporo, Japan

[2] Department of Orthopedic Surgery, Hokkaido University, Sappro, Japan

In performing surgery, we intended to preserve bone stock as much as possible and inserted thin tibial components. If there was a deep bony defect on one compartment of the tibia plateau, we cut the upper tibia at the higher level of the base line of the bony defect and grafted bone onto it.

In principle, we chose the posterior cruciate retention (type II) for knees with a functional posterior cruciate ligament, the stabilizer (type III) for absent or insufficient posterior cruciate ligament, and the rotating hinge (type IV) for severe deformity, narrow range of motion, or severe instability. The anteriorly joined type (type I) was indicated for knees with a functional anterior and posterior cruciate ligament. Type I was used for three knees, type II for 145 knees, type III for 36 knees, and type IV for 17 knees (Fig. 1). The patella was resurfaced in all of the patients.

Two hundred and one knees were evaluated 2–6 years 8 months postoperatively (average follow-up, 3 years 3 months) and the first 92 knees 4–6 years 8 months postoperatively (average follow-up, 5 years 1 month).

The knee-rating system described by Ewald [1] was used (Table 1). A score of 90–100 points is considered to be excellent, 80–89 points good, 70–79 points fair, and 60–69 points poor.

Overall varus or valgus angulation of the knee was measured on the radiographs both preoperatively and postoperatively. The radiolucent lines beneath the tibial component were investigated. Radiolucency of more than 1mm in width was presented as a positive case.

## Results

The average postoperative flexion, by diagnosis, was 104° (range, 30°–140°) in rheumatoid arthritis and 112° (range, 65°–150°) in osteoarthritis. The average postoperative extension was 4° (range, 0°–30°) short of full extension in rheumatiod arthritis and 3° (range, 0°–15°) in osteoarthritis. The average postoperative range of motion was 100° in rheumatoid arthritis and 109° in osteoarthritis (Fig. 2). The overall average postoperative flexion was 106°, and extension 4°. The preoperative and postoperative scores are shown in Fig. 2. In the 101 rheumatoid knees, 31 (31%) were rated excellent, 57 (56%) good, 9 (9%) fair, and 4 (4%) poor. The average preoperative score was 33 points (range, 11–56 points) and average postoperative score, 85 points (range, 60–96 points). In the 100 osteoarthritic knees, 45 (45%) were rated excellent, 43 (43%) good, 7 (7%) fair, and 5 (5%) poor. The average preoperative score was 40 points (range, 13–52 points), and postoperative score 87 points (range, 60–100 points) (Fig. 3). The average postoperative score for all 201 knees was 86 points, with 176 knees (88%) having a good or excellent result.

In the first consecutive 92 arthroplasties, the average preoperative score was 30 points (range, 13–56 points), and postoperative score 82 points (range, 52–96 points), with 69 knees (75%) having a good or excellent result. The percentage of excellent or good results, by type of prosthesis, was: types I and II 85%, type III 76%, and type IV

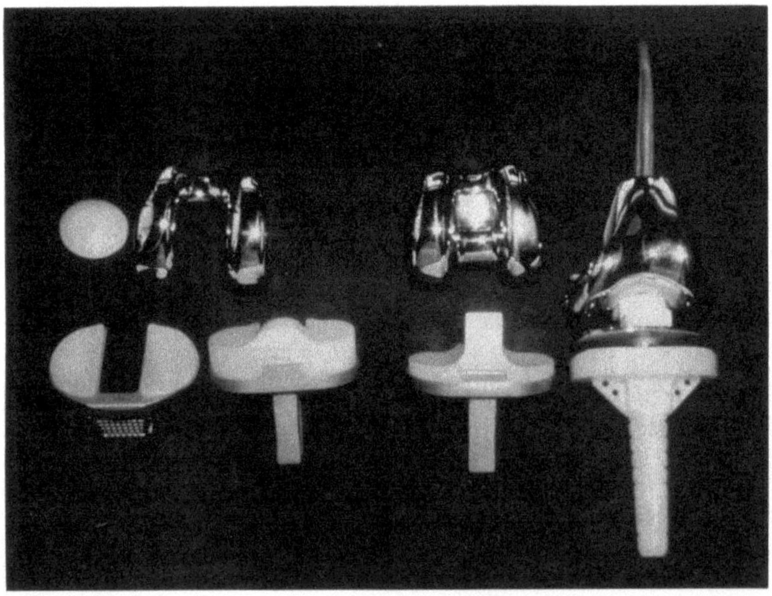

**Fig. 1.** From *left* to *right*, the prostheses are anteriorly joined (type I), posterior cruciate retention (type II), stabilizer (type III), and rotating hinge (type IV)

**Table 1.** Knee-rating system (after Ewald)

| | Points |
|---|---|
| Pain | |
| None, or patient ignores it | 50 |
| Slight on ascending or descending stairs or on prolonged walking (no compromise in activities of daily living) | 45 |
| Moderate pain when ascending or descending stairs or getting out of chair; no pain with level gait; occasional pain medication | 40 |
| Pain with level gait with more pain on stairs, especially down; no pain at rest; daily pain medication | 25 |
| Pain at rest or at night in addition to pain on walking; pain medication taken regularly | 10 |
| Continuous pain regardless of activity | 0 |
| Disabled because of pain | 0 |
| Total | _____ |
| Function | |
| Limp, antalgic | |
| None | 6 |
| Slight | 4 |
| Moderate | 2 |
| Marked | 0 |
| Total | _____ |
| Distance walked | |
| Unlimited | 6 |
| 4 to 6 blocks | 4 |
| 2 to 3 blocks | 2 |
| Indoors only | 1 |
| Bed to chair | 0 |
| Unable to walk | 0 |
| Total | _____ |
| Support | |
| None | 6 |
| Cane on long walks or only outside | 5 |
| Cane full time | 3 |
| Two canes or two crutches | 1 |
| Walker or unable to walk | 0 |
| Total | _____ |
| Stairs | |
| Normally | 6 |
| Needs banister | 5 |
| One stair at a time, up or down, or both | 3 |
| Banister plus cane or crutch, one stair at a time up or down | 1 |
| Two crutches | 0 |
| Unable to climb stairs | 0 |
| Total | _____ |

| | | Points |
|---|---|---|
| Rising from a chair | | |
| Normally | | 6 |
| Needs arm assistance | | 5 |
| Difficult using two arms | | 3 |
| Needs assistance | | 1 |
| Unable to rise | | 0 |
| Total | | _____ |
| Deformity | | |
| Permanent flexion contracture | | |
| 0 to 6 degrees | 5 | |
| 6 to 15 degrees | 3 | |
| >15 degrees | 0 _____ | |
| Varus angulation in stance | | |
| <5 degrees | 1 | |
| >5 degrees | 0 _____ | |
| Valgus angulation in stance | | |
| <10 degrees | 1 | |
| >10 degrees | 0 _____ | |
| Medial and lateral collateral ligaments | | |
| Stable | 2 | |
| Moderate or marked instability | 0 _____ | |
| Anteroposterior stability with knee flexed 90 degrees | | |
| Stable | 1 | |
| Moderate or marked instability | 0 _____ | Total _____ |
| Motion | | |
| Flexion | | |
| 110 degrees or more | | 10 |
| 100 to 109 degrees | | 8 |
| 90 to 99 degrees | | 6 |
| 70 to 89 degrees | | 4 |
| <70 degrees | | 0 |
| Total | | _____ |
| Patient's sum total | | _____ |

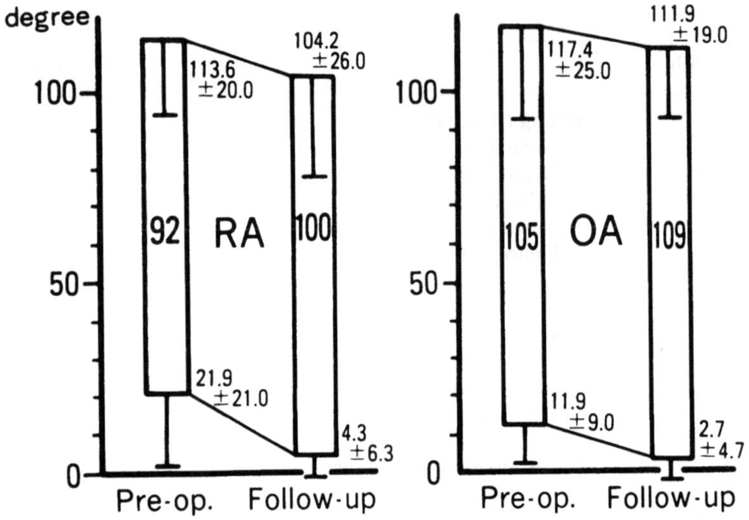


**Fig. 2.** Average preoperative (*Pre-op.*) and follow-up (*Follow-up*) flexion angle ± SD (*upper value*) and extension angle ± SD (*lower value*) are shown in rheumatoid arthritis (*RA*) and osteoarthritis (*OA*). *Figures in column* refer to the preoperative and follow-up range of motion

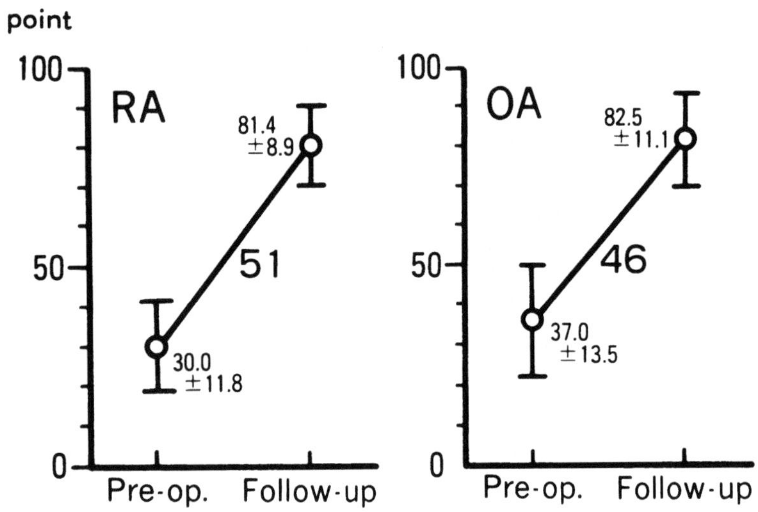


**Fig. 3.** Average preoperative (*Pre-op.*) and follow-up (*Follow-up*) score ± SD are shown in rheumatoid arthritis (*RA*) and osteoarthritis (*OA*). *Large figures* refer to improved scores after surgery

42%.

The average preoperative alignment in the rheumatoid knees was 2° ± 7° of valgus angulation, and in the osteoarthritic knees 11° ± 8° of varus angulation. Postoperatively, the alignment in the rheumatoid knees had been corrected to an average of 2° ± 5° of valgus angulation, and in the osteoarthritic knees an average of 2° ± 5° of valgus angulation.

Eight of 153 knees (5.2%) examined on standardized radiograms had radiolucent lines beneath the tibial component. There were six radiolucent lines in the medial condyle and two in the lateral condyle.

Ten knees (ten patients) had major surgical complications. There were three loosenings (1.5%), consisting of two rheumatoid knees (one tibial component, one femoral component) and one osteoarthritic knee (femoral component). There were two fractures (rheumatoid only), two dislocations of the patella (one rheumatoid, one osteoarthritic), two ruptures of the knee extension mechanism (osteoarthritic only), and one impingement due to recurrence of synovitis (rheumatoid). The overall complication rate was 4.9%.

## Discussion

There has been controversy as to whether it is better to preserve the anterior cruciate ligament and the posterior cruciate ligament in total knee replacement. We examined the functional status of the ligaments of 79 knees for which there was an indication of total knee replacement [4]. It was found that both the anterior cruciate ligament and the posterior cruciate ligament were functional for 22 knees, only the posterior cruciate ligament was functional for 29 knees, and neither the anterior cruciate ligament nor the posterior cruciate ligament was functional for 28 knees. The type I prosthesis, with which both the anterior cruciate ligament and the posterior cruciate ligament are preserved, was inserted only in 3 of 201 knees. This was because preservation of the anterior cruciate ligament would make osteotomy of the upper portion of the tibia and insertion of the component difficult and, moreover, it becomes difficult to obtain proper stability and favorable mobility postoperatively. The type II prosthesis, with which the posterior cruciate ligament is preserved, was inserted in 145 of 201 knees (72%). Various investigators, including the present writers [8], and Westin et al. [7] have published papers concerning the significance of preservation of the posterior cruciate ligament. The most significant advantage of preservation of the posterior cruciate ligament is that wide range of motion and good stability can be obtained simultaneously. Thus, the posterior cruciate ligament is the most basic stabilizer of knee joints and the structure of the artificial joint can be approximated to that of the nonconstrained type by preserving it. Moreover, the roll-back movement required for flexion of the knee can be retained. The second advantage of preservation of the posterior cruciate ligament is that the excessive stress applied to bone under certain mechanical circumstances can be dispersed. It is expected that this dispersion of stress is effective in decreasing the occurrence of loosening and sinking. In view of these facts, we consider that the posterior cruciate ligament should be preserved as far as possible. The type III prosthesis is of the semiconstrained type, with which anterior and posterior instability is prevented by the central spine, which is on the upper side of the tibial component. The type III prosthesis was inserted in 36 knees showing absence or functional insufficiency of the anterior and posterior cruciate ligaments and severe flexion contracture with excessive amount of osteotomy of the tibia. When this type of prosthesis is used, the redistribution of stress between components is extremely small and stress distribution within the tibia during walking poses a problem. Therefore, it is considered that in long-term results the incidence of loosening and sinking is increased. The type IV prosthesis is indicated for cases with severe instability in the anteroposterior and lateral directions, those with narrow range of motion or ankylosis, and those with marked deformity. With the type IV prosthesis, axial rotation is possible [6]. However, it is of the constrained type and a greater amount of osteotomy is required than with prostheses of types I, II, and III. The type IV prosthesis was inserted only in 17 of 201 knees (8.5%), nine knees of which were revision cases.

Even among knees for which total knee replacement is indicated, pathological conditions differ widely. In knees which had been in relatively good condition before the operation, the postoperative results after insertion of the prosthesis are naturally good. The results obtained in cases in which the type IV prostheses had been inserted were poorer than those obtained in cases in which prostheses of types I, II, and III had been inserted [3]. In the present study, we reviewed the results of all of our cases in which there was an indication for total knee replacement. Although the postoperative follow-up period was relatively short (mean, 3.3 years), the clinical results were satisfactory and rated as excellent and good in 88% of the cases of rheumatoid arthritis and osteoarthritis. In our previous paper, we reported the results of 105 knees treated by using the kinematic knee system (series I) in comparison with those obtained in the knees treated using prostheses chosen from the anametric type, total condylar type, and GUEPAR type (series II). Despite the fact that the follow-up period was similar for both groups, the ratio of results rated as excellent or good was 81% for series I and 59% for series II, showing significant superiority for the former series [3]. Moreover, the incidence of major complications was apparently lower for series I than with series II [5]. These results show clearly that the kinematic knee system is superior to this set of prostheses consisting of three different types.

The long-term results (mean follow up period, 5.1 years) of early 92 cases revealed a slight reduction in the ratio of excellent and good results to 75%. This reduction in the treatment success rate may be attributable to occurrence of complications, recurrence of synovitis in patients with rheumatoid arthritis, and influences from other deteriorated joints.

Ewald et al. reported 2- to 4-year-results obtained in cases of type II. According to their results, a score of 49 points was obtained after the operation, with a postoperative mean flexion angle of 106° and a mean extension angle of 2° [2]. These results almost correspond to those obtained by us (Fig. 4). This fact indicates that equivalent results can be obtained when the kinematic knee system is used even with different surgeons and in patients with different body structure and life style.

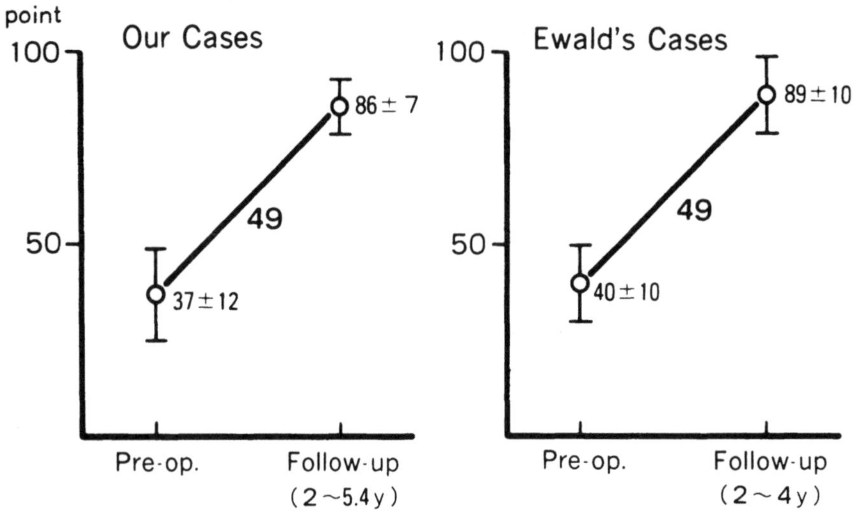


**Fig. 4.** Average preoperative (*Pre-op.*) and follow-up (*Follow-up*) score ± SD are shown in our study (*Our Cases*) and Ewald's series (*Ewald's Cases*). *Large figures* refer to improved scores after surgery. Figures *in parentheses* refer to follow-up period

## References


1. Ewald FC (1979) Rheumatold arthritis: III. Surgery of the knee in rheumatoid arthritis. Instructional Course Lectures, American Academy of Orthopaedic Surgeons, vol 28. Mosby, St. Louis, pp 285–298
2. Ewald FC, Jacobs MA, Mlegel RE, Walker PS, Poss R, Sledge CB (1984) Kinematic total knee replacement. J Bone Joint Surg 66-A: 1032–1040
3. Kurosawa H, Sasaki T, Yagi T, Monji J, Yasuda K, Minami M, Tsuge H, Kanno Y (1986) Follow-up on kinematic total knee replacement in 120 knees after a minimum of two years., Jpn Rheumatism Joint Surgery 5: 513–520
4. Sasaki T, Matsuno S, Yagi T, Monji J, Yasuda K, Hikino K, Tanji H, Minami M, Tsuge H (1984) Kinematic knee system; a report of 105 cases. Seikeigeka 35: 1613–1620 (in Japanese)
5. Sasaki T, Matsuno S, Yagi T, Yasuda K, Tsuge H (1986) Complications following total knee replacement. J Jpn Orthop Ass 60: 35–49
6. Walker PS, Emerson R, Potter T, Scott R, Thomas WH, Turner RH (1982) The kinematic rotating hinge: Biomechanics and clinical application. Orthopedic Clinics North America 13: 187–199
7. Westin CD, Clarke IC (1984) Should the cruciate ligaments be saved in total knee replacement? Orthopaedic Review XIII: 89–97
8. Yasuda K, Sasaki T (1986) Stress analysis after total knee arthroplasty with posterior cruciate ligament-resection type and -retention type prosthesis. With special reference to the significance of retaining the posterior cruciate ligament. J Jpn Orthop Ass 60: 547–562

# A Prospective Comparison of the Cemented Kinematic II and Cementless PCA Total Knee Replacements

R.B. Bourne, C.H. Rorabeck, and L. Nott[1]

**Summary.** One hundred and sixty consecutive primary total knee joint replacements (110 cemented Kinematic II and 50 noncemented porous coated anatomic (PCA) form the basis of the this review. All patients were operated upon by two surgeons with a minimum follow-up of 24 months. Each patient was seen pre- and postoperatively at 6 weeks, 3 months, 6 months, 12 months, and 24 months. The Hospital for Special Surgery (HSS) score was recorded by an independent third party at each visit to minimize interobserver variance. In addition, standing X-rays of the knees were made at each follow-up visit. Results were compared according to the HSS score at follow-up, the HSS scores for osteoarthritis and rheumatoid arthritis, pain relief, range of motion, radiographic assessment, and complications.

This study has demonstrated that at a minimum 24-month follow-up the average HSS score for the cemented Kinematic II is 10 points higher ($P < 0.01$) than the noncemented PCA implant (88 vs. 78). In addition, at the same follow-up period, the arc of motion of the cemented Kinematic II is greater ($P < 0.02$) than the noncemented PCA (106° vs. 97°). Finally, the reoperation rate for the cemented Kinematic II was 3.6% compared with 12% for the cementless PCA.

On the basis of this prospective nonrandomized clinical review, the authors conclude that the cemented Kinematic II gives superior results to the cementless PCA at a minimum 24-month follow-up; however, the superior results may be related to the difference in the design of the prosthesis and/or limited weight bearing offered to the cementless implant group rather than to the use of cement itself.

**Keywords:** Prospective comparison—Cemented TKR—Cementless TKR

## Introduction

Since Gunston's description of the first low-friction total knee arthroplasty in 1971, hundreds of total knee replacement designs have emerged [1–3, 5, 8, 10, 13]. Clinical experience has demonstrated the superiority of the condylar surface replacement over other designs [2, 3, 13–15, 19]. Insall et al. [14] described the 5- to 9-year follow-up of their first 100 Total Condylar I total knee joint replacements. Sixty-four patients were excellent, 27 good, 2 fair, and 7 poor. In this same group, seven patients required reoperation, one for sepsis, four for pain, and two for subluxation [13]. Improvements have been made to the Total Condylar design in terms of increasing the number of implant sizes, adding metal backing to high-density polyethylene components, providing better instrumentation (both for insertion and alignment) and improving cementing techniques [3, 19].

With the success of the condylar type of total knee joint replacement, the age indications for this procedure have steadily decreased. Life expectancy charts have suggested that a 60-year-old patient might anticipate 17 (male) to 22 (female) more years of life (Table 1). It has been felt that perhaps a cemented arthroplasty would not stand up to this prolonged use. The advent of porous ingrowth total knee replacements has been associated with a hope for increased longevity of the im-

**Table 1.** Life expectancy at birth and at age 60 by sex in Canada, 1931–1976

| Year | Males (years) | | Females (years) | |
|---|---|---|---|---|
| | At birth | 60 years | At birth | 60 years |
| 1931 | 60.0 | 16.3 | 62.1 | 17.2 |
| 1941 | 63.0 | 16.1 | 66.3 | 17.6 |
| 1951 | 66.3 | 16.5 | 70.8 | 18.6 |
| 1956 | 67.6 | 16.5 | 72.9 | 19.3 |
| 1961 | 68.4 | 16.7 | 74.2 | 19.9 |
| 1966 | 68.8 | 16.8 | 75.2 | 20.6 |
| 1971 | 69.3 | 17.0 | 76.4 | 21.4 |
| 1976 | 70.2 | 17.2 | 77.5 | 22.0 |
| Gains (1931–1976) | 10.2 | 0.9 | 15.4 | 4.8 |

Source: Statistics Canada, Life Tables (1930–1932 to 1975–1977)

[1] Division of Orthopaedic Surgery, University Hospital, University of Western Ontario, Ontario, Canada

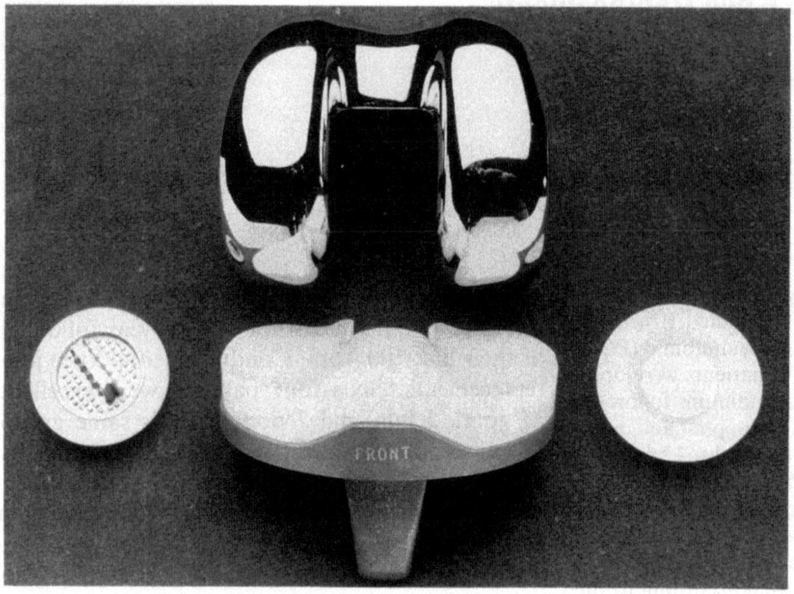


**Fig. 1.** The femoral, tibial, and patellar components of the Kinematic II total knee replacement

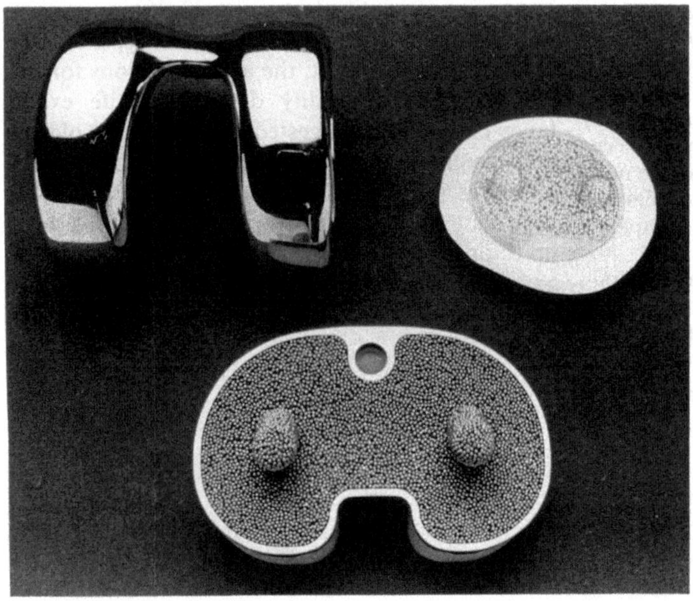

**Fig. 2.** The femoral, tibial, and patellar components of the PCA total knee replacement

plant [10]. There is ample experimental evidence that bony ingrowth is possible and, indeed, an ever increasing number of cementless total knee replacements is emerging [6, 7, 10–12, 17]. What is not clear is whether or not the cementless total knee replacement is as clinically successful as its cemented counterpart. The purpose of this paper is to compare two contemporary total knee replacements, namely the cemented Kinematic II total knee replacement (Fig. 1) and the cementless PCA implant (Fig. 2).

## Method

One hundred and sixty consecutive primary total knee replacements were analyzed. One hundred and ten patients were treated by means of cemented Kinematic II total knee replacements. This population group was compared with 50 patients in which cementless PCA total knee replacements were inserted. Patients were selected to enter one of the two groups on the basis of age and/or bone stock. The two groups were *not* identical and *not* randomized. No patient was lost to follow-up.

This study was performed by two surgeons (RBB and CHR), using the same operating room, horizontal laminar air flow, body exhaust suits, prophylactic antibiotics, the original universal instrumentation, and comparable surgical techniques. Continuous passive motion (CPM) machines were used beginning on the 2nd postoperative day. Initially, each CPM machine (Kinetec 3080, Richard Mgf. Inc., Memphis, TN, USA) was set at 0°–30° at a rate of 3.34 min/cycle. The arc of motion was increased by 10° daily and the rate turned up to 2.30 min/cycle, depending on patient comfort. Each patient utilized the CPM machine a mean of 15 (7–21) h on day 2, but increased out-of-bed activities reduced this to 7 (5–14) h by day 7.

Each patient was assessed preoperatively, as well as 6 and 12 weeks and 6 and 12 months postoperatively, then yearly by an independent observer (Nott). Prospective analysis employed the Hospital for Special Surgery (HSS) knee rating scale which gave 30 points for pain, 22 points for function, 10 points for strength, 10 points for stability, 10 points for lack of flexion deformity, and 18 points for range of motion (Fig. 3). In addition, X-ray parameters and complications were sought. Standing anteroposterior, lateral, and 60° skyline radiographs were taken at each postoperative visit. These films were analyzed for implant alignment, radiolucent lines, change in orientation, and restoration of the joint line.

## Results

The results of the two groups were compared and analyzed according to the following parameters: (a) HSS scores (Kinematic II vs. PCA), (b) osteoarthritis (OA) versus rheumatoid arthritis (RA) HSS scores (Kinematic II and PCA), (c) pain relief, (d) range of motion, (e) radiographic assessment, (f) complications.

Though the study was prospective with no exclusions, the groups were not randomized. The minimum follow-up was 24 months and the maximum 36 months. The average age of patients with the Kinematic II total knee joint replacement was 71 years (52–88 years) compared with an average age in the cementless group of 62 years (22–82 years). Females outnumbered males in both groups, the ratio being 3:2. Osteoarthritis was the primary diagnosis in both groups with the ratio of osteoarthritic to rheumatoid arthritic patients being approximately the same in both groups. In the cemented Kinematic II group, there were 92 patients with osteoarthritis and 18 with rheumtoid arthritis, while in the cementless PCA group there were 44 patients with osteoarthritis and six with rheumatoid arthritis. In addition to differences in age, there was also a significant difference between the two groups in average body mass. The average mass of the cemented Kinematic II total knee joint patients was 76 kg versus an average for those with the cementless PCA total knee joint replacement of 86 kg ($P < 0.001$).

### Hospital for Special Surgery Scores (Kinematic II vs. PCA)

An analysis of the HSS knee rating scores (Table 2) demonstrated that the cemented Kinematic II patients had higher scores than the noncemented PCA total knee joint replacement patients at 2 year follow-up (88 vs. 78 points, $P < 0.01$). This observation is significant considering that the preoperative scores for both groups were identical: 49 in the cemented Kinematic II and 48 in the cementless PCA patients. Though both groups had approximately the same HSS scores at 3 months, at 6, 12, and 24 months the HSS scores for the cemented Kinematic II prosthesis began to outdistance the HSS scores for the cementless PCA prosthesis (88 vs. 78). Further examination of the data demonstrated that the HSS scores seemed to be improving over time with the cemented Kinematic II prosthesis; however, this was not the case with the cementless PCA prosthesis.

### Osteoarthritis Versus Rheumatoid Arthritis HSS Scores (Kinematic II and PCA)

Although the number of patients with rheumatoid arthritis in both groups was small, a comparative analysis of the data suggested that the results for osteoarthritis versus rheumatoid arthritis were somewhat different when the cemented Kinematic II was compared with the cementless PCA prosthesis (Tables 3, 4). The HSS scores for the cemented Kinematic II prosthesis at 24 months' follow-up were virtually identical when the osteoarthritis patients were compared with those with rheumatoid arthritis (87 vs. 88). However, when the results of the cementless PCA total knee arthroplasty in osteoarthritis versus rheumatoid arthritis were examined (Table 4), the HSS scores at 24 months for the osteoarthritics were better than for rheumatoid arthritics (81 vs. 69). It is important to note however, that the number of rheumatoids in the PCA group was small and the data were not statistically significant at the 0.05 level.

University Hospital
Owned and Operated by
London Health Association

## H.S.S. KNEE ASSESSMENT SHEET

KNEE: R L | DATE: D / M / Y

P R1 R2 R3 | SURGEON: R.B.B. C.H.R.

NAME: ______________

CHART NUMBER ______________

FOLLOW-UP 0 / .16 / .25 / .50 / 1 / 2 / 3 Yrs.

**PAIN** — ADD POINTS

ACTIVITY
- no pain on walking/ignores ... 15
- mild pain on walking (ASA) ... 10
- moderate pain on walking (Codeine) ... 5
- severe pain on walking (Severe Limitations) ... 0

REST
- no pain at rest/ignores ... 15
- mild pain at rest ... 10
- moderate pain at rest ... 5
- severe pain at rest ... 0 /30

**FUNCTION**

STAIRS
- climb stairs ... 5
- climb stairs with support ... 2
- unable ... 0

TRANSFER .. chair
- transfer activity ... 5
- transfer activity with support ... 2
- unable ... 0

WALKING
- walking and standing unlimited ... 12
- walking 5 – 10 blocks and standing intermittent more than ½ hour ... 10
- walking 1 – 5 blocks and standing ability up to ½ hour ... 8
- walk less than 1 block/indoors only ... 4
- can't walk ... 0 /22

**MUSCLE STRENGTH**
- very good (can't break quadraceps power) ... 10
- good (can break quadraceps power) ... 8
- fair (moves through arc of motion) ... 4
- poor (can't move through arc of motion) ... 0 /10

**INSTABILITY**
- none ... 10
- mild (0 5) ... 8
- moderate (6 15) ... 5
- severe (16 or more) ... 0 /10

**FLEXION DEFORMITY**
- no deformity ... 10
- few degrees ... 8
- 5 10 degrees ... 5
- 11 degrees or more ... 0 /10

**R.O.M.**
(1 point given for each 8 degrees of arc of motion) /18

STATE RANGE OF MOTION ______________

**SUPPORT** — SUBTRACTION POINTS
- 2 crutches/walker ... 3
- 1 crutch/2 canes ... 2
- 1 cane ... 1

**EXTENSION LAG**
- 5 degrees ... 2
- 10 degrees ... 3
- 15 degrees or more ... 5

**VALGUS OR VARUS DEFORMITY**
- 5 degrees or more ... 1

minus ______________

TOTAL POINTS ______________/100

Ortho 2(06/86)1 NS

**RADIOGRAPHIC FINDINGS:**

**FEMUR**
RADIOLUCENT LINES: NONE N/C B W
LOOSENING No Poss. Prob. Def.
MIGRATION No Yes
SUBSIDENCE No Yes

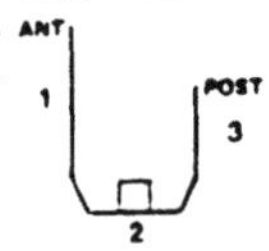


**PATELLA**
RADIOLUCENT LINES: NONE N/C B W
LOOSENING No Poss. Prob. Def.
MIGRATION No Yes
SUBSIDENCE No Yes

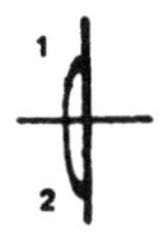


**TIBIA**
RADIOLUCENT LINES: NONE N/C B W
LOOSENING No Poss. Prob. Def.
MIGRATION No Yes
SUBSIDENCE No Yes

**NON-CEMENTED**

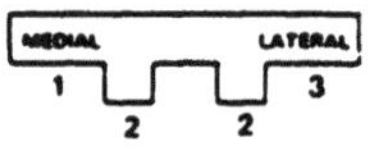

AP

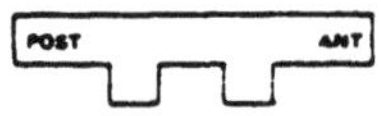

LATERAL

**CEMENTED**

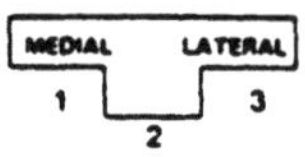

AP

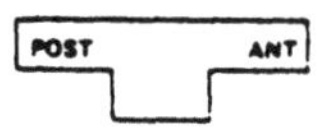

LATERAL

**COMMENTS:**

Number of operations since last TKA ______________
Complications Y N Details:

EXAMINER ______________

**Fig. 3.** The modified Hospital for Special Surgery knee rating scale used in this study

**Table 2.** Hospital for Special Surgery Scores

| | Kinematic II (110) | PCA (50) |
|---|---|---|
| Preoperation | 49 | 48 |
| 3 months | 79 | 78 |
| 6 months | 84 | 79 |
| 12 months | 86 | 81 |
| 24 months | 88 | 78 |

**Table 3.** HSS scores in osteoarthritic patients treated with Kinematic II and PCA prostheses

| | Kinematic II (92) | | PCA (44) | |
|---|---|---|---|---|
| | HSS score | ROM | HSS score | ROM |
| 3 months | 81 | 3°–98° | 78 | 4°–91° |
| 6 months | 83 | 2°–102° | 79 | 3°–92° |
| 12 months | 86 | 2°–107° | 81 | 3°–96° |
| 24 months | 87 | 1°–107° | 81 | 3°–99° |

*ROM* range of motion

**Table 4.** HSS socres in rheumatoid patients treated with Kinematic II and PCA prostheses

| | Kinematic II (18) | | PCA (6) | |
|---|---|---|---|---|
| | HSS score | ROM | HSS score | ROM |
| 3 months | 87 | 3°–101° | 71 | 5°–88° |
| 6 months | 88 | 1°–104° | 85 | 5°–100° |
| 12 months | 88 | 3°–107° | 84 | 8°–115° |
| 24 months | 88 | 1°–104° | 69 | 13°–88° |

**Table 5.** Pain relief in activity and at rest afforded by Kinematic II prosthesis

| | Activity | Rest |
|---|---|---|
| Preoperation | 1 | 5 |
| 3 months | 14 | 14 |
| 6 months | 14 | 14 |
| 12 months | 14 | 14 |
| 24 months | 14 | 15 |

No pain = 15 points

**Table 6.** Pain relief in activity and at rest afforded by PCA prosthesis

| | Activity | Rest |
|---|---|---|
| Preoperation | 1 | 5 |
| 3 months | 13 | 14 |
| 6 months | 12 | 13 |
| 12 months | 12 | 14 |
| 24 months | 13 | 14 |

No pain = 15 points

**Table 7.** Preoperative and postoperative knee range of motion in patients treated with Kinematic II and PCA prostheses

| | Kinematic II (110) | PCA (50) |
|---|---|---|
| Preoperation | 6°–110° | 9°–104° |
| 3 months | 3°–98° | 4°–91° |
| 6 months | 2°–103° | 3°–92° |
| 12 months | 2°–107° | 4°–97° |
| 24 months | 2°–106° | 5°–97° |

## Pain Relief

Pain was evaluated in all patients by assigning a maximum of 15 points for rest pain and 15 points for activity-related pain. The results of the two operative procedures in terms of achieving pain relief are illustrated in Tables 5 and 6. Preoperatively, both groups had severe activity-related pain and the average preoperative pain score for activity was 1 in both. Preoperative rest pain was scored at 5 for both groups. Postoperatively, both the cemented Kinematic II total knee joint replacement and the cementless PCA total knee joint replacement gave excellent pain relief. It is important to note, however, that a slight difference in these data emerged when pain relief with activity was compared between the cemented Kinematic II and the cementless PCA prostheses. In addition, it can also be seen from Tables 5 and 6 that the cemented Kinematic II patients attained pain relief earlier than the noncemented PCA patients.

## Range of Motion

Table 7 documents the range of motion preoperatively and postoperatively in each of the two groups. The preoperative range of motion in the cemented Kinematic II group was similar although not identical to that in the cementless PCA group (average 6°–110° vs. 9°–104°). The post-operative data demonstrated that the cementless PCA total knee joint patients consistently had less motion at each follow-up than the cemented Kinematic II knee joint replacement patients. At 2-year follow-up, the cemented Kinematic II prosthesis had an average arc of motion of 2°–106°, whereas the cementless PCA total knee arthroplasty had an average arc of motion of 5°–97° ($P < 0.02$). Though the difference in range of motion at 24-month follow-up between the two groups was only 9°, this was extremely significant in terms of common activities of daily living, such as climbing stairs, rising from a chair, and tying shoe laces.

## Radiographic Assessment

Radiographic assessment of all patients in both groups included antero-posterior (AP) and lateral X-rays in the recovery room followed by standing AP, lateral, and 60° skyline postoperative X-rays taken at 6 weeks, 3, 6, 12, and 24 months follow-up. From the postoperative X-rays, measurements were made of the angle of insertion of the components, the presence or absence of radiolucent lines, migration of one or other components, subsidence of the component, as well as patellar position, and tilting. Postoperatively, the average anatomical valgus angulation in both groups was 6°. The average alignment of the tibial component to the tibia was 3° of varus for the cemented Kinematic II group and 2° of varus for the cementless PCA group (Fig. 4). Using a modification of the criteria of Harris and McCarthy for definite, probable, and possible loosening of hip implants, there was no evidence of loosening in any of the patients in the cemented Kinematic II group [9]. Nonprogressive lucent lines, however, were demonstrated in six patients on the tibial side (Fig. 5); they were obvious by 6 months and did not change over the next 24-month follow-up. Radiographic assessment of the cementless PCA components demonstrated that three of the tibial components changed their orientation with respect to the tibia by subsiding anteriorly (Fig. 6); however, the change in X-ray appearance did not correlate with changes in the HSS score, range of motion, or pain. Bony apposition (ingrowth) to the cementless PCA prosthesis seemed to be complete in all without radiological evidence of apparent stress protection.

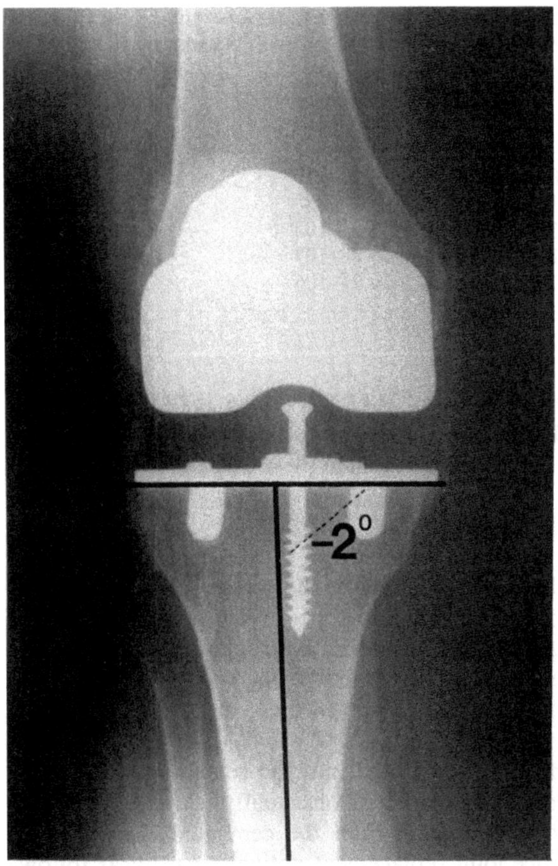


**Fig. 4.** Alignment of the tibial component of a PCA knee replacement to the long axis of the tibia (*2*° varus)

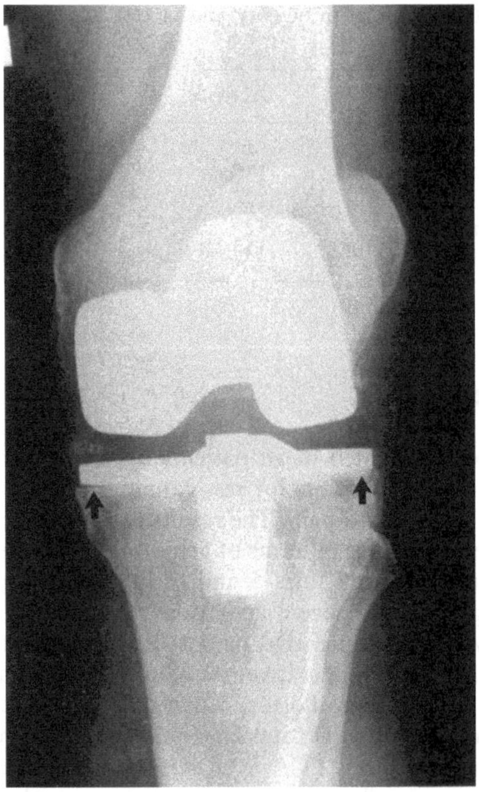

**Fig. 5.** Nonprogressive bone-cement lucent line under the tibial component of a Kinematic II total knee replacement

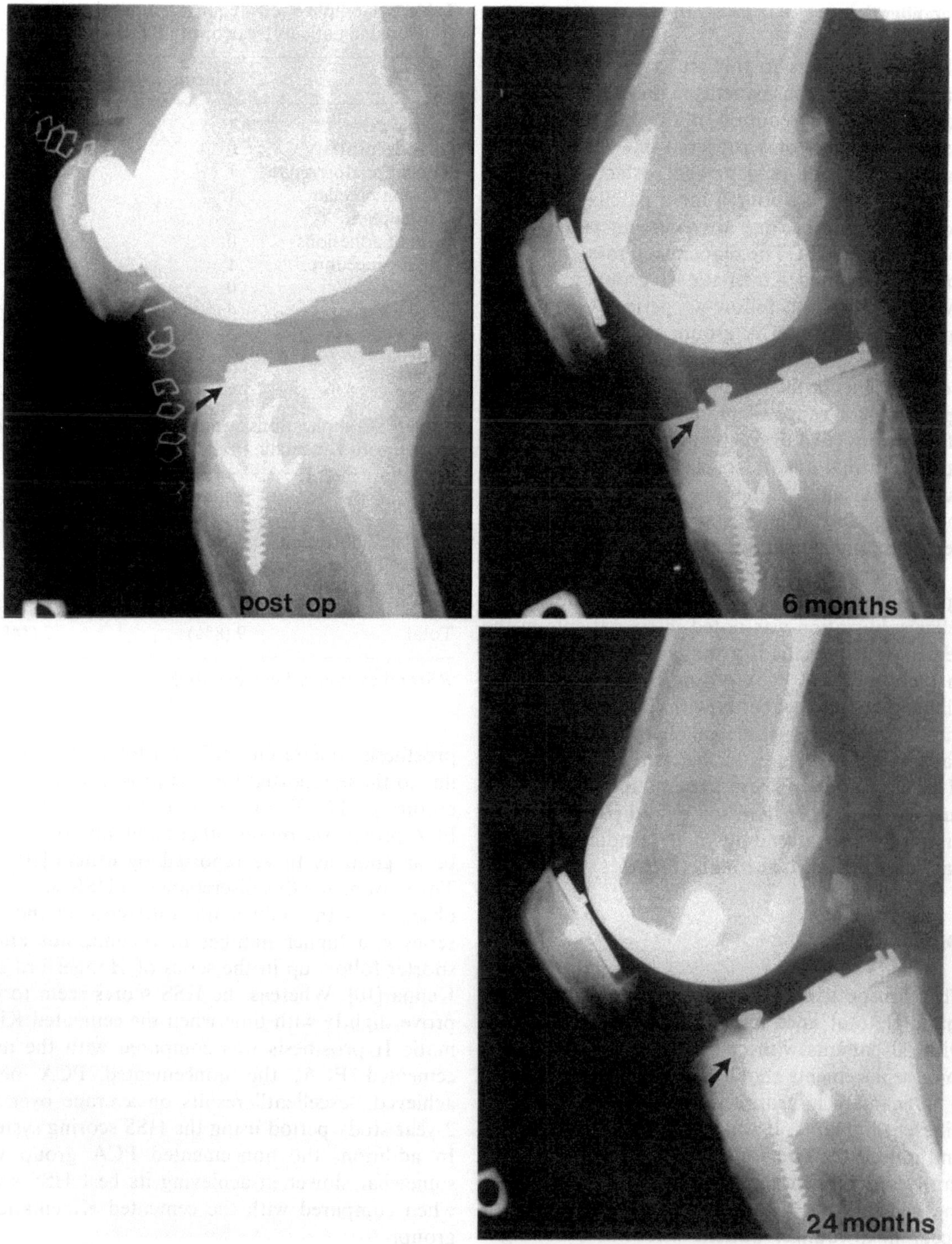


**Fig. 6a–c.** Anterior subsidence of a PCA tibial component in a 6′6″ (1.98 m), 250 pound (114 kg) patient treated with large components **a** 0, **b** 6, and **c** 24 months follow-up

## Complications

The complications in this study are presented in Tables 8 and 9. Four patients in the cemented Kinematic II group required re-operation—one for deep sepsis, one for a ruptured patellar tendon, a third for excision of a patellar osteophyte which was painful, and a fourth for a patellar stabilization procedure because of recurring patellar dislocation (Table 8). The reoperation rate, therefore, for the cemented Kinematic II group was 3.6% over the 24-month follow-up period. Conversely, in the cementless PCA group, six patients (12%) required reoperation within the follow-up period. Four patients in the cementless group required reoperation for range of motion, three having lysis of adhesions (two through an arthroscope) and the other a formal quadricepsplasty. Two patients required revision of the patellar component for loosening, and in both a second patellar component was cemented in successfully (Fig. 7).

Less serious complications (not requiring reoperation) occurred as presented in Table 9. Patellar subluxation was noted in six patients in the cemented Kinematic II group and in three patients in the cementless PCA group, however this complaint seemed to get better with time. Of interest, is that two patients (three patellae) were noted to have patellar fractures in the cemented Kinematic II group. None of these patients required further surgery, and other than some mild patellofemoral discomfort on ascending or descending stairs all patients functioned normally (Fig. 8).

**Table 8.** Complications requiring surgical correction encountered in patients treated with Kinematic II and PCA

| | Kinematic II (110) | PCA (50) |
|---|---|---|
| Deep sepsis | 1 | 0 |
| Quadricepsplasty | 0 | 1 |
| Patellar tendon repair | 1 | 0 |
| Excision patellar osteophyte | 1 | 0 |
| Lysis of adhesions | 0 | 3 |
| Trillat procedure | 1 | 0 |
| Revision | 0 | 2[a] |
| Total | 4 (3.6%) | 6 (12%) |

[a] Patella

**Table 9.** Complications not requiring surgery in patients treated with Kinematic II and PCA

| | Kinematic II (110) | PCA (50) |
|---|---|---|
| Patellar subluxation | 6 | 3 |
| Tibial subsidence | 0 | 3 |
| Patellar fracture | 3 | 0 |
| RSD | 0 | 1 |
| Total | 9 (8%) | 7 (14%) |

*RSD* reflex sympathetic dystrophy

## Discussion

This prospective review of 110 cemented Kinematic II total knee joint replacements compared with 50 patients with cementless PCA total knee joint replacements should be recognized for what it is, namely a prospective comparison of two different implants. It was not a randomized study and indeed the two study populations are significantly different in age and weight. Inclusion into the cementless PCA group was more likely to occur in a younger patient who was overweight with good bone stock; however, occasionally, the decision to do a cementless PCA replacement was made intraoperatively on the appearance of the bone after the initial saw cuts were made. Despite the fact that the groups are not identical, it is felt that some important observations can be made from this study.

The HSS scores for the cemented Kinematic II prosthesis, at a minimum 2-year follow-up are similar to those reported for this prosthesis in the literature [3, 19]. The HSS scores for the cementless PCA prosthesis, on the other hand, do not seem to be as good as those reported by others [10–12]. The reasons for this discrepancy in HSS scores are obscure, as the only major difference in the two series is a higher number of rheumatoids and a shorter follow-up in the series of Hungerford and Kenna [10]. Whereas the HSS scores seem to improve slightly with time when the cemented Kinematic II prosthesis was compared with the noncemented PCA, the noncemented PCA never achieved "excellent" results on average over the 2-year study period using the HSS scoring system. In addition, the noncemented PCA group was somewhat slower in achieving its best HSS score when compared with the cemented Kinematic II group.

The ultimate range of motion achieved at 24-month follow-up was significantly different between the cemented Kinematic II and the noncemented PCA prosthesis (106° vs. 97°). The results of this study for range of motion in the noncemented PCA patients are at some variance with these reported in the literature [10]. Hungerford and Kenna reported an average range of motion

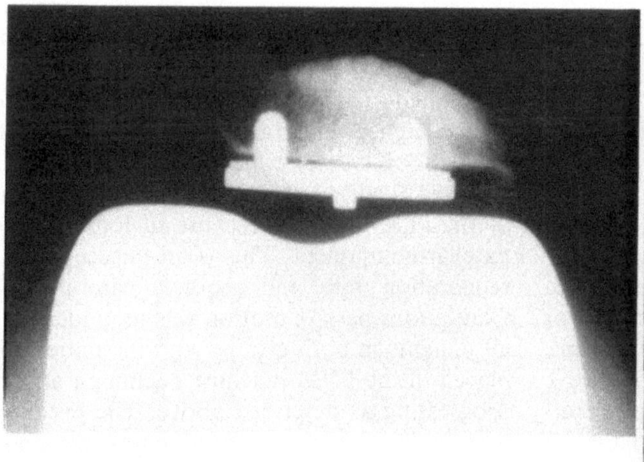
a

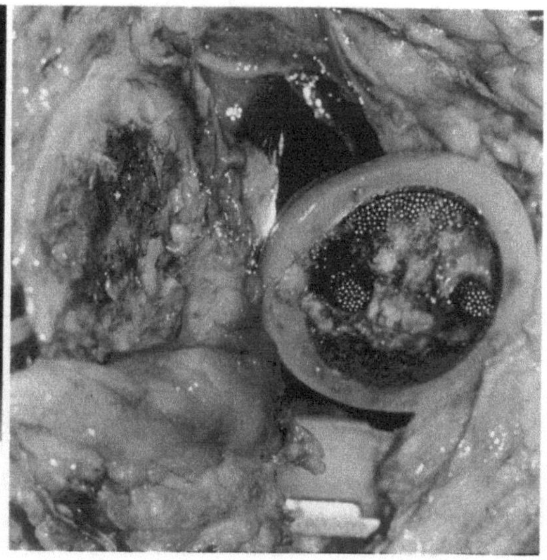
b

**Fig. 7a, b.** Loose PCA patellar component **a** radiographically and **b** intraoperatively successfully salvaged with a cemented patellar implant. Only fibrous ingrowth was noted on the patellar implant

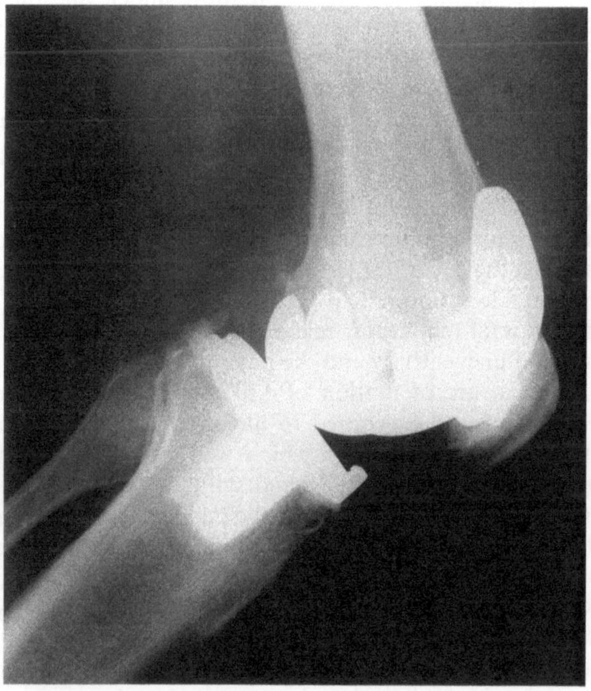

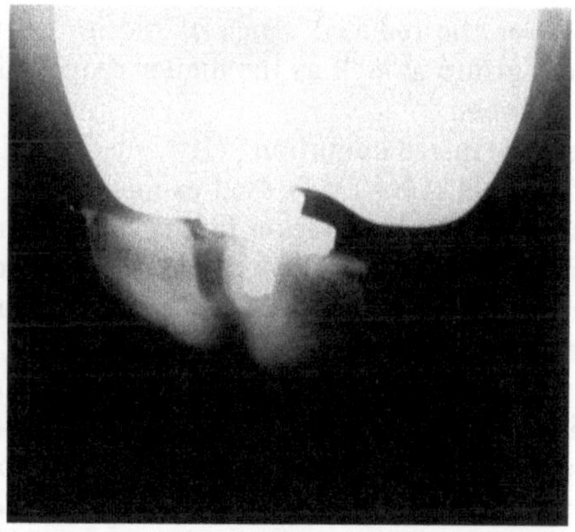

**Fig. 8.** Lateral and axial patellofemoral radiographs demonstrating the value of axial films in depicting longitudinal patellar fractures. This patient continues to function well

postoperatively of 107° with the cementless PCA and also stated that only one patient of the 63 reported had less than 90° of flexion at follow-up [10]. The current study does not support their observations.

Conversely, the ultimate range of motion achieved with the cemented Kinematic II prosthesis (107° average) correlates well with that reported in the literature in most series [3]. The difference in the final average arc of motion between the cemented Kinematic II and the noncemented PCA prosthesis is extremely important from a functional standpoint. The extra 9° of flexion allowed the patient to rise more easily from a chair and ascend and descend stairs one step at a time [1, 18]. This observation has been noted by others [18].

From a functional standpoint, therefore, the cemented Kinematic II group was much better than the cementless PCA group. The postoperative physical therapy routine differed significantly for the cementless PCA patients and may explain the poorer motion in this group. For the first 6 weeks, the patients were kept on crutches and allowed up to 50% weight bearing on the operated knee. For the next 6 weeks, weight bearing was increased to full with one point of external support (crutch or cane). Physical therapy itself, in both groups, began the night before surgery with preoperative instruction and quadriceps strengthening exercises, which were continued beginning on the 1st postoperative day. On the 2nd postoperative day, a continuous passive motion machine and physical therapy, consisting of range of motion, hamstring, and quadriceps tightening exercises, was instituted in both groups. The only difference, therefore, in the groups was with regard to the amount of weight bearing and the timing of initiation of full weight bearing. These factors may be partially responsible for the reduced range of motion in the cementless group as well as the higher reoperation rate for stiffness.

Universal Instrumentation (Howmedica Inc, Rutherford, NJ, USA) was used exclusively in all patients. This instrumentation favors an anatomical orientation of the tibial component in the frontal plane, thereby forming a 2°–3° varus angulation with the mechanical axis. Hungerford et al. suggest that the joint is more parallel to the ground in walking if orientated in this position [12]. Using these instruments, the alignment of the tibial component radiologically in both groups was approximately the same (3° varus cemented Kinematic II vs. 2° varus cementless PCA). The Universal Instrumentation, however, did not allow for any posterior inclination in the sagittal plane, but rather the tibial implant was inserted perpendicular to the anatomical axis of the tibia in the sagittal plane. Once again, there did not seem to be any difference in orientation of the tibial component in the sagittal plane when the cemented Kinematic II group was compared with the cementless PCA group. One, therefore, cannot attribute the different results to peculiarities of the instrumentation.

Three patients in the cementless PCA group were noted to have some subsidence of the tibial component anteriorly in follow-up X-rays, thereby changing the sagittal orientation of the prosthesis with regard to the sagittal axis of the tibia. A critical review of these three patients demonstrated that the prosthesis did not have good cortical contact anteriorly at the time of insertion but was resting upon cancellous bone. The small degree of subsidence which occurred in these patients did not affect their final HSS scores and range of motion.

The higher reoperation rate in the cementless PCA group was of concern as six patients (12%) required further surgery, four because of stiffness of the knee and two because of loosening of the patellar component. This is an unacceptably high reoperation rate and requires careful analysis. Continuous passive motion was used identically in all patients in both groups with the patients being placed in the CPM machine beginning at 30° and progressing as described above. The preoperative motion in the three patients reoperated upon for stiffness was not greatly different from the average pre-operative motion for the rest of the cementless PCA patients; however, two of the three requiring reoperation were Workers' Compensation Board patients. Hungerford and Krackow [11] recommend that those patients who have not achieved 90° of flexion by the 12th postoperative day should be submitted to manipulation under anesthesia followed by continuous passive motion and active flexion exercises. This was not done in these three patients and perhaps it is something that should be performed more frequently in those patients with delayed achievement of postoperative range of motion.

The reoperation rate for the cemented Kinematic II group (3.6%) was similar to that reported in the literature [3]. The patient with the patellar tendon rupture had rheumatoid arthritis and had a lateral retinacular release. The rupture was repaired uneventfully and the patient went on to attain a final arc of motion of 110°. Two patients (three patellae) were noted to have patellar fractures at follow-up, none of which was symptomatic and none of which interfered with the patients' outcome. Of interest is that the patellar fractures were not seen on the routine lateral X-ray of the knee but were only apparent on the skyline view, which should form part of all routine follow-up X-rays (Fig. 8).

On the basis of this prospective, nonrandomized, clinical review comparing the cemented Kinematic II with the cementless PCA prosthesis, the authors conclude that the cemented Kinematic II gives superior results to the cementless PCA; however, those superior results may be related to a difference in the design of the prosthesis and/or limited weight bearing offered to the cementless implant group rather than to the use of cement itself. Nevertheless, in a carefully controlled environment, the results of the cementless PCA component were not as good and the reoperation rate was substantially higher, making its indications for use more controversial. This cementless implant, if it is to be used at all, should probably be utilized mainly in osteoarthritic patients with good bone stock. It is imperative when using this prosthesis that great care and attention must be given to the accuracy of the saw cuts, but even if this is done the results do not seem to be as good. Time alone will allow us to discover the role of the noncemented implant in a patient with arthritis of the knee. Based on this review, however, it is our recommendation that the noncemented PCA total knee arthroplasty should be used with caution until longer term results are forthcoming.

## References


1. Andriacchi, TB, Galante JO, Fermier RW (1982) Influence of total knee replacement design on walking and stair climbing. J Bone Joint Surgery 64A: 1328–1335
2. Cloutier JM (1983) Results of total knee arthroplasty in non-constrained prostheses. J Bone Joint Surg 65-A: 906–919
3. Ewald FC, Jacobs MA, Miegel RE, Walker PS, Poss R, Sledge CB (1984) Kinematic total knee replacement. J Bone Joint Surg 66-A: 1032–1040
4. Figgie HE III, Goldberg VM, Heiple KG, Moller HS III, Gordon NH (1986) The influence of tibial-patellofemoral location on function of the knee in patients with the posterior stabilized condylar knee prosthesis. Bone Joint Surg 68-A: 1035–1040
5. Freeman MAR, McLeod H, Levai JP (1983) Cementless fixation of prosthetic components in total arthroplasty of the knee and hip. Clinical Orthopaedics Related Research 176: 88–94
6. Galante JO, Rostoker W (1973) Fiber metal composites in the fixation of skeletal prostheses. J Biomed Materials Research 7: 43–61
7. Galante JO, Rostoker W, Lueck R, Ray RD (1971) Sintered fiber composites as a basis for attachment of implants to bone. J Bone Joint Surg 53-A: 101–114
8. Gunston FH (1971) Polycentric knee arthroplasty prosthetic simulation of normal knee movement. J Bone Joint Surg 53-B: 272–277
9. Harris WH, McCarthy JC, O'Neil DA (1982) Femoral component loosening using contemporary techniques of femoral cement fixation. J Bone Joint Surg 64-A: 1063–1067
10. Hungerford DS, Kenna RV (1983) Preliminary experience with the total knee prosthesis and porous coating used without cement. Clin Orthop Related Research 176: 95–107
11. Hungerford DS, Krackow KA (1985) Total joint arthroplasty of the knee. Clinical Orthopaedics Related Research 192: 23–33
12. Hungerford DS, Krackow KA, Kenna RV (1984) Total knee arthroplasty: A comprehensive approach. Williams and Wilkins, Baltimore p. 126
13. Insall JN, Hood RW, Flawn LB, Sullivan BJ, Bernstein AH (1983) The total condylar prosthesis in gonarthrosis: A five year clinical and radiographic follow-up. J Bone Joint Surg 65-A: 619–628
14. Insall J, Scott WN, Ranawat CS (1979) Total condylar knee prosthesis. A report of 220 cases. J Bone Joint Surg 61-A: 173–180
15. Insall J, Tira AJ, Scott WN (1979) The total condylar knee prosthesis: The first five years. Clin Orthop Related Research 145: 68–77
16. Kettelkamp DB (1976) Gait characteristics of the knee: Normal, abnormal and post reconstruction. American Academy of Orthopaedic Surgeons, Symposium on Reconstructive Surgery of the Knee. St. Louis, Mosby, pp 47–57
17. Landon GC, Galante JO, Maley MM (1986) Noncemented total knee arthroplasty. Clinical Orthopaedics Related Research 205: 49–57
18. Laubenthal KN, Smidt GL, Kettelkamp DB (1972) The quantitative analysis of knee motion during activities of daily living. Physical Therapy 52: 34–42
19. Scott RD, Volatile TB (1986) Twelve years' experience with posterior cruciate-retaining total knee arthroplasty. Clinical Orthopaedics Related Research 205: 100–107

## *Discussion*

*Hasting* (Wellesley Hospital): I would like to ask you about range of motion: We encountered similar problems when we changed from the Kinematic to the PCA. The PCA button is considerably bigger than the Kinematic button and we had to resect a much greater amount of patella in order to obtain a good range of motion. From your slides, I see that your patellar resection was more or less the same in the Kinematic and PCA. I think that this well be a factor in reducing the range of motion.

*Bourne* (University of Western Ontario): I think that may well be a factor. Since we performed this study, we have been measuring the thickness of the patella preoperatively and then checking this with the trial patellar button before cementing or impacting so as to be certain that the patellar height is consistent.

*Etoh* (Nagoya Red Cross Hospital): Could you please comment on clinical experience of bone ingrowth with the PCA.

*Bourne*: As you will have noted, several of our cementless patients underwent reoperation. There was no evidence of loosening on either the tibial or fibial side. However, on the two patellar buttons that were obviously loose and could easily be displaced simply by inserting an osteotome under the implant, there was no evidence of bony ingrowth whatsoever; there was simply fibrous ingrowth. In other cases, there was no observable motion and so I cannot really comment on whether bony ingrowth was present. As you know, there is a great deal of evidence, particularly from groups such as that of Dr. Hadad in the USA, concerning prostheses retrieved for failure. Doubt has been cast as to whether indeed we do obtain good bony ingrowth on the tibial side.

*Krackow* (John Hopkins University): You did not comment on the postoperative weight-bearing routine with the uncemented knees. I saw some X-rays that did not have fixation screws in the tibial components. There also appeared to be one or two fixation screws that could have been AO screws rather than vitallium screws. We feel that it is extremely important in uncemented knees that patients be at profoundly limited weight bearing for the first 6 weeks or more and that the presence of a fixation screw is very very important. I think that while on the one hand you stress that the study is not well controlled, you are still leaving the audience with a relatively strong statement about the "poorer" kind of results in a group of younger, healthier, more active, heavier patients. These patients were 10 kg heavier than average. A more obese leg does not even bend as far owing to subcutaneous fat. Our findings are rather different: Our patients gain range of motion with time rather than lose it.

*Bourne*: I think that your points are valid. I tried to be very honest in stressing that this was not a randomized population. There is some room for a randomized study; whether this is ethical or not, that remains to the investigator. The patients that had PCA implants were indeed a different category in terms of age and weight. In terms of the fixation, we began with the molybold, but we were not very satisfied with this. We then went over to using a screw, initially with the AO screw and then later with the vitallium screw. In terms of the postoperative routine, we followed your protocol exactly initially, although we have deviated from it since this study.

*Goldie* (Karolinska Institutet): As for the selection of method you used the criterion of so-called bone stock. How was that measured? Would this not introduce an element of prejudice in the judging of your results? Did you have a statistician help you in the selection of the groups?

*Bourne*: As I said, this was not a randomized study. I think a randomized study should be carried out. With regard to your second point, we did not use a statistician because the study was not randomized.

# Value of the Total Condylar Knee Arthroplasty

Y. Eto, I. Nagaya, and S. Saito[1]

**Summary.** In 55 cases, 75 joints were followed up clinically and radiologically. Clinical evaluation was carried out according to the scale of the Japanese Orthopedic Association and radiological evidence at the bone-cement interface of the tibial plateau was noted using fluoroscopy and a skyline view of 45° was also employed. With the visualization using the fluoroscopic method, it was quite clear that the bone-cement interface was eliminated.

**Keywords:** Rheumatoid arthritis—Osteoarthritis—Knee joint—Total replacement arthroplasty—Total condylar knee prosthesis

## Introduction

The total condylar knee prosthesis is a conventional type of tricompartment arthroplasty. Many kinds of prosthesis have been developed recently. New biological and biomechanical concepts for surgical techniques and materials have been developed in the field of artificial joints within the last decade. These advances were produced by accurate surgical techniques, cementing methods, and uncemented prostheses. Some of the newly designed prostheses are as yet unacceptable for clinical use. Considerable study is needed before a decision between the cemented and uncemented prostheses for clinical use can be made. For these reasons, total condylar knee replacement was evaluated clinically and radiologically in this research. Patella resurfacing is still a problem because patellar prostheses are subject to stresses from the extensor dynamic mechanism. The strength of the patella, wear of the patellar dome, and blood circulation of the patella are still unknown. Gliding of the patella and X-ray changes in the patellar dome are also examined to establish the work and durability after operation.

[1] Department of Orthopedic Surgery, Nagoya National Hospital, Nagoya, Japan

## Material and Method

During the period 1978–1985, 367 total condylar knee replacements were carried out in 256 patients. In this series, 55 cases (75 joints) were evaluated over 5 years postoperatively. The clinical results were evaluated and employed on the protocol of the scale of Japanese Orthopedic Association. For the scale of the radiological evaluation, the grading system at the Hospital for special surgery (New York, USA) was employed. The skyline view of the patella was also examined.

The follow-up time was 5–8 years and the average follow-up time was $6\frac{1}{2}$ years. The diagnosis was osteoarthritis in eight cases (nine joints) and rheumatoid arthritis in 47 cases (66 joints) The age of patients ranged from 38 to 79 years and the mean was 60 years at the time of operation.

## Operative Technique

A medial parapatellar incision was used on the knee joint. A capsular incision was made on the edge of the patella. The groove of the vastus medialis and rectus femolis of the extensor mechanism was excised. Periosteum from the medial tibia was released. Bony osteophyte was removed from the femur and tibia. The anterior and posterior cruciate ligaments were released. After balancing of the soft tissues, cutting of bone was performed on the femoral side initially and then the tibial part was cut. After checking the femorotibial alignment and ligament balance, cementing of both sorts of the prosthesis and patella resurfacing were performed simultaneously. Lateral release was carried out when patellar gliding was not smooth or the patella-femoral joint was subluxated. After reduced tourniquet pressure, bleeding of the soft tissue was coagulated. After the insertion of drainage, the wound was closed after operation, and a compression bandage was applied.

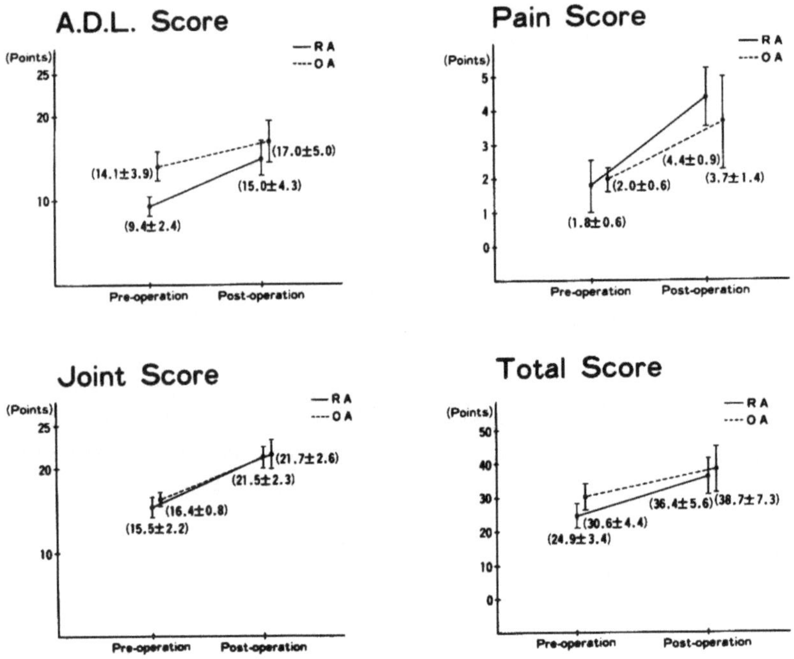


Fig. 1. Clinical results of total condylar knee replacement

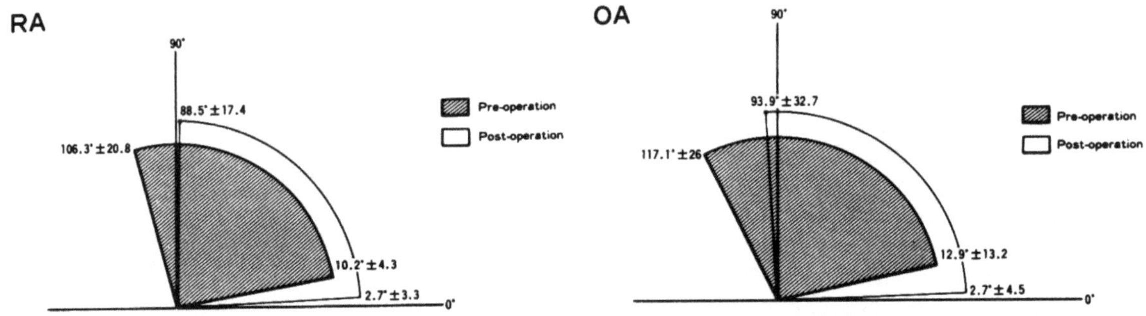


**Fig. 2.** Range of movement (*ROM*) of patients with rheumatoid arthritis (*RA*) and osteoarthritis (*OA*)

## Results

Relief of pain was most significant. Preoperatively, most patients had severe pain with an average score of 1.8 in rheumatoid arthritis (RA) and 2.0 in osteoarthritis (OA). Postoperatively, the average score was 4.4 in rheumatoid arthritis and 3.7 in osteoarthritis. Most patients experienced little or no pain (Fig. 1). The preoperative flexion averaged 106.3° in RA and 117.1° in OA. The average postoperative flexion was 88.5° in RA and 93.9° in OA (Fig. 2). The average preoperative flexion contracture was 10.2° in RA and 12.9° in OA. The average postoperative flexion contracture was 2.7° in RA and OA. Figure 3 shows the differences of X-ray findings between the simple anteroposterior (AP) view on the left and fluoroscopy on the right.

By means of fluoroscopy, accurate detection of the radiolucent zone is possible. This method is optimal except for the risk of irradiation to the doctor. The X-ray evaluations were usually made four times in the tibial AP and lateral views (Fig. 4).

All of the radiolucent zones were assessed. The radiolucent zone grading is divided into four groups (Fig. 5). Grade IV was found in the AP view as shown in Fig. 6. The patellar lateralization rate was investigated according to the schema (Fig. 7). The average values are 2.7% with the patellar dome, 10.2% without patella shaving, and 13.8% in patella shaving. Lateralization of the patella

**Fig. 3a, b.** Comparison of X-ray findings. **a** Simple AP view; **b** using fluoroscopy

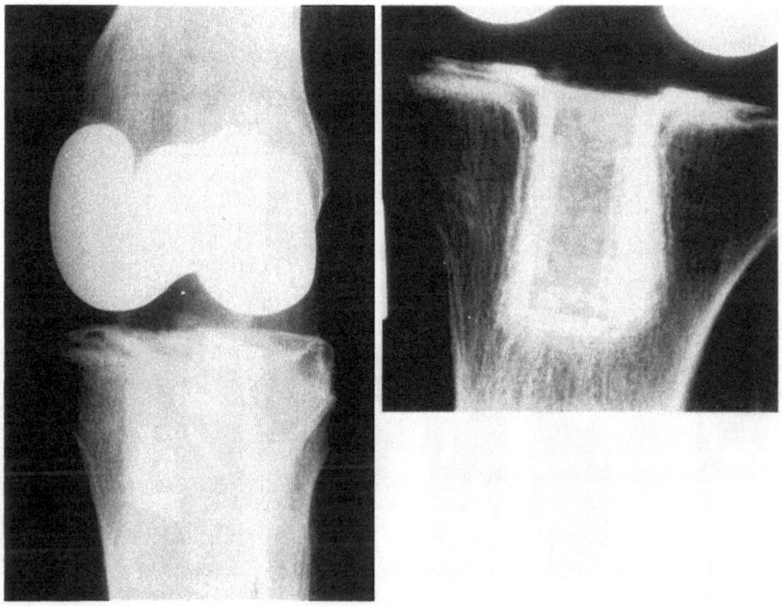

a b

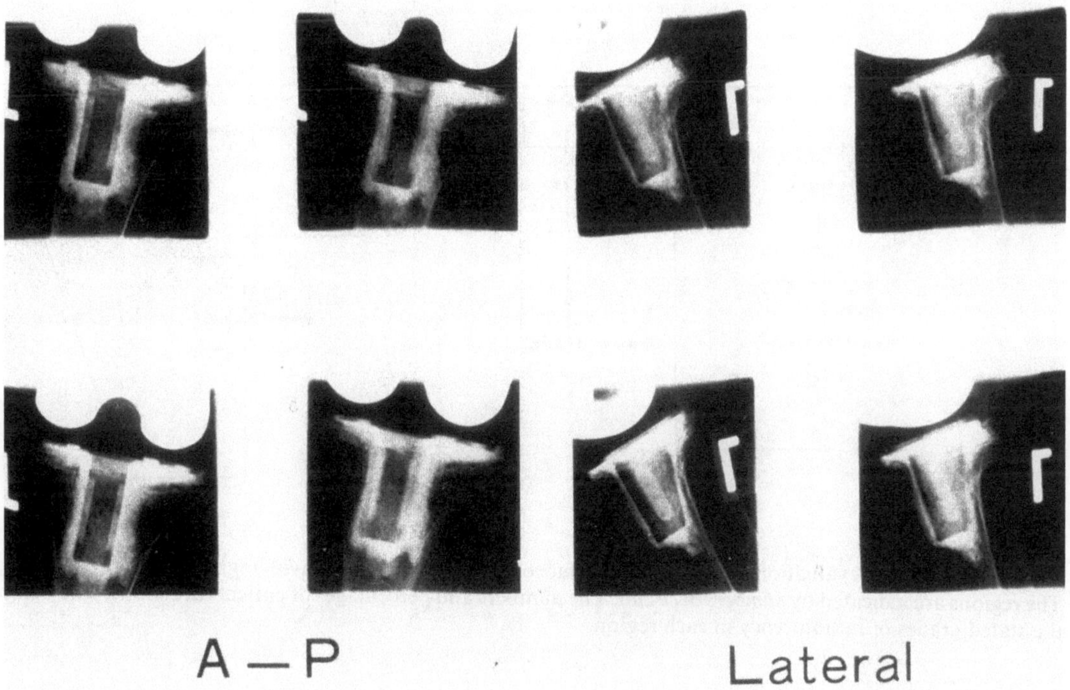


**Fig. 4.** X-ray images used for evaluation

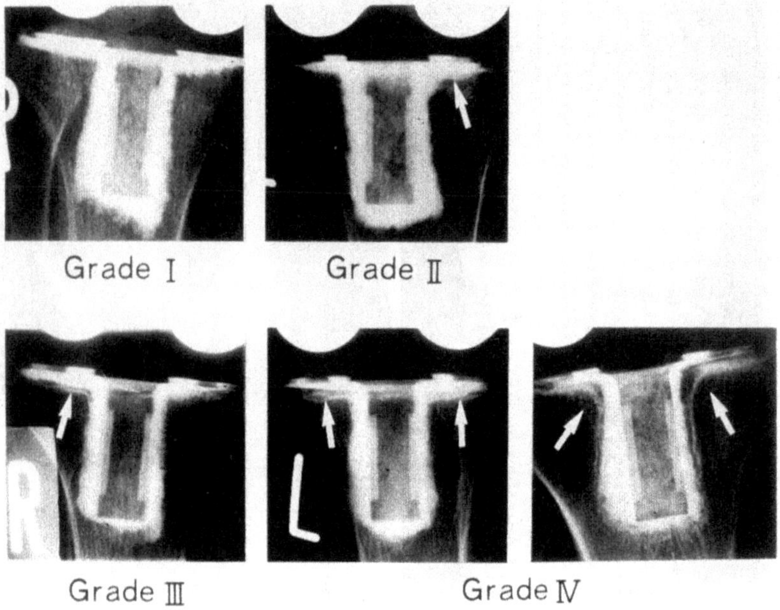


**Fig. 5.** Grade of Cement-bone demarcation [3]

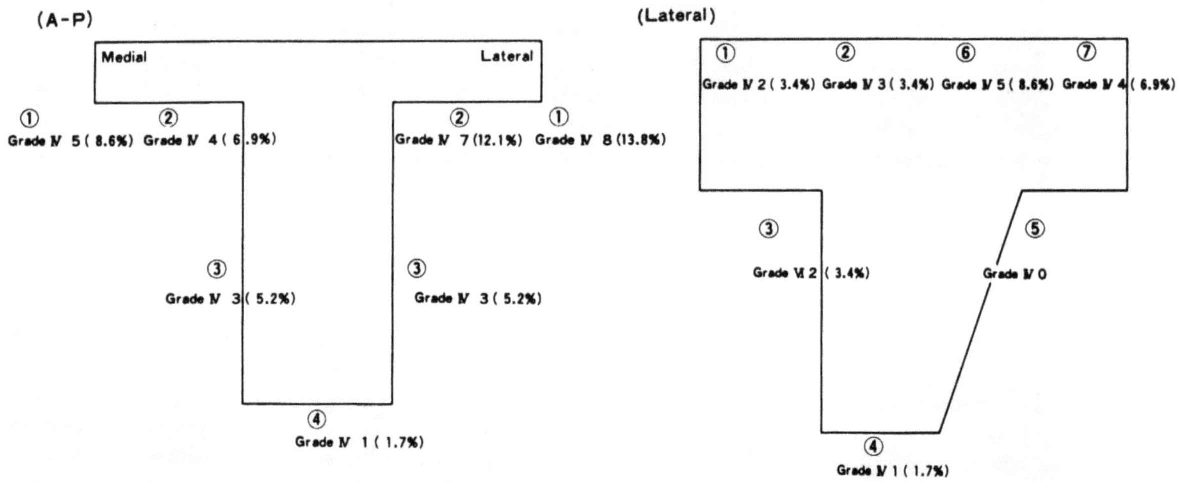


**Fig. 6.** Radiological evaluation of fixation using fluoroscopy from 40 cases involving 58 joints—a 5-year experience. The regions are indicated by *numbers in circles*. The numbers and percentages of patients are shown who demonstrated the stated grades of radiolucency in each region

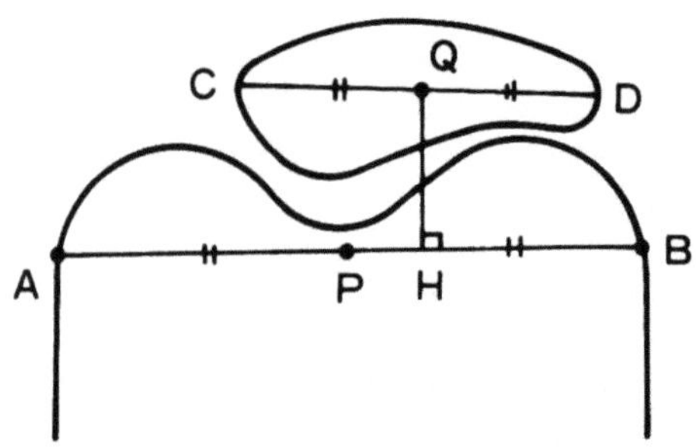


**Fig. 7.** Lateral deviation of patella.

$$\text{Lateral deviation (d)} = \frac{PH}{AB} \times 100(\%)$$

In patients receiving a patellar dome d = 2.7 ± 3.3(%). In patients without a patellar dome d = 10.2 ± 4.3. For patients treated by patella shaving d = 13.8 ± 9.5

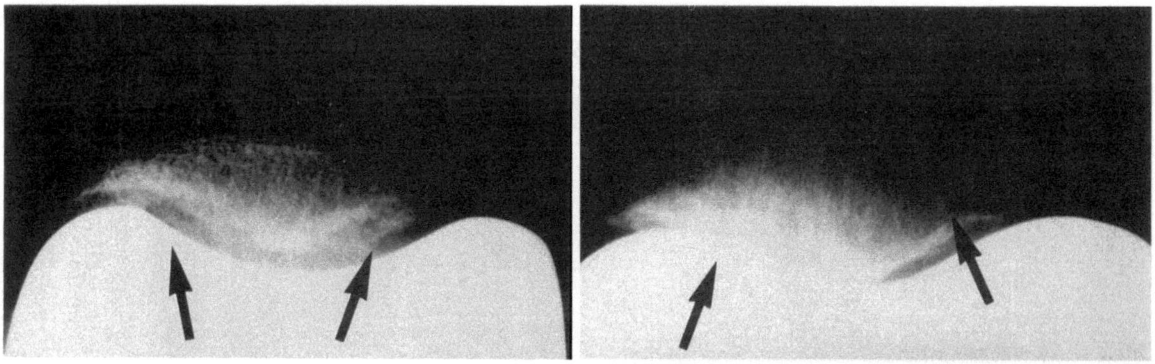

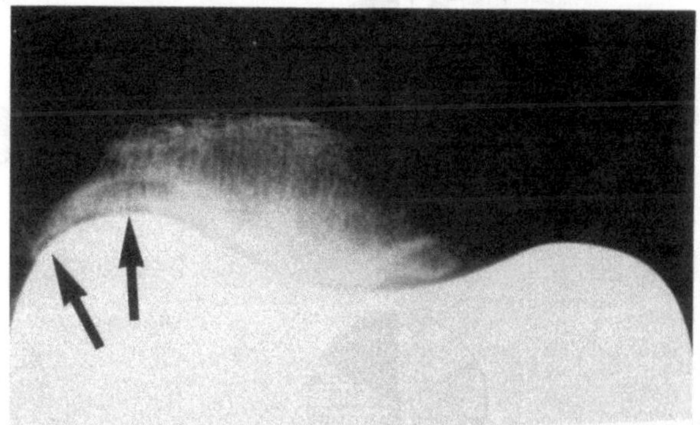

**Fig. 8a–c.** X-ray change in patellar dome (−). **a** Erosion; **b** lateral erosion, medial atrophy; **c** lateral osteophyte, lateral cyst

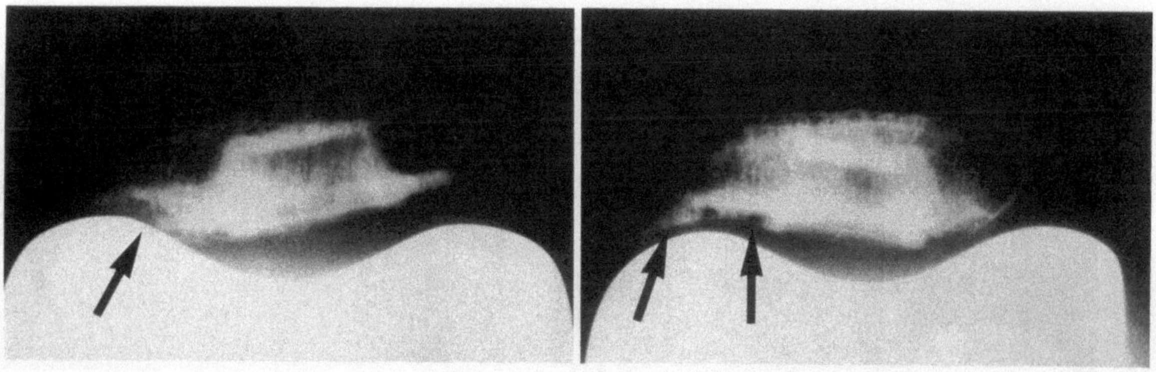

**Fig. 9a, b.** X-ray change in patellar dome (+). **a** Medial erosion; **b** lateral osteophyte, lateral cyst

was much more significant in patients who had undergone patella shaving. In X-ray, changes in the facet in the skyline view were evident (Figs. 8, 9). Bone changes were much less frequent in the patellar dome group than in the group without the patellar dome.

Sclerotic, erosive, and cystic changes were recognized in patients without the patellar dome or who had undergone patella shaving (Fig. 10). The changes in trabecular pattern were investigated (Fig. 11). In the upper X-ray, the trabecular pattern was dominant in the lateral facet and the medial facet had atrophy. In the lower X-ray, the trabecula surrounding the peg of the patellar dome was recognized, but in part of the perimeter of the patellar dome was recognized, but in part of the perimeter of the patellar dome the trabecular pattern was not evident. Where the patella had been shaved there was severe deformity in all cases postoperatively; deviations were usually present and also osteophyte and cystic formation (Fig. 12). However, in some cases the X-ray showed the patella to be quite stable irrespective of whether the patellar dome was present or not (Fig. 13c, d). In Fig 13a, b, the bone-cement interface was advanced and the perimeter of the peg band has the appearance of an umbrella.

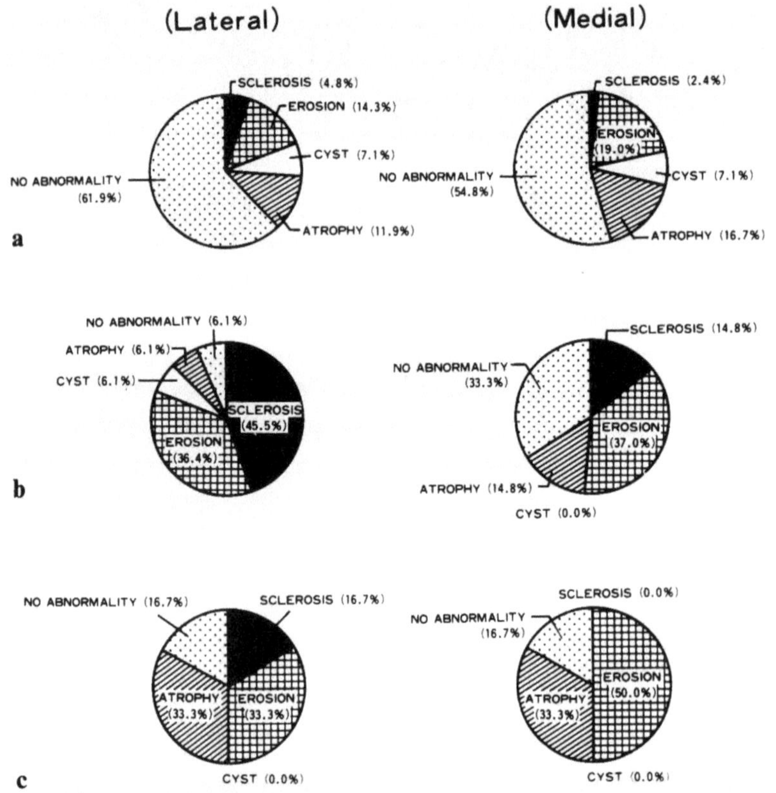


**Fig. 10a–c.** X-ray change in facet. **a** With patellar dome (43 joints); **b** without patellar dome (29 joints); **c** patella shaving (6 joints)

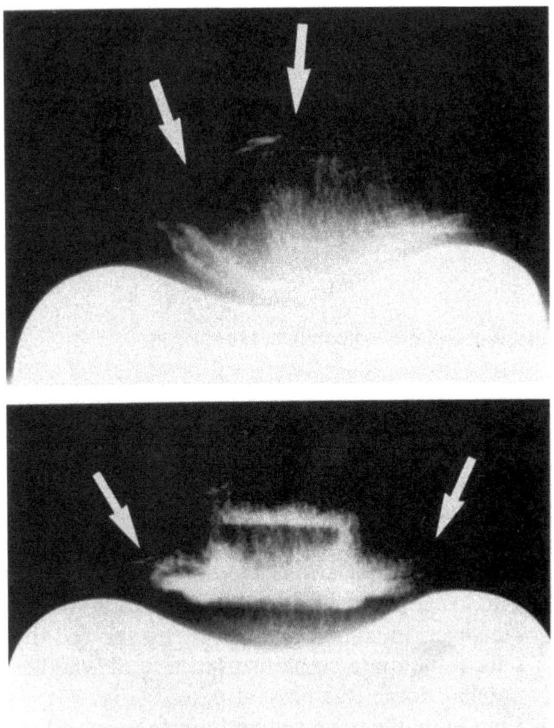

**Fig. 11.** Change in trabecular pattern

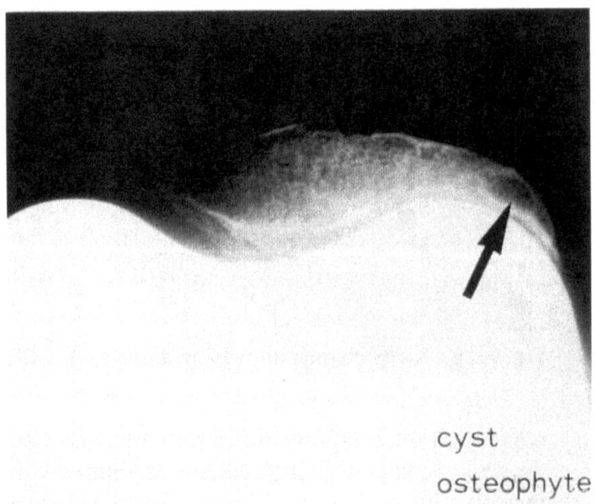


**Fig. 12.** Patellectomy

**Fig. 13a–d.** X-ray assessment of patellar instability

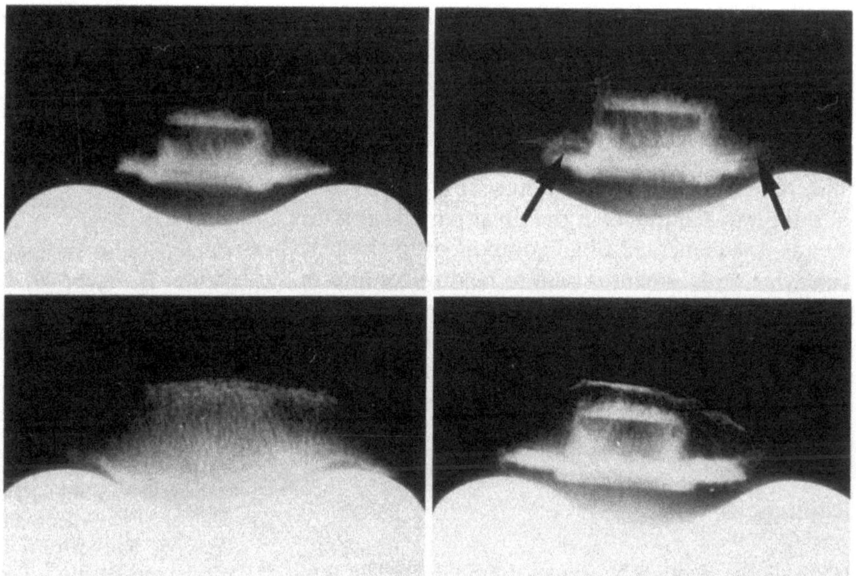

## Dicussion

Various types of knee prostheses have been developed by many surgeons and physicians. Different kinds of technical and mechanical failures have been analyzed and evaluated [2, 8]. Hinge prostheses and some surface implants in young patients were found to be unacceptable for clinical use [4]; this was due not only to prosthetic design but also to inadequate operative techniques. Surgical instruments have now become more sophisticated and the concept of soft-tissue release and bony resection and bone grafting for tibial defects have also been established in recent years. Advances in technical concepts have been important in obtaining good results in this area. The condylar type of prosthesis was established by Ranawat and Townley [6] and this has led to great advances in knee arthroplasty, especially in the design of the femoral component. The total condylar femoral component is the most common, reliable, and durable design for tricompartment arthroplasties. The design of the tibial component of the total condylar prosthesis has some problems concerning the presence or absence of metal backing [8].

Optimal evaluation of the X-ray is important in assessing the value of a prosthesis. Usually, postoperative X-rays are insufficient for evaluating the radiolucent zone. The fluoroscopic method is a better way of analyzing the radiolucent zone. In our series, the radiolucent zone was recognized in part of zone I mainly in the AP view. The bone-cement interface in zone IV has a very narrow radiolucent zone. In the lateral view, grade IV did not have a recognizable radiolucent zone. The X-ray evaluation showed that the peg is useful in achieving stability and hence durability in the fixation of the tibial component.

The patellar dome was routinely inserted when the total condylar knee was introduced except in the initial cases. When the patellar dome was inserted, a gliding test was performed. If the patella was unstable or subluxated, lateral release was carried out. We check the patellar dome in the 45° skyline view postoperatively [3]. The changes in the trabecular pattern are quite significant. The trabecular pattern of the patella is recognized on the peg part on the patellar dome and other part of the patella as bony atrophy or cystic change. The trabecular pattern is located on the weight-bearing area and disused or non-weight bearing area usually shows some atrophic change. In our series, some cases with a patellar dome showed deformity on the perimenter of the patella. The shape of the deformity resembled an umbrella. After the X-ray evaluation of the patella, it was considered that the peg part of the patellar dome was able to transmit the quadriceps muscle force to the original patella but that the circumference of the peg had inadequate strength to transmit this force. The patellar dome of the total condylar knee prosthesis can transmit the load only by means of the peg; the perimeter of the patellar dome cannot transmit the load adequately. The umbrella-like deformity of the patella was considered to be some kind of creep deformity; a quite subjective conclusion is that the strength of the patellar dome is still insufficient. Improvement is needed so that the strength of the patella dome is sufficient to transmit the load due to the extensor muscles.

## Conclusion

The radiolucent zone in fluoroscopy can be visualized quite accurately in the tibial part. Using this means, the cemented tibial component of the total condylar replacement is seen to be durable and reliable. In some cases, the patellar component is seen to have a creep deformation in the perimeter of the patella. This is still a hypothetical conclusion, but strength is needed at the base of the patella to avoid this deformity.

## References

1. Insall JN, Scott WN, Ranawat CS (1979) The total condylar knee prosthesis. A report of two hundred cases. J Bone Joint Surg 61-A: 173–180
2. Lewis JL, Michael JA, Donald PJ (1982) A comparative evaluation of tibial component designs of total knee prosthesis. J Bone Joint Surg 64-A: 129–135
3. Ranawat CS (1986) The patellofemoral joint in total condylar knee arthroplasty. Clin Orthop 205: 93–99
4. Riley J, Woodyard JE (1985) Long term results of geomedic total knee replacement. J Bone Joint Surg 67-B, 548–550
5. Rosenqvist R, Bylander B, Knutson K, Rydholm U Rooser B, Egund N, Lidgren L (1986) Loosening of the porous coating of bicompartmental prostheses in patients with rheumatoid arthritis. J Bone Joint Surg 68-A: 538–542
6. Townley CO (1985) The anatomic total knee arthroplasty. Clin Orthop 192: 82–96
7. Winsor RE, Insall JN, Sculco TP (1986) Bone grafting of tibial defects in primary and revision total knee arthroplasty. Clin Orthop 205: 132–137
8. Walker PS, Greene D, Reilly D, Thatcher J, Ben-Dov M, Rutherford, Ewald FC (1981) Fixation of tibial components of knee prostheses. J Bone Joint Surg 63-A: 258–267

# Total Condylar Knee Arthroplasty: 8- to 11-Year Follow-Up

C.S. RANAWAT and O. BOACHIE-ADJEI[1]

**Summary.** This study deals with total condylar knee arthroplasties in 87 consecutive patients with 112 knees. Of 87 patients, 72 (90 knees) were available for clinical and radiographic assessment with an 8- to 11-year follow-up. Eight patients (12 knees) died and seven (ten knees) were lost to follow-up. Results were excellent to good in 93%, fair in 3%, and poor in 4%. Radiographic evaluation revealed well-fixed components in 36 knees (40%). Radiolucencies of varying degree were present in 54 knees (60%). Of the 54 knees, seven had radiolucency under the tibial condyle in zones I–IV and partially along the peg in zones V or VI. Two knees had component loosening—one with a loose patella and the other with a loose tibial component. Both patients were symptomatic.

Variables such as the patient's age, sex, diagnosis, alignment and position of prosthesis, and the level of bone cut did not influence the development of radiolucencies at the cement-bone interface. There was a correlation between body weight and the presence or absence of radiolucencies ($P = 0.001$).

We conclude that the total condylar knee arthroplasty is a predictable and durable operation at 8–11 years of follow-up.

**Keywords:** TKR—Follow-up—Evaluation—Surgical technique—Cement

## Introduction

The total condylar prosthesis, which was designed and developed at The Hospital for Special Surgery, was first implanted in March 1974 and remains the oldest unmodified total knee replacement design presently in extensive use [3]. Favorable clinical and radiographic results with the total condylar knee arthroplasty have been reported by Ranawat and Rose [11] and Insall, et al. [3, 6].

[1] Department of Orthopaedics, Cornell University Medical College, New York Hospital and The Hospital for Special Surgery New York, NY, USA

## Materials and Methods

The study consisted of the first 112 consecutive primary total condylar knee arthroplasties in 87 patients performed by the senior author between March 1974 and December 1977. All patients had radiographic and clinical evaluations at 1 to 2 year intervals. There were 18 men and 69 women in the study group with ages ranging between 31 and 79 years, with an average of 65 years. The preoperative diagnosis was osteoarthritis in 47 knees and rheumatoid arthritis in 65 knees. Twenty-five patients underwent one-stage bilateral procedures and all but one (two knees) had patellar resurfacing. The average weight of the patients was 69.1 kg with a range of 45–97 kg.

Radiographic evaluation was done on standing antero-posterior and lateral radiographs of each knee to assess tibio-femoral alignment, component position, and radiolucent zones along the cement-bone interface of the tibial component.

The zones under the tibial component and around the peg were numbered 1 through 7. Zones I, II, III, and IV and under the tibial condyle, from medial to lateral; zones V and VI are on either side of the peg, while zone VII lies under the peg itself. The width of the radiolucencies was graded 1 through 4. Grade 1 represented no radiolucency, grade 2.1 mm or less, grade 3.1–2 mm, grade 4 represented global radiolucency around the tibial component with or without component shift. Grade 4 radiolucency was considered a failure of fixation of the component. The patella was evaluated with a skyline view with the knee flexed at 60°. The femoral component was not amenable to critical radiographic assessment due to difficulties in recognizing the cement-bone interface.

At last follow-up, eight patients (12 knees) had died and seven patients (ten knees) could not be reached for follow-up. Thus, 90 knees in 72 patients were included in the clinical and radiographic results. There were 15 males and 57 females with an age-range of 31–79 years and an average age of 65 years. There was osteoarthritis in 47 knees and

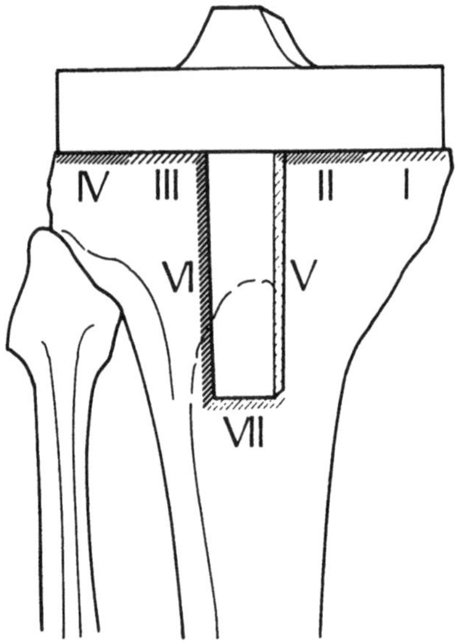


**Fig. 1.** Zone distribution of radiolucency under tibial component

rheumatoid arthritis in 65 knees. Twenty-five patients had one-stage bilateral procedures and all but one patient (two knees) had patellar resurfacing. The average weight was 70 kg with a range of 45–97 kg.

There were 40 knees in varus with a maximum deformity of 35°. Forty-one knees were in valgus with a maximum deformity of 38°. Biplanar deformities in either varus or valgus associated with flexion contracture were present in 29 knees. The maximum flexion contracture was 40°. Two knees were in neutral alignment. All patients were examined by the authors and rated according to the Hospital for Special Surgery Knee Disability Score Sheet [12], which takes into account activity, pain relief, range of motion, and stability. A score of 85–100 points represents an excellent result, 70–84 a good result, 60–69 a fair result, and less than 60 a poor result.

The techniques involved in this total condylar knee arthroplasty included proper patellar tracking, proper release for fixed deformities, balancing the ligaments, and restoration of the mechanical axis, which have been previously reported [5–7].

## Clinical Results

Seventy-two patients with 90 knees had an average follow-up of 9.5 years. The average postoperative score was 83.3. There were 48 excellent results (53.3%), 35 good (39%), 3 fair (3.3%), and 4 poor (4.4%). A patient with excellent results had no pain at rest and was able to walk an unlimited distance and go up and down stairs without the help of a railing. In rheumatoid patients unlimited walking was defined as that the operated knee did not interfere with the walking ability. A patient with good results had no rest pain, occasional ache on walking, and could go up and down steps but often required minimum assistance with a railing when going down steps. A patient with fair results had mild pain, some pain at rest, and was unable to walk any significant distance due to poor general health. Poor results were obvious failures.

The average range of motion was 95°. The range of motion was more than 90° in 86 knees, and of these 50 knees had a range of motion of 100°–120°. Four knees had 70° of motion. The knees were stable in both planes in 91 knees. Twenty-two knees had a few millimeters of medial/lateral laxity on passive testing. In seven knees antero-posterior and/or medial-lateral laxity varied between 5 and 10mm; none of these required bracing or revision. There were no subluxations or dislocations either of tibiofemoral or patellofemoral joints. Three knees in two patients were rated fair: One patient with multiple medical problems including cardiopulmonary compromise had limited function and use of the replaced knees; the other patient had rheumatoid arthritis with multiple joint involvement, severe disability, and limited function. Both patients experienced mild pain in the replaced knee.

Four arthroplasties in the study were rated poor. One was due to an infection at 9 years postoperation. The second failed arthroplasty occurred in an overweight female with osteoarthritic involvement of multiple joints and limitation of function with knee pain; this patient had to use a wheelchair. The third poor result was due to a loose patellar component. This patient has refused revision surgery. The fourth poor result was due to a loose tibial component. Thus, the four poor results were due to poor general health, infection, loose patella, and loose tibial components.

## Radiographic Results

The postoperative range of alignment of knees varied between 3° of varus and 10° of valgus. Ten knees were between 0° and 3° of varus and 17 knees between 0° and 4° of valgus. The rest were between 5° and 10° of valgus. The tibial component was placed at 90° ± 6°, to the long axis of the tibia, while the femoral component measured ± 5° of valgus. Of the knees, 40% ($n = 36$) remained well fixed without evidence of radiolucency. The remaining 54 knees (60%) had radiolucencies (Table 1). The width of radiolucency was less than 1 mm (grade II) in 37 knees, between 1 and 2 mm (grade III) in 16 knees, and one knee exhibited over 2 mm (grade IV) shift of component position was present in one knee. Thirty-six knees were well fixed and had no radiolucency (grade I). The zonal distribution of the radiolucencies of 54 knees was as follows. The distribution was in all seven zones in one (the knee with grade IV; Table 1). It was in zones 1–5 or 6 in nine knees, four of these were symptomatic. In 44 knees, it was under the tibial condyle, i.e., in zones 1, 2 or 3 or 1–4. Thus, 80 of 90 knees had stable function: The ten knees which did not have stable fixation consisted of one with a loose tibial component and nine with radiolucency under zones 1–4 and partially along the peg or in zones 5 or 6. No correlation was noted between radiolucency and variables such as age, sex, diagnosis, alignment, and level of tibial bone cut. Only body weight was found to influence the development of radiolucencies under the tibial component. Excess weight accounted for 14% of the variance in radiolucencies. The body weight of patients whose knees had no radiolucency was 63.5 kg on average as against 74.9 kg in patients whose knees had radiolucency; this was significant ($P = 0.001$).

In 13 knees, bone defects of the tibial plateau were filled with cement or cement with screw fixation. Of these, 11 knees developed radiolucency of 1–2 mm; the remaining two knees had no radiolucencies.

## Complications

Wound drainage occurred in 5% of the knees; these were managed with local wound care and immobilization. None of these developed late infection. Two patients developed uncomplicated myocardial infarctions and three patients developed nonfatal pulmonary emboli. No immediate postoperative deaths or infection occurred. One patient had an infection 6 months postoperation. A revision procedure was undertaken and the patient did well. The patient died 7 years after surgery and is not included in the 72 patients. One patient had peroneal nerve palsy, which improved slowly within 6 months.

**Table 1.** Percentage of knees showing lucency in specific zones (see Fig. 1)

| Zones | Percentage |
|---|---|
| 0 | 36 |
| 1 or 4 | 14 |
| 1, 2, or 4 | 13 |
| 1–4 | 17 |
| 1–4, 5, or 6 | 9 |
| 1–7 | 1 |

## Discussion

The clinical results were excellent to good at 8–11 years of follow-up in 93% of 72 patients with 90 knees. The average follow-up was of 9.5 years. These results are quite similar to other published reports on total knee arthroplasty [1–4, 6, 7, 9–11, 14] of shorter duration.

Radiolucency of different grades under the tibial condyle was noted in 60% (54 knees). This rate is quite similar to that reported by Laskin [7] and higher than that reported by Insall et al. [6]. The length of follow-up of these two reports was shorter. The patients with no radiolucency in our study (34 knees) had an average weight of 63.5 kg, while the patients with radiolucency (54 knees) had an average weight of 74.9 kg. These numbers were statistically significant ($P = 0.001$). The development of radiolucency may be related to the cementing technique [8, 13]. The present series which covers the period 1974–1977 did not utilize modern cement techniques for knee arthroplasty. With the modern technique of cementing, which utilizes proper bone preparation, thorough cleaning with pulsatile water lavage, proper drying of the bone, and the use of soft or low-viscosity cement to penetrate into the cancellous bone, the incidence of appearance of radiolucency has been reduced to 19% [11]. With modern cement technique [8, 11, 13], it is possible to achieve 2–5 mm of cement penetration into the cancellous bone for excellent microinterlock between the cancellous bone and the cement. It is therefore reasonable to assume that total condylar knee arthroplasty is a safe, durable and predictable procedure which could last for a long time. The arthroplasty does fail at times due to early or late infection, mechanical loosening, and, occasionally, due to instability and fractured patella.

## References

1. Buchanan JR, Greer RB, Bowman CS, Shearer A, Callahan K (1982) Clinical experience with the variable-axis total knee replacement. J Bone Joint Surg 64-A: 337
2. Ewald FC, Jacobs MA, Miegel RE et al. (1984) Kinematic total knee replacement. J Bone Joint Surg 66-A: 1032
3. Insall JN, Hood RW, Flawn LB, Sullivan DB (1983) The total-condylar prosthesis in gonarthrosis: A 5 to 9 year follow-up of the first 100 consecutive knee replacements. J Bone Joint Surg 65-A: 619
4. Insall JN, Lachiewicz PF, Burstein AH (1982) The posterior stabilized condylar prosthesis: A modification of the total-condylar system. J Bone Joint Surg 64: 1317
5. Insall JN, Ranawat CS, Aglietti P, Shine J (1976) A comparison of four models of total knee replacements prostheses. J Bone Joint Surg 58-A: 754
6. Insall JN, Scott WN, Ranawat CS (1979) The total condylar prosthesis: A report of two hundred cases. J Bone Joint Surg 61-A: 173
7. Laskin RS (1981) Total-condylar knee replacement in rheumatoid arthritis. J Bone Joint Surg 63-A: 29
8. Lee AJC, Ling RSM, Vangala SS (1978) Some clinically relevant variables affecting the mechanical behavior of bone cement. Arch Orthop Traumat Surg 92: 1–18
9. Malory TH, Smalley D, Danyi J (1982) The Townley anatomic total knee arthroplasty using a total tibial component with cruciate release. Clin Orthop 169–197
10. Murray DG, Webster DA (1981) The variable-axis knee prosthesis: A two year follow-up study. J Bone Joint Surg 63-A: 687
11. Ranawat CS, Rose HA (1985) Clinical and radiographic results of total-condylar knee arthroplasty: A 3 to 8 year follow-up. In: Ranawat CS (ed) Total-condylar arthroplasty: Technique, results and complications. Springer, New York, p. 140
12. Ranawat CS, Insall JN, Shine J (1976) Duo-condylar knee arthroplasty: The Hospital for Special Surgery Design. Clin Orthop 120: 76
13. Ranawat CS (1981) Fixation failure of tibial components: Causes and prevention. Instructional Course Lecture 30: 397
14. Scott RD (1982) Duo-patellar total knee replacement: The Brigham experience. Ortho Clinics No Am 12(1): 89

# *Discussion*

*Miller* (McGill University): Firstly, do you still use the Total Condylar in preference to other knees? Second, what was the range of motion? Third, could you describe very briefly what "modern cement technique" signifies?

*Ranawat* (Cornell University Medical College): I still use the original Total Condylar prosthesis for total knee arthroplasty. Second, the average range of motion in this series was 95°; two-thirds of the knees had over 100° and 50 knees had more than 115°. I cannot remember exactly, but I think about ten knees had less than 90°; four knees had 75°–85°.

I would credit two surgeons with the introduction of the modern cement techniques—Clive Lee and the person who is asking this question, Jo Miller. The technique I use is as follows. I do not use low-viscosity cement; I use Simplex in a doughlike state for about 2–4 min, depending on the humidity and room temperature. I would prepare the bone appropriately, i.e., cut the bone within 2–3 mm of the subchondral plate in rheumatoid patients and up to 5–6 mm in osteoarthritic patients on the normal side of the subchondral plate. We clean the bone with a saline solution. If there is hard bone on the site of deformity, I make multiple holes—above five to ten, 2–3 mm in diameter. At 3 min of cement setting, I pressurize the cement manually. I then put the cement under the tibial plateau and bring it in contact at 3–4 min. I pressurize finally with the implant at about 5–6 min of cement setting and remove the excessive cement. With this method, 2–5 mm of cement penetration into the cancellous bone can be achieved in the majority of knees.

*Hastings* (Wellesley Hospital): I agree with you that the cemented total knee is the best form of treatment. I notice that most of your emphasis on loosening was on the tibial side; did you in fact look as carefully on the femoral side? Secondly, do you think there is any place for a noncemented femoral component? Thirdly, in your 11- to 12-year results, did you notice any evidence of stress shielding, loss of bone, or osteoporosis in the distal femur?

*Renawat*: With respect to the femur, we often see radiolucency in the posterior condyle and femoral part of the patello-femoral groove. It is difficult to assess the radiolucency where it matters, i.e., in the load-bearing area, and therefore I have not reported on it. We have not revised any cases and so I do not know if there has been any loosening. Femoral loosening does occur, but it is very uncommon compared with the tibial side. With the patella, radiolucency is often present at the periphery, but it also is very uncommon.

With regard to shielding of the femoral condyle, there is loss of bone substance from the periphery, the area not under the condyle. However, I do not think this is a problem as we have not seen any fractures, detachment of the ligaments, or other gross abnormalities. But from the X-ray, the bone density appears to be less. So shielding does occur, though as to whether it is of clinical importance at the present follow-up time, I would think not; perhaps with a longer follow-up time it may become important.

You also asked about noncemented devices; yes, I believe there is a place for them, especially with porous-coated implants. Perhaps they are more applicable to hips than to knees. I think this area deserves a great deal more study.

*Goodfellow* (Oxford University): You said that the outcome is better than with total hip replacement. I noticed that there was a heavy preponderance of rheumatoid cases among the knee arthroplasties; I doubt whether this was true of the total hip replacements. Perhaps then the comparison is not really justified. In my experience, the outcome of total hip and total knee replacements is far better in the long term in rheumatoid than in osteoarthritic patients.

Secondly, are you satisfied with the method of presenting results in the form of point scores? I find that this obscures details of the outcome very considerably. For example, we learn that there are 90% excellent results, but what proportion of those patients could climb and descend stairs?

*Ranawat*: Both your points are quite valid. In the

total hip series, there were two reports. One set of patients was 55 years of age and under and was non-rheumatoid patients. This study was conducted to assess the quality and durability of the hip arthroplasty in young and active people. The second series involved bilateral hip replacement arthroplasty and included rheumatoid patients. You may well be right that in a controlled study taking all parameters into account the data could be somewhat different. However, we all know that any longterm study with a follow-up is very difficult. I revise more total hips than I revise total knees, and so it is my strong feeling that the hip fails more than the knee.

With respect to the points system, I would not say it is a good one, but it is the best we have. The Knee Society is working very hard on a system which could eliminate points, taking into consideration pain, function, and an objective assessment of range of motion, muscle strength, and stability. In the present study, two-thirds of patients were able to go up and down stairs without any difficulty. The remainder required assistance coming down stairs; after total knee replacement, a large number of patients often lack the confidence to go down stairs without support and prefer to hold on to the rail I agree that in total knee replacement in spite of good motion a significant number of patients hesitate to walk down stairs, which is perhaps due to loss of the cruciate ligament and feedback from the joint in descending.

# Panel Discussion

*Walker* (Harvard Medical School): Dr. Sasaki, you reported the results of Kinematic replacement using types I–IV. Your best results appeared to have been with type III, the Kinematic stabilizer; is that correct?

*Sasaki* (Hokkaido University): No, that is not what I meant to imply. Types I and II are used for good cases based on X-ray assessment; type III is used for cases with strong instability or deformity but with no varus or valgus problems; and type IV, the rotating hinge, is used for cases with strong instability or ankylosis. The scores before operation differed greatly and so no conclusions can be drawn as to which gave the best results.

*Walker*: Do you still believe it is necessary to have a range of implants for the different indications? Do you still use the device that preserves both cruciates and do you still use the rotating hinge?

*Sasaki*: For patients without cruciate ligaments, we use the rotating hinge,, but for patients with intact cruciates we use type II or III.

*Walker*: Dr. Ranawat, how often do you use a device other than the Total Condylar?

*Ranawat* (Cornell University Medical Collage): We recently examined this and found that in the 3000 knees we had replaced, we used an implant other than Total Condylar I or posterior stabilizer type in less than 3%. The other device we use is the Total Condylar III or its variant and we use this in revision surgery where the mediolateral ligaments have been compromised to the extent that we cannot balance them appropriately. The second indication is if at the time of surgery the medial collateral ligament is cut, either inadvertently or otherwise, and stability cannot be achieved. The third indication is in an arthrodesis or a very ankylosed knee, such as in juvenile rheumatoid arthritic patients.

*Walker*: Dr. Sasaki, using the evaluation scales for the rotating hinge, clearly the preoperative condition of these patients is very much worse than if you are using the Condylar. Is it useful to examine different aspects, e.g., is range of motion after implanting the rotating hinge equal to condylar replacement?

*Sasaki*: As I indicated in the earlier slides many of the postoperative parameters, including range of motion, are poor. In the case of the rotating hinge, the preoperative condition was likewise poor.

*Walker*: I think that with the whole issue of a graduated knee system, there is probably some disagreement as to the percentage of different types used by different surgeons, which may be due to experience or preference. It is necessary to look with great care at the follow-ups with the different types, for example, the Posterior Stabilized versus the Total Condylar. I think that Dr. Bourne's study is particularly good because it is a direct comparison of two different designs by the same surgeons. A principal difference that came out in your study was range of motion. However, I feel that the way range of motion is reported leaves a lot to be desired: It is not measured very accurately. Do you not think it would be better to quote range of motion as a pre- to postoperative ratio rather than as an absolute value?

*Bourne* (University of Western Ontario): Yes, I think your points are well taken. At our institute, we found that there was an average of a 10° difference in the assessment of range of motion by different individuals. So after this, we decided to use one observer only, preferably someone not directly concerned with the study.

The other observation I would like to make relates to what Dr. Ranawat was discussing with regard to the Hospital for Special Surgery knee rating. For an 8° difference in range of motion, only one point is allotted, but I think that many of us would agree that 8° are very important, particularly in the 90°–100°.

In this particular study, although the PCA group had on average a lower preoperative range of motion, it was not statistically significant.

With regard to your question about pre- to postoperative ratio, I think it is certainly well worth investigating, though I must admit we did not do so.

*Walker*: Looking at some of your X-rays in the mediolateral view, there were two things I noticed: Some of the tibial trays were tilted anteriorly, and the femoral component was located rather anteriorly on the tibia. I would like to ask you about the technique for the insertion of these prostheses which preserve the posterior cruciate ligament. It seems to me that not enough attention is paid to the correct tension of the posterior cruciate with the knee in flexion. Do you think this is the case?

*Bourne*: Obviously this is important. It is very difficult to restore soft tissue tension with the condylar-type implants that we have. I think this is probably why Dr. Ranawat sacrifices it in many cases. I would agree with you that it is an area we have ignored. Obviously, we try to ensure in preoperative planning, intraoperative instrumentation, and in our trial prostheses before we cement or impact into place that there is stability in tension as well as in flexion, but the way of assessing this is very crude. The meniscal system has 1 mm increments, whereas many of the implants that we employ with the condylar-type series often have several millimeters between sizes.

*Walker*: Is this a failure of the techniques rather than the implant? For example, if the femoral and tibial bones are cut independently of each other and only balance in extension to obtain the correct tightness and extension is this not fundamentally different from the Total Condylar idea, where the object is to achieve a tight result in flexion and extension?

*Bourne*: Logically, it would seem that it does matter. However, as you know, many of the popular systems of instrumentation do not take into consideration the so-called flexion space and extension space. Clinical results have not really shown a difference.

*Ranawat*: There should be no doubt as to the fact that normally functioning posterior and anterior cruciate ligaments are essential to a well-functioning knee, irrespective of whether the joint is artificial. This is evidenced by thc observations of John Goodfellow: When both cruciates are present and functioning well, there is better range of motion. With the unicondylar knee replacement, where the posterior cruciate is present and at the appropriate tension because the opposite condyle maintains the tension in all degrees of motion, the patients have better range of motion.

When preserving the posterior cruciate ligament, three possibilities exist: (a) The tension is correct and there is good posterior roll-back as a result; if there is no excessive peripheral pain, a good range of motion should result. (b) An attempt is made to preserve the right tension but this fails and it becomes too tight; there is then less range of motion because of pain and binding in flexion. (c) This, the most frequent case with these knees, is where the posterior cruciate ligament is preserved but does not function because too little attention is paid to tension in flexion and the design of implants does not allow the posterior cruciate to function properly both in tension and in flexion. I believe that it should be released, capped, and the implant should be spaced in flexion and extension appropriately; it is then possible to rely on new scar formation and the dish of the component to provide anteroposterior limitation of laxity.

*Walker*: Dr. Nagaya, you alluded to patellar remodeling, remodeling of the trabecular bone. Are you saying that there is significant bone resorption, which could lead to subsequent loosening?

*Nagaya* (Nagoya National Hospital): This study has only started in recent years and so detailed data are not yet complete.

With respect to loosening, in my 6-year series there has been thus far no case of revision, which indicates that there has been no clear case of loosening. However, by comparison with total hip replacement and cemented cases I would guess that loosening might result in the later cases.

*Walker*: Dr. Nagaya, you started off with a preoperative range of motion in most of your patients with approximately 10° flexion contracture to about 105°–110° and after the operation you had about 0°–90°. I always thought that Japanese surgeons had to have a very large range of motion and yet you are using a Total Condylar, which even though it has a very low failure rate does have a very poor range of motion. Why do you not use a prosthesis with TCL preservation to obtain more motion?

*Nagaya*: This report includes cases that data back to 1982 and so covers the early experience. As you say, in Japan the range of motion has to be large; however, most of my patients are rheumatoid arthritic patients, and in these weight bearing and pain relief are of greater importance than the range of motion. Therefore, we used a tight insertion.

*Sasaki*: In rheumatoid arthrititis or osteoarthritis of the knee, even though the disease might be advanced there is a great deal of variation from case to case and so devices that can meet each individual case must be developed. This is why we have worked on the Kinematic knee system. The same prosthesis cannot be used for every case and so there is a need for flexibility. We should also be able to use the devices developed by other people.

*Bourne*: I certainly think that fixation is very important. In whatever new design we have looked at, if the patellar and tibial components are fixed with cement we have achieved greater range of motion. The thickness of the patella with the component pre- and postoperatively is of great importance. The alignment of the prosthesis in the anteroposterior and mediolateral planes is important; it is possible to be out by 5° and it does not appear, as least in our hands, to affect range of motion. What we have not addressed is rotation: It is fairly easy to malrotate a tibial component by plus or minus 5° upon insertion.

*Nagaya*: To increase the range of motion, I think it is necessary to work on a good biomechanical design. I also think that development is required in biomaterials to produce a stronger surface, it may be possible to preserve the anterior cruciate ligament, not just the posterior. But as Dr. Sasaki mentioned, in terms of indication it is not necessary to stick purely to range of motion.

*Walker*: Dr. Ranawat could you give us your opinion of the advantages and disadvantages in trying to achieve a very large range of motion?

*Ranawat*: A good range of motion depends on many factors: design of the implant, size of the implant for a given bone size, soft tissue handling at the time of surgery, bleeding episodes during and after surgery, anticoagulation, amount of physiotherapy. I will refer to the ones I think are most important. If there is residual pain in the patellofemoral joint or due to the implant fixation, such as in press-fit, range of motion will be limited despite all other good factors. In the design, I would think that there should be a posterior slope in the component to clear the femur and tibia by 3–4 mm in the sagittal plane. The point of contact should be slightly posterior in a normal articulating surface. The joint line of the artificial joint should be as close to the original as possible so that there is no binding of the collateral ligament capsule. One should not close the quadriceps system under a lot of tension, which means that one should be liberal with lateral release if it is needed for proper closure of the incision.

With regard to whether a large range of motion is harmful, with some designs it has been harmful to some degree. In the GUEPAR, there is a fixed hinge in which the external rotation was posterior and superior, allowing the femur to clear from the tibia very well at the cost of the patellofemoral joint; the latter is under great pressure and may dislocate, loosen, or cause pain. A similar case is seen to a lesser extent in the rotating hinge, though here the axis of rotation is slightly better than in the GUEPAR. The Posterior stabilized knee is the best of the three systems, but it produces posterior displacement, opens anteriorly, and gives rise to more tension on the quadriceps. So all three designs give more motion at the cost of the patellofemoral joint. The optimal situation in my opinion is to head for a combination whereby posterior roll is preserved, with or without the posterior cruciate ligament, by changing the design of the implant, contact area, slope, and joint line and go for a range of motion not exceeding 110°–115°.

*Koshino* (Yokohama City University): I would like to ask the panel about limb alignment shown in the slides. Is this standing or lying alignment? Some alignment is lost, a few degrees toward valgus, when the patient stands up.

*Sasaki*: All the cases I presented today were of measurement at the time of standing; we have not observed loosening. There was 2° in valgus in the osteoarthritic and rheumatoid arthritic patients. In the cases of Dr. Walker, valgus was 5°–8°; our own extent of valgus was somewhat less.

*Bourne*: There are two points here: There is the anatomical axis of the femur to the tibia, and there is the axis of the tibial component to the long axis of the tibia. Obviously, the anatomical axis has to be taken in the standing position and that is how we assess it postoperatively, though this is, of course, difficult to do in the operating room. The alignment of the tibial component to the tibia can be done in a non-weight-bearing film. I think perhaps we are a little more forgiving with metal backing and better cementing techniques and that studies such as those suggested by Dr. Ranawat—instead of 5- to 8-year follow-up, 10 or more years—are required to see with certainly whether these so-called improvements are indeed improvements.

*Nagaya*: Our object in correcting the angle of the femorotibial alignment is about 170°–175° in valgus. We see some shift in weight bearing. The degree changes slightly with time, but I do not know as yet the best way to meet this challenge.

*Ranawat*: I would agree that the alignment axis of ambulation is what matters, not what you judge from the patient lying down. This is dependent on the deformities, torsional or angular, from the foot to the knee and the knee to the hip. The ultimate load should come from the center of the hip through the middle of the knee to the middle of the ankle; this is what we are striving toward. This can change by 5° from patient to patient.

In cemented knees, it does not make any difference if the component position is within 5° of varus, valgus, or tilt, both of the femur and of the tibia, as long as the overall alignment of the knee is toward the valgus plane. It is my feeling that it is better to err toward valgus than toward neutral.

# Part 2
# Cemented Total Knee Replacement II

# Keio Total Knee Arthroplasty: Concept, Design, and Clinical Results

F. Iseki, T. Takeda, and K. Fujikawa[1]

**Summary.** The concept, design, and clinical results of the Keio total knee prosthesis are presented. This prosthesis is of the semiconstrained surface type and is designed both to reproduce a movement similar to that of the normal knee joint and to give sufficient stability. Between 1977 and 1986, 150 Keio total knee arthroplasties were performed. Of the 150 knees, 94 knees in 70 patients had RA, 56 knees in 46 patients had OA. Follow-up data were available on 130 knees in 99 patients with an average follow-up of 72.6 months.

Relief of pain was the most significant result in our series. Walking ability also remarkably increased, particularly in the OA patients. Thus, the clinical results have been somewhat satisfactory.

However, serious complications such as infection, loosening, and fracture occurred in 18 knees. Among these, 14 knees required revision or arthrodesis. Further studies for decreasing the complications must be continued.

**Keywords:** Total knee arthroplasty—Semiconstrained design—Clinical trial

In the past 30 years, various designs of total knee prosthesis have been developed [2–4]. They are classified according to the degree of mechnical constraint provided by the prosthetic design. The degree of constraint given to the ideal knee prosthesis is difficult to determine because of the complexity of both the anatomical structures and movement of the knee joint.

We began developing a semiconstrained knee prosthesis in 1973 and completed the Keio total knee in 1976 [2]. In this paper, we present the concept, design, and clinical results of the Keio total knee arthroplasty.

## Concept

Anatomically, the knee is classified as a hinge joint; however, the movement of the knee is not that of a simple hinge but an extremely complex one. Flexion and extension of the knee consist of a rolling, gliding, and slipping motion between the femoral and tibial condyles, and the movement is polycentric. In addition to flexion and extension, internal and external rotation, and abduction and adduction occur simultaneously.

A more detailed explanation is as follows. The movement of the normal knee joint consists of the following three major phases from the functional point of view (Fig. 1): (a) Slipping (hinge) phase—range of motion of over 60° of flexion, where the femoral condyles slip on the tibial table; (b) rolling phase, range of motion of 15°–60° of flexion, where the femoral condyles roll over the tibial table with a different slipping factor in each condyle; (c) gliding (screw-home) phase range of motion of 15° of flexion to full extension, where the lateral condyle glides on the tibial table, which is a pivotal turn, while the medial condyle rolls over the tibial table.

The knee bears the heaviest load of all the joints in the human body; firm stability is, therefore, required. Since the stability provided by the geometry of the articular surface itself is very weak, the surrounding soft tissues, such as muscle, capsule and ligaments must play both a dynamic and static role to fulfil the contradictory requirements of adequate stability and wide range of motion. In particular the ligaments must work to prevent abnormal movement and guide the physiological movement.

In knee joints requiring total knee arthroplasty in patients with osteoarthritis (OA) or rheumatoid arthritis (RA), not only the articular surface but also the ligaments are severely damaged. Therefore, a total knee prosthesis providing both excellent mobility and adequate stability is required. The Keio total knee was designed not only to induce normal knee joint movement but also to give sufficient stability.

[1] Department of Orthopaedics, School of Medicine, Keio University, Tokyo, Japan

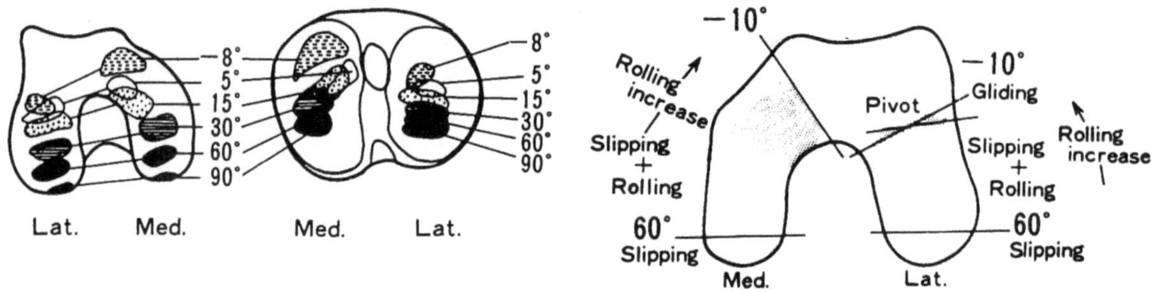


**Fig. 1.** Movement of the femorotibial contact area and the three phases of knee motion

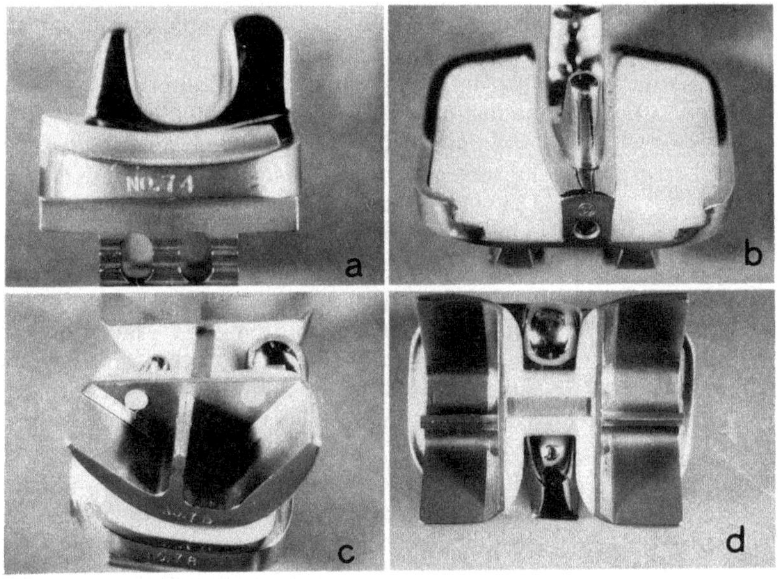

**Fig. 2a–d.** Profile of Keio total knee. **a** Lateral view of tibial component **b** Anterior view of tibial component **c** Prosthesis articulated as viewed from top and side. **d** Prosthesis articulated as viewed from top

## Design

The Keio knee is of the semiconstrained surface type consisting of a femoral and a tibial component. The femoral componet has no anterior flange for the patella and is common to both left and right sides. The tibial component is of a metal tray design with a high-density polyethylene (HDP) surface and different components are required for the left and right sides. There are two eminences in the central part of the tibial component, and the transverse axle of the femoral component is inserted into the hollow between them (Fig. 2).

This mechanism gives sufficient stability and also restricts non-physiological movements in all directions. However, there is a small amount of play at this part so that a certain degree of rotation can be given. Between 20° and 60° of flexion, approximately 20° of rotation is permitted, with greater rotation in a more flexed position.

Figure 3 shows the torque-rotation curve obtained from the knee joint of a cadaver with the Keio knee, which shows that an approximately 10° internal and external rotation is allowed at 30° of flexion.

Figure 4 shows the contact pattern between the two components. This pattern is very close to the femorotibial contact pattern of the normal knee joint shown in Fig. 2. The contact moves over almost the whole area of the surface of the HDP tibial component, which is an advantage with respect to abrasive wear. Since the contact surface of the tibial component and the transverse axle of the femoral component are covered by the HDP, all the contact is metal to HDP.

As shown in Fig. 5. this prosthesis requires resection of only a very small portion of bone and uses only a small amount of bone cement in the operation. Therefore, even if a salvage operation becomes necessary, it can be easily performed.

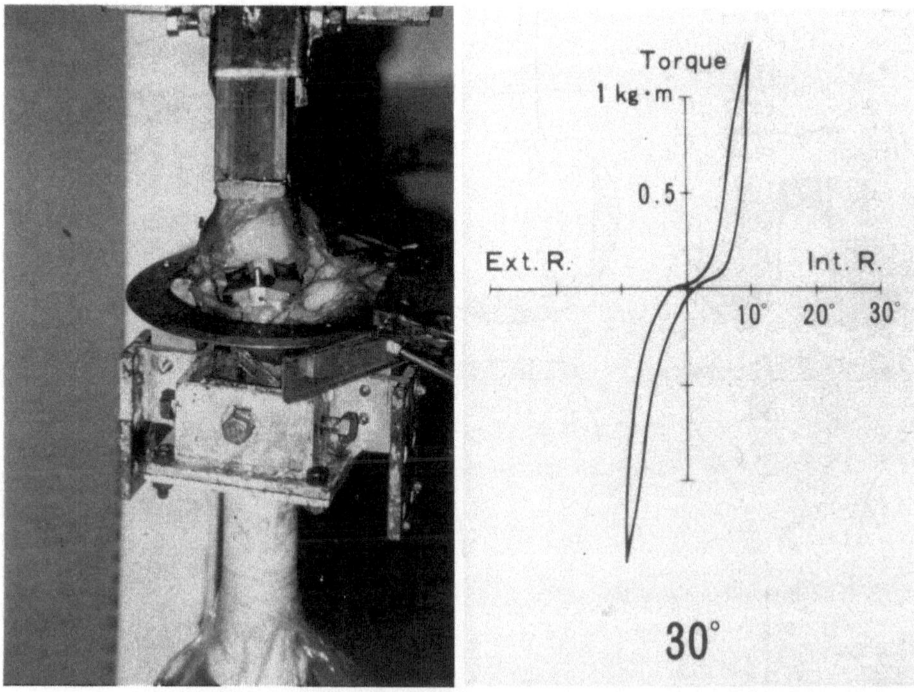


**Fig. 3.** Torque-rotation curve obtained from the cadaveric knee joint replaced by Keio total knee when flexed to 30°

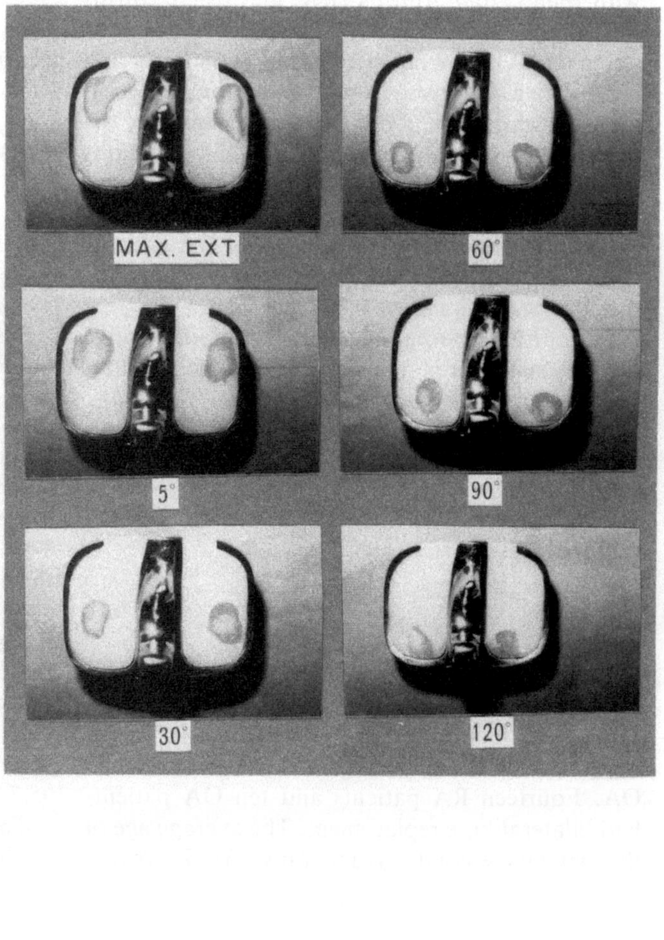


**Fig. 4.** Movement of contact between both components. This pattern is very close to the femorotibial contact pattern of the normal knee joint

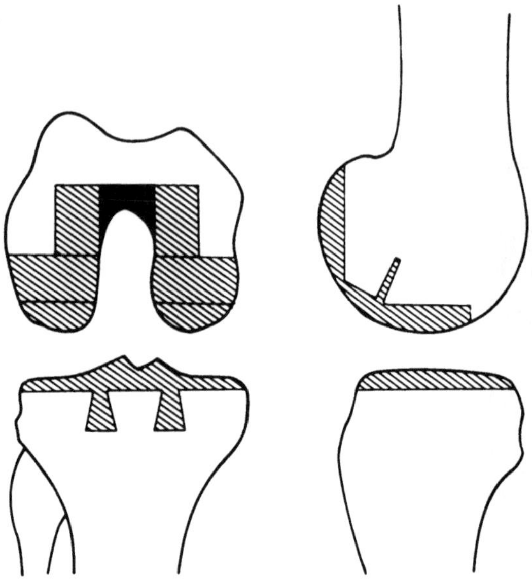

Fig. 5. The area of bone resection

**Table 1.** Pre- and postoperative pain

| | Preoperation | | Postoperation | |
|---|---|---|---|---|
| | No. | Percent | No. | Percent |
| RA | | | | |
| None | 0 | | 29 | 41.4 |
| Minimal | 0 | | 31 | 44.3 |
| Mild | 0 | | 6 | 8.6 |
| Moderate | 18 | 25.7 | 4 | 5.7 |
| Severe | 52 | 74.3 | 0 | |
| OA | | | | |
| None | 0 | | 31 | 62 |
| Minimal | 0 | | 14 | 28 |
| Mild | 0 | | 4 | 8 |
| Moderate | 11 | 22 | 1 | 2 |
| Severe | 39 | 78 | 0 | |

The cases of arthrodesis and revision with other types of prosthesis are excluded

## Indications

Keio knee arthroplasty is indicated for patients with rheumatoid arthritis (RA) and osteoarthritis (OA). However, OA is our main concern since patients with OA are in better general condition and more active than patients with RA. However good the short-term results of OA patients may be, the possibility of development of late complications is increasing annually. Therefore, in principle we operate on OA patients over 60 years of age. In contrast, we operate on some younger RA patients depending on their condition. Among our patients, the youngest was a 31-year-old female.

Since the Keio total knee has no anterior flange for the patella, it is not indicated in knees with a severely damaged patellofemoral joint.

The following are the clinical results of operations performed between 1977 and 1986.

## Clinical Results

### Materials

Since 1977, we have operated on 116 patients and carried out 150 knee arthroplasties using the Keio total knee. Of the 150 knees, 94 knees in 70 patients had RA, and 56 knees in 46 patients had OA. Fourteen RA patients and ten OA patients had bilateral knee replacement. The average age of the patients was 60.2 years (range 31–77 years). There were six deaths of RA patients due to unrelated causes. Twelve knees in 12 patients were lost to follow-up; thus, follow-up data for 130 knees in 99 patients were available. All these patients have been followed up and evaluated by the authors. The minimal follow-up period was 6 months, ranging to 119 months, with an average of 72.6 months.

### Results

#### Pain

Knee pain was the predominant complaint in all patients, and relief of pain was clearly the most significant postoperative improvement in this series. All of the knees had preoperative pain graded as moderate or severe. Pain was relieved in more than 90% of both OA and RA patients (Table 1). Several patients (about 10%) complained of pain around the patellofemoral joint and the infrapatellar area. Of these patients, only one required further surgery (partial patellectomy). The remaining patients required no treatment as the pain was mild and tolerable.

#### Range of Motion

In the knees of patients with RA, the average range of motion was 88.3° preoperatively and 90.1° postoperatively; in the knees of patients with OA, these values were 100.1° preoperatively and 95.7° postoperatively.

Thus, a significant increase in average range of motion was not seen in either the RA or OA

**Table 2.** Pre- and postoperative range of motion

| | Preoperation | | Postoperation | |
|---|---|---|---|---|
| | Average | Range | Average | Range |
| RA | 88.3° | 17.2°–105.5° | 90.1° | 6.0°–96.1° |
| OA | 100.1° | 11.4°–111.5° | 88.9° | 3.3°–99° |

group. However, the flexion contracture apparently improved (Table 2).

**Walking Ability**

We evaluated walking ability on the basis of the following criteria: (a) unlimited; (b) minimally limited, more than 500 m; (c) moderately limited, 100–500 m; (d) markedly limited, less than 100 m or unable to walk outdoors; (e) unable to walk. Postoperative walking ability markedly improved by the relief of pain and obtaining stability. Walking ability seemed to increase more in the group with OA than in the group with RA. The reason may be that rheumatoid patients often present with more or less generalized rheumatoid manifestations (Fig. 6).

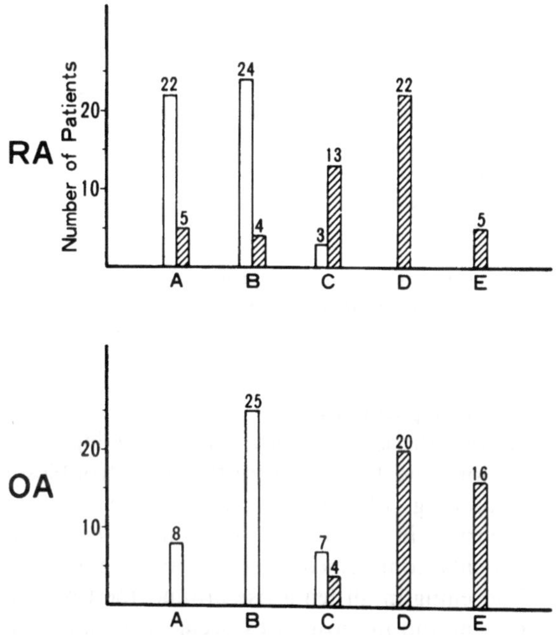


**Fig. 6.** The walking ability preoperatively and postoperatively for both OA and RA. Cases of arthrodesis and revision with other types of prosthesis are excluded. *Unshaded columns* show preoperative number, *shaded columns* show postoperative values. *A* unable to walk, *B* markedly limited, *C* moderately limited, *D* minimally limited, *E* unlimited

## Complications

Table 3 shows the list of complications; among these, 18 knees needed further surgery or revision (Table 4). The complications are discussed in the following.

**Table 3.** Complications

| Complication | Number of knees |
|---|---|
| Early | |
| Deep infection | 1 |
| Superficial infection | 1 |
| Delayed wound healing | 5 |
| Peroneal palsy | 3 |
| Patellar impingement | 1 |
| Dislocation | 8 |
| Late | |
| Loosening | 10 |
| Progressive radiolucent zone | 3 |
| Fracture of upper tibia | 3 |
| Late infection | 4 |

**Early Complications**

There were eight cases of posterior dislocation between both components. (Fig. 7). All these dislocations occurred during a relatively early stage of the postoperative course when repair of the soft tissues was not sufficient in those patients whose quadriceps muscle strength was markedly weakened. All patients were treated by immobilization with a plaster cast for 3 weeks after manual reduction. The dislocations showed scarcely any effect on the clinical results at the time of follow-up. Furthermore, to prevent such dislocation, the tibial component is now improved by making the forward eminence higher than in the previous model.

All three cases of peroneal palsy were caused by a plaster cast which was put on in the initial postoperative period; in no case was peroneal palsy caused by the surgical procedure itself. Of these three patients, two recovered fully and one incompletely.

In the patellar impingement case, pain was caused by the anterior margin of the femoral component snagging the patella. The superficial infection and delayed wound healing were resolved without any problem.

In the immediate postoperative period, deep infection due to *Staphylococcus aureus* occurred in one knee in a patient with RA. Eventually, arthrodesis was performed in this case.

**Table 4.** Reoperation after Keio total knee replacement

| | Number of knees |
|---|---|
| Arthrodesis | 5 |
| Partial patellectomy | 1 |
| Wound closure | 1 |
| Reduction | 1 |
| Neurolysis | 1 |
| Replacement with another prosthesis | 5 |
| Replacement of tibial component | 4 |

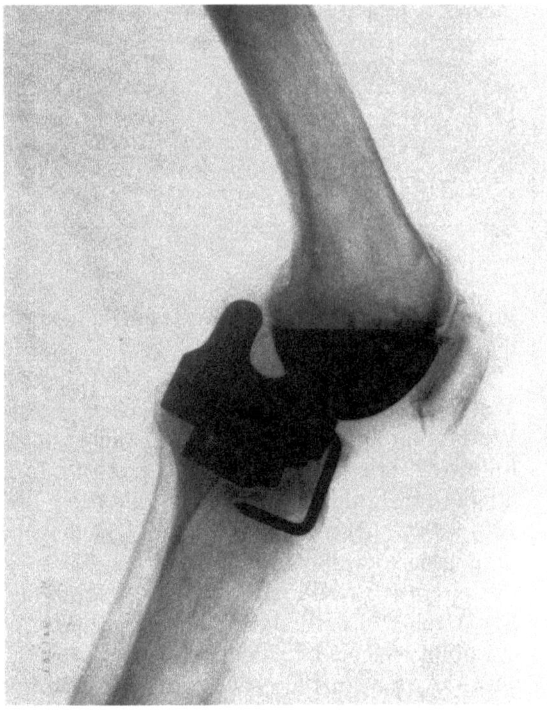

**Fig. 7.** Lateral view of dislocation between both components

**Late Complications**

Among the late complications, loosening, late infection, and fracture were the most troublesome. Loosening of the prosthesis with symptoms occurred in ten knees in seven patients. These patients complained of pain on weight bearing. Loosening in all ten arose around the tibial component and in most cases occurred within 3 years after surgery. Eight of the knees were in RA patients, including three bilateral cases. The treatment for loosening was as follows: replacement of the prosthesis in three cases, replacement of the tibial component in two cases, arthrodesis is one case, and conservative treatment in four cases. In two patients, the tibial component was replaced by the stem type (Fig. 8). In three cases, the prosthesis was replaced with another type.

Late infection developed in four knees (Table 5). They were all RA patients, and the latest case occurred 60 months after surgery. The organisms were *Staphylococcus aureus* in three knees and *Escherichia coli* in one. Arthrodesis was performed in three of these four knees. All three cases showed successful bony fusion with little shortening of the lower limb. In one case, a total knee was reinserted after closed suction irrigation with no subsequent evidence of recurrence.

All three fractures were at the upper end of the tibia and occurred in patients with OA. Two were treated by replacing the tibial component with the stem type and the other was treated by replacing with another type of prosthesis.

## Discussion

### Design of Prosthesis

#### Mobility and constraint of prosthesis

It has frequently been pointed out that the ideal total knee prosthesis should satisfy the following conditions: (a) guiding function of normal range of motion in all planes of knee motion; (b) adequate stability and constraint function against nonphysiological movement; (c) materials nontoxic to the human body; (d) materials nonabrasive and unbreakable; (e) easy surgical procedure involving minimal invasion.

However, such a prosthesis has not yet been designed. The various knee prostheses which have been reported can be classified according to the degree of mechanical constraint provided by their design. The hinge type and the nonconstrained surface type are two extremes from the mechanical constraint point of view. The hinge types have very strong stability but the movement is constrained to be uniaxial allowing only flexion-extension. Therefore, the stresses caused by rotational and varus-valgus movement are transmitted to the prosthesis-bone interface or link parts of the prosthesis. Thus, the hinge types are likely to have serious complications such as loosening, breakage of the prosthesis, and fracture. They also require a large amount of bone to be resected to allow insertion. On the other hand, complications such as instability and dislocation, in addition to loosening and sinking, have often been reported for the nonconstrained surface replacement types.

For these reasons, at present the most popular

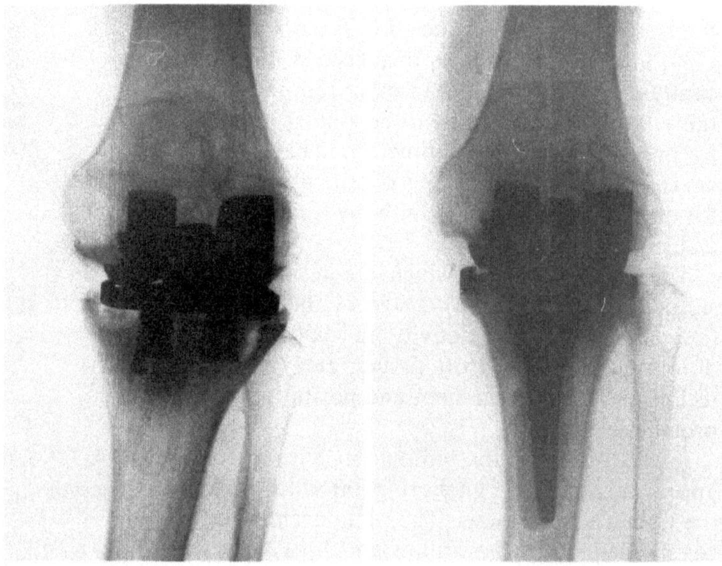

**Fig. 8. a** Radiograph showing loosening of the tibial component. **b** Radiograph after revision with a stem-type component

designs are the semiconstrained types. However, the amount of constraint that should be given to the total knee prosthesis is an unsolved problem because mobility and stability are inversely related. However, we believe that the Keio knee satisfies the contradictory criteria of good mobility in all planes and firm stability.

**Need for patellofemoral replacement**

The Keio knee does not provide a patellofemoral compartment. This is not due to neglecting the clinical role of the patellofemoral joint but to the following reasons. When the femoral component with an anterior flange is replaced (a) even a slight inclination of the inserting axis, especially in the transverse or coronal plane, causes patellofemoral malalignment; (b) if the patella is replaced with an HDP surface having the HDP on the convex side and metal on the concave side is disadvantageous with respect to abrasive wear, while making the patella thinner to insert the HDP unit might cause complications such as patellar fracture; (c) if the patella is not replaced, the cartilage surface is always in contact with the metal flange; (d) a larger amount of bone resection is necessary than for the component without the flange.

According to many reports, the frequency of patellofemoral complaints with first generation prostheses that have no patellofemoral component (such as the Geomedic type) is less than 15%, and the complaints are mainly patellofemoral pain and sometimes patellar impingement. This frequency is not significantly different from that with patellofemoral replacement. Furthermore, the complications in patients with patellofemoral replacement were usually more serious, such as dislocation and fracture of the patella [5]. In the Keio knee arthroplasty, approximately 10% of the patients have continued to complain of patellofemoral pain, but we have not experienced any of the above serious complications.

**Table 5.** Clinical data on four knees with infection

| Diagnosis | Time post-operation (months) | Treatment |
|---|---|---|
| 1. RA | 6 | Arthrodesis |
| 2. RA | 12 | Arthrodesis |
| 3. RA | 13 | Arthrodesis |
| 4. RA | 60 | Replacement with another prosthesis |

Currently, patellofemoral replacement is usually performed for the condylar type prostheses, however we cannot agree with the opinion that patellofemoral replacement should be performed routinely in all cases.

## Complications

Among the complications with Keio total knee arthroplasty, infection and sterile loosening were very servious and troublesome. The overall results are greatly affected by these complications. Of course, infection is the most serious complication since it may require removal of the prosthesis. In this series, there were one (0.1%) early and four (3%) late infections. This incidence is not significantly different from that in other reports. Regrettably, at present, it seems to be almost impossible to prevent infection completely. Therefore, decreasing the loosening rate is of critical importance for obtaining good results with the Keio total knee arthroplasty.

The various factors which are responsible for sterile loosening are: (a) design of the prosthesis; (b) patient factors—activity in daily life, conditions of bone and soft tissues, etc; (c) surgical technique—axial alignment and positioning of the prosthesis.

In this series, all the radiolucent lines started to appear around the anchoring interface between the tibia and prosthesis. The radiolucent lines can be divided into the following three groups—progressive, nonprogressive, and improving.

The progressive type eventually proceeds to loosening. Such a progressive type was found mainly in patients with RA. The reason could be that usually, in RA cases, there is not only advanced bone atrophy but also functional deficiency of the ligaments and muscle weakness, so all the stresses are directly transferred to the anchoring interface without a buffer. In some cases, loosening was obviously due to axial malalignment and malposition of the prosthesis. Design of the prosthesis is one of the most important factors in sterile loosening. In general, the frequency of loosening is higher in the highly constrained prosthesis than in the nonconstrained one. The frequency of loosening with the Keio knee is less than 10%, which is comparable with that in the other highly constrained types [6] and is much lower than that of the hinge type.

We shall continue our efforts to reduce the frequency of loosening. At present, we are considering altering the anchor design of the tibial component from the dovetail type to the meduallary stem type shown in Fig. 9. Although the latter has the advantage of obtaining firm anchoring and being easily aligned and positioned accurately, it has the disadvantages of requiring a large amount of bone cement for fixation and injuring the bone marrow.

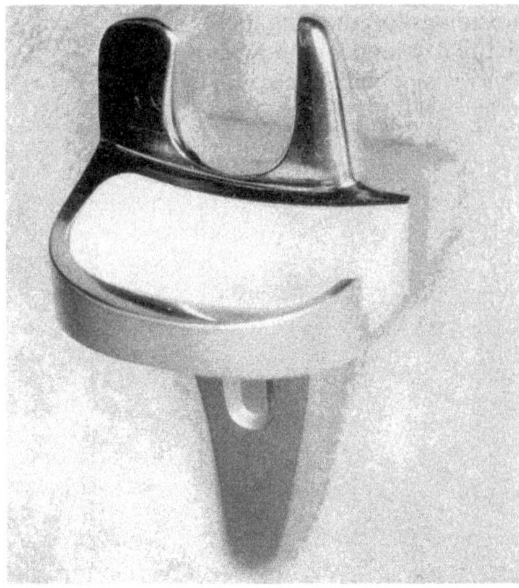

**Fig. 9.** Tibial component with a medullary stem

## References

1. Bryan RS, RAN JA (1982) Revision total knee arthroplasty. Clin Orthop 170: 116–112
2. Fujio I, et al. (1977) Functional endoprosthesis for the knee (Keio type). Keio J Med 26: 179–185
3. Gunson FA (1973) Polycentric knee arthroplasty. J Bone Joint Surg 53B: 272–279
4. Savastano AA (1980) Total knee replacement. Appleton-Century-Crofts, New York
5. Scott RD (1982) Toroff N, Ewald FC Stress fracture of the patella following Duopatellar total knee arthroplasty with patellar resurfacing. Clin Orthop 170: 147–151
6. Wilson FC, Venters GC (1976) Results of knee replacement with the Walldius prosthesis. Clin Orthop 120: 39–46

# *Discussion*

*Hoshino* (Tokyo Medical and Dental University): Compared with the results of the Total Condylar and Kinematic knee replacements, these results would appear to be inferior, but I do not think that this is in fact the case. Of 150 cases, you had ten cases of loosening. Loosening occurs with most prostheses to a very high percentage and does not always signify revision.

*Yamamuro* (Kyoto University): You said that changing to the stem type improved the number of revision cases. Why did you not use the stem type from the beginning? Was it because of fusion?

*Iseki* (Keio University): Yes, we originally tried to minimize the amount of bone resection and patellofemoral lesions were an indication against use of the implant. We first used the stem type in revision cases and revision or loosening occurred in about 10% of cases. With use of the stem type, infection may occur, making further revision difficult.

We attempt physiological reconstruction, if that is not possible we use a prosthesis; but these prostheses cannot be used in cases requiring a great deal of bone resection. It may be possible to replace cartilage and if loosening can be minimized this is ideal. In the current biomechanical concept and from interface studies, I think that may be quite difficult.

*Yamamuro*: You seem to have a relatively high rate of loosening; so perhaps at the moment the stem would seem to be desirable. Perhaps in the future we will be able to replace the surface only, which would be ideal.

*Iseki*: This prosthesis was inserted for the first time in 1970. In Oxford, there is the linked type prosthesis, which is similar to our model with an attached stem. Dr. Takeda of our group would like to change to the stem type. However, the length of the stem and biomechanical issues should be considered. Perhaps a length of 3–4 cm would be suitable. Complications were observed and if the numbers increase perhaps the stem could be used for the tibial side. We have to be careful, however, because in revision cases we cannot change to another type of prosthesis.

*Kurosawa* (The University of Tokyo): Did you use a patellar button?

*Iseki*: No. We made a preoperative selection of patients: Those given the PF had a panarticular condition; lesions of the meniscus and ligaments are not indications for the patellofemoral joint. We use the rotatory hinge in severe lesions.

*Kurosawa*: So when the patellar surface is damaged you do not implant this prosthesis?

*Iseki*: No. In these cases, the patellar surface is shaved. The damage to the patellofemoral joint PF itself is small. In our cases, the femorotibial joint is the main cause. The PF is treated only in serious cases with extensive damage present.

# Distal Femoral and Proximal Tibial Segmental Interchangeable Hinge Knee Prosthesis

C.-T. CHENG and C.-W. HSU[1]

**Summary.** A personal experience is recounted of internal prosthetic replacement of a long segmental bony defect about the knee joint after en bloc resection for an extensive bone tumor. Three patients with two distal femoral and two proximal tibial bone tumors were treated with resection and replacement by hinged knee replacement prostheses and followed up for more than 10 years. One patient underwent amputation because of the extensive recurrence of the giant cell tumor 5 years after the joint replacement and finally died of multiple lung metastases 5 years later. The others were followed up for 10 and 11 years respectively. Each has a painless stable knee with a useful range of motion.

**Keywords:** Bone tumor—Femur—Total knee replacement—Two-stage procedure—Tibia

## Introduction

With the development of human biomechanics and improvement of the resurfacing total knee prosthesis, the constrained total knee prosthesis is gradually becoming less popular. The constrained type is now reserved for use in knees with severe bone loss or marked ligamentous laxity and in certain revision procedures.

A radical en bloc resection is an accepted procedure for low-grade and certain high-grade malignant lesions, such as giant cell tumor, parosteal osteogenic sarcoma, chondrosarcoma and chondromyxoid fibroma, and certain other definitely benign primary lesions, such as enchondroma, chondroblastoma neurilemmoma, nonosteotic fibrous dysplasia, and angiomatous osteolysis of undue size or recurrence after curettage. When an en bloc resection involves the distal femur and/or proximal tibia there are problems of preservation of the leg length, joint function, and stability [1–4, 7–10].

After initial experience with a custom-made proximal tibial internal prosthesis in 1973, having to wait for the prosthesis to be fabricated suggested the idea of a distal femoral and proximal tibial interchangeable hinged knee replacement system to avoid these problems.

The present paper is a report of our early cases, which have been followed up for more than 10 years.

## Case Report

**Case 1.** A 20-year-old female with a 14-month history of soreness of the right knee sustained a fracture of the right lower femur 6 months later and was treated with a spica cast for 3 months. After removal of the cast, the X-ray showed a bone tumor occupying the whole of the femoral condyles with extension of the tumor upward through the medullary canal, over the fracture line, and out of the cortex. The patient was then transferred to us. A biopsy was taken, and a giant cell tumor identified.

Because of the extent of the tumor, the resection had to include all ligamentous constraints at the knee joint. Following discussion of the design of the replacement prosthesis with engineers, we used the hinged knee prosthesis as the basic design model. The wide excision of the distal femur measured 6 in. (15 mm) in length and, supported by a fibular graft, was done as a first-stage operation. The distal femoral segmental replacement hinge knee system was completed 8 months later and the second-stage operation for prosthetic replacement was done in August 1976. The patient could walk without support 6 weeks after the replacement, and at follow-up 11 years later the range of motion (ROM) was 0°–100° and the patient was stable when walking (Fig. 1).

**Case 2.** A 40-year-old female came to us because of a recurrent and progressive pain associated with a localised growing mass over the left upper tibia over a period of 3 years. The patient had suffered from

[1] Department of Orthopedics, Chung Shan Hospital, Taipei, Republic of China
[2] Taipei Medical Collage, Taipei, Republic of China

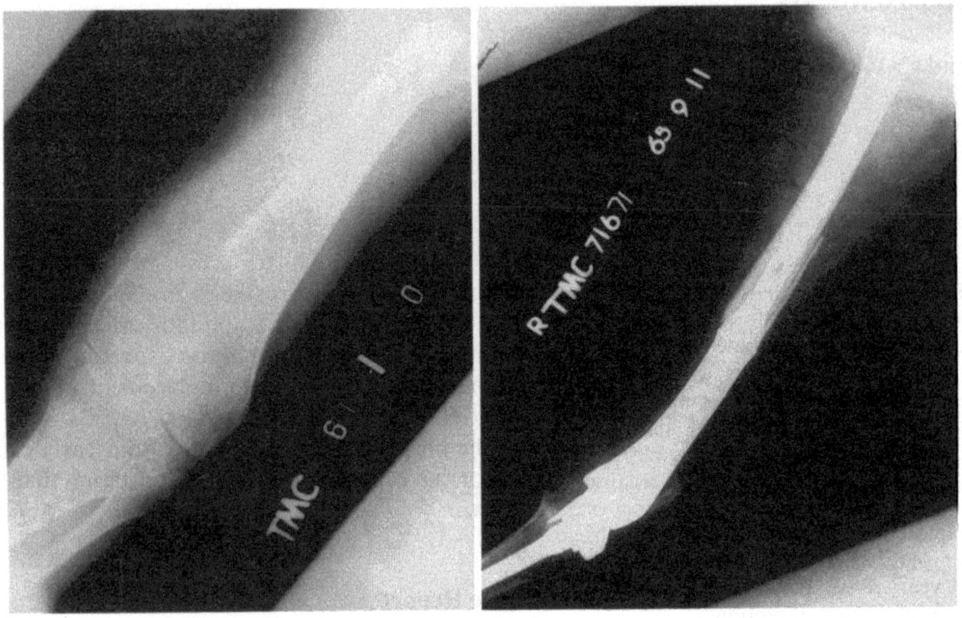

a b

**Fig. 1a, b.** Case 1 **a** Radiograph showing giant cell tumor and supracondylar fracture. **b** Postoperative radiograph of distal femoral segmental replacement hinged knee prosthesis

pain on the left upper tibia since 1973. Curettage and bone grafting had been performed at another hospital. The pathological investigation revealed a giant cell tumor. Recurrence of the tumor under the operation scar was noted 2 years later and local excision of the mass was done again at the same hospital.

Wide resection and prosthetic replacement were carried out in May 1976, and the patient could flex her left knee to 120° degrees 1 month after the surgery. Unfortunately local recurrence of the tumor developed 3 years after replacement and the limb had to be amputated through the midthigh 5 years after prosthetic replacement surgery. The patient developed multiple lung metastases and died 10 years after the replacement (Fig. 2).

**Case 3.** A 24-year-old male sustained a left knee injury in a car accident in 1977. He was treated by a bone-setter for 1 month. Because of persistent pain, he was admitted to hospital and an X-ray examination revealed different bone tumors in both the distal femur and proximal tibia with pathological fracture in the lower femur. He was transferred to our department and resection of the distal femur and proximal tibia (4 in. each) was carried out with replacement by a segmental interchangeable hinged knee prosthesis.

Pathological investigation revealed enchondroma in the distal femur and giant cell tumor in the proximal tibia. The patient could walk without support and flex his knee to 80° at 1 month, and at 10 years ROM was 0°–100° (Fig. 3).

## Surgical Technique

**Incision.** Under a pneumatic tourniquet, the operation was carried out through an anterior midline or curvilinear incision to include excision of the route of the previous biopsy.

**Excision of bone.** This was always carried out through the muscle, taking care not to strip the periosteum from the bone.

**Insertion of prosthesis.** After test seating of both components, the prosthesis was fixed with bone cement under pressure. Making a central mark on the bone before the excision facilitated the rotational orientation.

**Closure.** The muscles and fascia were restored without attaching them to the prosthesis, and the wound was closed over a suction drain.

**After treatment.** The suction drain was removed after drainage ceased. The patient was allowed to sit up and start exercise as soon as possible. The stitches were removed after 14 days.

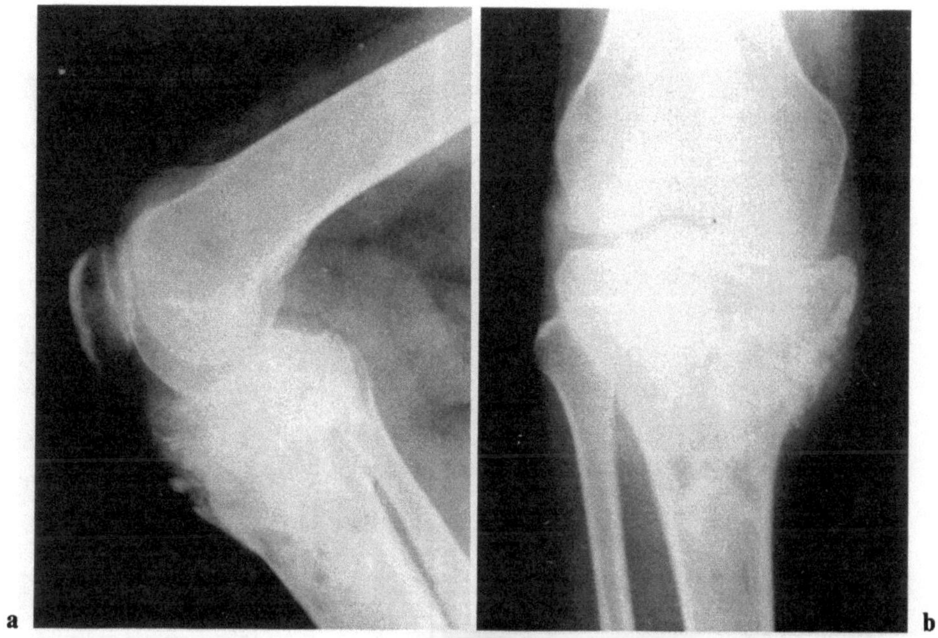

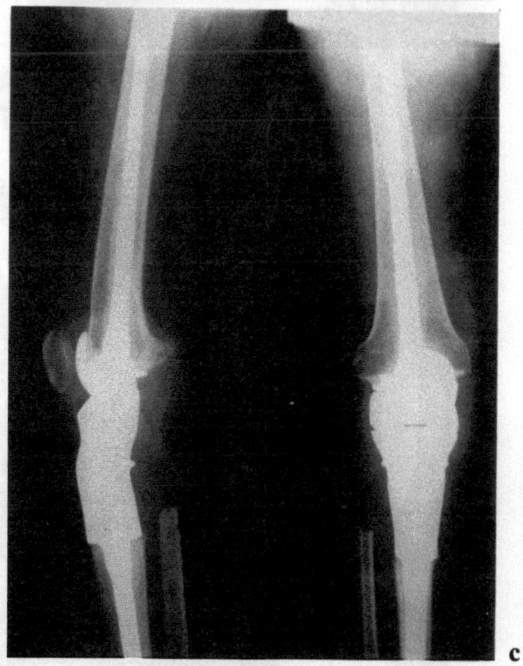

**Fig. 2a–c.** Case 2. **a, b** Radiograph showing upper tibia giant cell tumor postcurettege and bone graft. **c** Upper tibial segmental replacement hinge knee prosthesis

**Phasing of operation.** The operation is preferably done in one stage. If the operation required two stages we would use a temporary spacer made of methylmethacrylate and an intramedullary rod to maintain limb length and also provide a good prosthetic bed [6, 9, 11]

## Complications

There were no perioperative complications. The second patient showed tumor recurrence, which resulted in amputation 5 years after implantation and the patient died of multiple metastasis 10 years after implantation. The possible complications

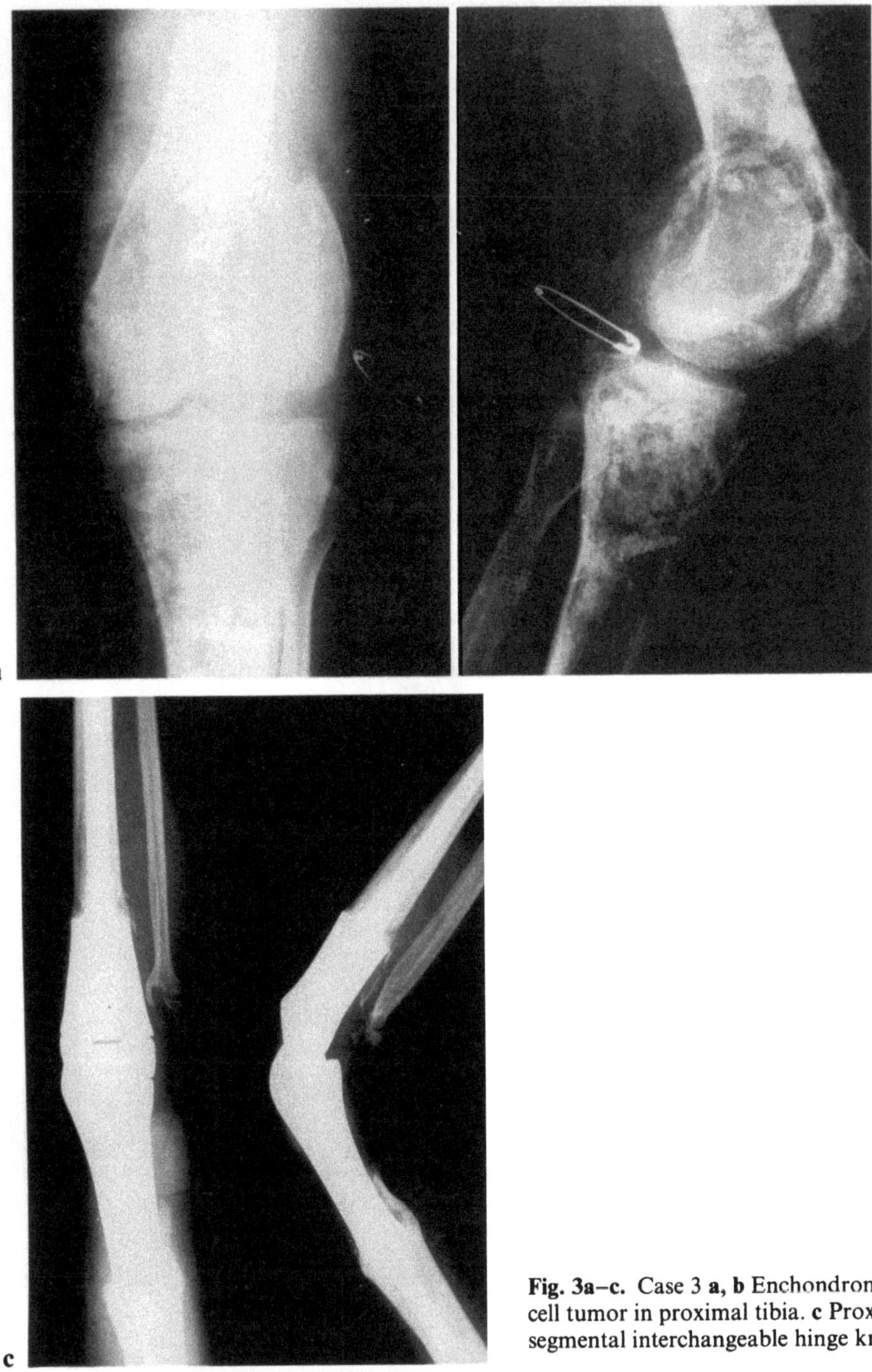

a b c

**Fig. 3a–c.** Case 3 **a, b** Enchondroma in distal femur and giant cell tumor in proximal tibia. **c** Proximal tibial and distal femoral segmental interchangeable hinge knee prosthesis

include thrombosis and thromboembolism, infection, hemorrhage, fracture, patellar tendon rupture, peroneal nerve injury, poor wound healing, component breakage, and tumor recurrence. These should be treated as in complications of total knee arthroplasty, except for tumor recurrence, which has to be widely excised again or amputated.

## Discussion

Replacement arthroplasty is best reserved for patients with total resectable lesions that are mostly benign and some malignant lesions when the patient refuses amputation.

Surgery for en bloc resection and prosthetic implantation can be done in one stage because the ready-made product can be chosen while planning the operation.

An important parameter in selecting a good functional prosthesis is the length of the segment resected. If a two-stage operation is scheduled, a temporary spacer made of methylmethacrylate incorporating a metal rod is an excellent method of maintaining the length of the limb and providing a good prosthetic bed.

Cemented fixation of the prosthesis is still the most important stabilization factor. To eliminate cement-bone loading, a rotating hinged knee prosthesis is used to replace the original fully constrained hinged knee prosthesis. The idea of bone ingrowth involving biological fixation in a segmental replacement has yet to be investigated.

## References


1. Wilson PD Lance EM (1965) Surgical reconstruction of the skeleton following segmental resection for bone tumor. J Bone Joint Surg 47-A: 1629–1656
2. Sih FH, Chao EYS (1979) Prosthetic replacement of the knee and a large segment of the femur and tibia. J Bone Joint Surg 61-A: 887-892
3. Burrows HJ, Wilson JN, Scales JT (1975) Excision of tumors of humerus and femur, with restoration by internal prostheses. J Bone Joint Surg 57-B: 148–159
4. Volz RE, Kloss J, Peltier LF (1980) The use of methylmethacrylate as a temporary spacer following en bloc resection of the distal femur. Clin Orthop 147: 185–187
5. Johnston JO et al. (1983) Limb salvage procedure for neoplasms about the knee by Spherocentric total knee arthroplasty and autogenous autoclaved bone graft. Clin Orthop 181: 137–145
6. Harrington KD et al. (1972) The use of methylmethacrylate as an adjunct in the internal fixation of malignant neoplastic fractures. J Bone Joint Surg 54-A: 1665–1676
7. Campanacci M, Costa P (1979) Total resection of distal femur and proximal tibia for bone tumors. J Bone Joint Surg 61-B: 445–463
8. Smith WS, Simon MA (1975) Segmental resection for chondrosarcoma. J Bone Joint Surg 57-A: 1097–1103
9. Enneking WF, Shirley PD (1977) Resection-arthrodesis for malignant and potentially malignant lesions about the knee Joint Surg 59-A: 223–235
10. Andersson G BJ Gaechten A, Galante JO Rostoker W (1978) Segmental replacement of long bone in baboons using a fiber titanium implant. J Bone Joint Surg 60-A: 31–40
11. Harrington KD, Sim FH, Enis JE, Johnston JO Dick HM, Gristina AG et al. (1976) Methylmethacrylate as an adjunct in internal fixation of pathological fractures. J Bone Joint Surg 58-A: 1047–1054

## *Discussion*

*Koshino* (Yokohama City University): At my university, the majority of giant cell tumors around the knee are treated by bone grafts. Only in a few cases, which involve very big tumors, do I use total knee replacement. What would be your comments to this?

*Cheng* (Taipei Medical College): In my country, many tumors are neglected or are recurrent cases involving subchondral bone. You can see in case 3, the articular surface is already decreased; in such a case, it would be difficult for a bone graft to improve the condition. In some giant cell tumors, if recurrence occurs or if the tumor is extensive, I prefer resection and replacement.

*Paul* (University of Strathclyde): In your surgical procedure do you undertake any myoplasty to preserve knee flexion or extension?

*Cheng*: No, because with giant cell tumors, we resect through muscle not through periosteum. Also, reconstruction of muscle to the prosthesis is very difficult. Patients with this kind of prosthesis can use the hip flexor and extensor and the hamstring to provide satisfactory compensation. The patients cannot do any violent motions in order to protect the joint.

*Goldie* (Karolinska Institute): I notice that most of your cases were giant cell tumors, would you advise your method for any type of tumor in the knee joint? Your case number 3 was a giant cell tumor which turned very malignant; was it truly a giant cell tumor? Do you use any cement with these prostheses?

*Cheng*: We use cement to fill the giant cell tumor if the tumor is not involved to the subchondral cortex. In my series, five patients had giant cell tumor and case 4 was enchondroma. I have also resected a proximal femur for hemangioma.

# Management of Problem Knees in Total Knee Replacement

D.K. BAE, S. LEE, and J.Y. AHN[1]

**Summary.** Eighty-six total knee replacements in 60 patients were performed during the period from August 1982 to August 1986. The first consecutive 43 knees in 30 patients were prospectively reviewed with a follow-up period of more than 2 years.

The average preoperative knee motion was 91°. The average postoperative knee motion improved to 110.2°. The improvements in pain and flexion contracture were significant. Hospital for Special Surgery knee scores improved from 39.5 to 87. Major complications included one deep infection and two knees with peroneal nerve palsy.

In total knee replacement, special considerations were needed for the management of problem knees. For successful results, management must be considered in relation to individual patients and specific prostheses.

The correct tightness in flexion was difficult to obtain after an extensive ligament release for the correction of severe deformity. In patients with severe flexion contracture and angular deformity, the posterior cruciate-sacrificing design seemed to be more useful, especially if bone cuts were needed before soft tissue release.

A patient who had severe knee range of motion restriction following total knee replacement was treated by the percutaneous release of adhesions under arthroscopic visualization. The source of pathology was intra-articular adhesion formation. Intra-articular release of adhesions under arthroscopic control was found to be very useful.

Late hematogenous infection that developed after total knee replacement with the Charcot knee was treated with debridement, suction drainage, and systemic antibiotics. In the Charcot knee with neurological dysfunction, posterior dislocation of the prosthesis developed about 7 months after infection. A brace was applied to prevent redislocation.

**Keywords:** Knee—Arthroplasty—Total replacement—Problems—Management

## Introudction

During the past decade, the design of total knee prostheses has undergone a continual evolution. The new generation of nonarticulating surface replacements, both cruciate retaining and cruciate sacrificing, have distinct design characteristics that are essential for correct usage. Whether cruciate-retaining prosthetic designs are better than cruciate-sacrificing designs has not yet been determined. Both concepts have theoretical advantages and disadvantages, but whether these are important in practical terms is not certain [7]. In knees with a lesser degree of deformity either design can be used according to the surgeon's preference and particular experience. There are some instances where cruciate retention is impossible and in these cases a cruciate-sacrificing design must be used. In patients with severe flexion contracture or angular deformity, we prefer to use the posterior cruciate-sacrificing design.

Surgical techniques must be considered in relation to individual patients and specific prostheses for successful results. The Insall-Burstein posterior stabilized prosthesis was designed to increase the range of motion and enhance anteroposterior stability [7, 8]. The Insall-Burstein constrained condylar knee provides added constraint over the posterior stabilized design. It also provides needed stability for patients who lack collateral ligaments or who cannot be stabilized by the usual soft tissue releases [7]. The cruciate-sacrificing designs were initally used routinely for all types of knees at our institution. Later, the cruciate-retaining design was employed to replace knees with lesser deformity and to preserve the posterior cruciate ligament.

After total knee replacement, restricted knee motion is a recognized complication [13]. Good range of motion is especially required from the view-point of the oriental life style, which requires the capability of squatting or sitting cross-legged.

## Materials and Methods

At Kyung Hee University Hospital, Seoul, Korea, 86 total knee replacements in 60 patients were performed during the period from August 1982 to

[1] Department of Orthopedic Surgery, Kyung Hee University Hospital, Seoul, Korea

August 1986. The first consecutive 43 knees in 30 patients were prospectively reviewed with a follow-up period of more than 2 years. The procedures were performed by the senior one of us (D.K.B.), and all patients were personally seen at follow-up. The maximum period of follow-up was 4 years and the average was 3 years. The average patient age at operation was 56.7 years (range, 26–75 years) and there were 27 woman and three men. The preoperative diagnosis was rheumatoid arthritis in 20 knees, osteoarthritis in 18 knees, post-traumatic arthritis in three, and other (including neuropathic arthropathy) in two.

Thirty-five posterior stabilized condylar prostheses, six Porous Coated Anatomic (PCA) knees, one Insall-Burstein constrained condylar knee, and one Guepar prosthesis were used in these patients.

Preoperatively, by radiographic measurement there were 22 knees with a varus deformity. The maximum varus deformity was 25°. Thirteen knees had a valgus deformity and the maximum valgus deformity was 18°. There were eight knees with neutral alignment. Thirty-two knees had a flexion contracture. The maximum flexion contracture that was corrected was 65°.

The surgical approach and the technique of knee replacement employed were as described by Insall [6] and Hungerford et al. [5]. Appropriate ligament and soft tissue releases were done before any bone cuts were performed except in one case where the knees had a flexion contracture of 65°. Perpendicular and parallel bone cuts to position the components accurately were performed using instruments. When using the PCA knee, we performed a 3° varus tibial cut to reproduce the mechanical axis and keep the joint parallel to the ground during stance.

Postoperatively, a Robert Jones bandage was used, sometimes reinforced with plaster splints when a flexion contracture was present before operation. Flexion was begun on the 2nd postoperative day. Walking with either crutches or a walker was started on about the 5th postoperative day. In this series, manipulation under anesthesia was not done. The Hospital for Special Surgery knee rating scale was used for patient evaluation. Using this rating, a score of 85–100 points represents an excellent result, 70–84 a good result, 60–69 fair, and less than 60 points poor.

We report three problem cases in this series where special management was required.

## Case Reports

### Case 1

The patient was a 47-year-old housewife with a history of rheumatoid arthritis since the age of 27 years. She was strictly confined to bed and wheelchair. The period of nonambulation was 11 years. The main complaint was pain and deformity which prohibited ambulation. The roentgenograms of both knee joints showed marked destruction and severe narrowing of the joint (Fig. 1). She had involvement of the upper extremities to lesser degrees. On examination, both knees revealed flexion contractures—about 65° on the right and 60° on the left. The patient had been treated with anti-inflammatory analgesics. Physical therapy and cast correction were done without improvement. Examination of the right knee revealed an 18° valgus deformity and flexion to 95°. The left knee had a 15° valgus deformity and further flexion to 80°. The hips had 30° flexion contracture bilaterally. There was severe muscle atrophy but muscle testing showed that she had good (grade II) knee flexor and fair (grade III) quadriceps strength bilaterally.

Both knees were operated on using a posterior stabilized condylar knee in each case. After the posterior femoral condyles were removed, the posterior capsular recess was recreated by stripping the capsule from the femoral condyle. A posterior capsulotomy was done from one side of the knee to the other. Because excision of the cruciate ligaments had already removed the central portion, the capsulotomy was mainly performed anterior to the two heads of gastrocnemius, which themselves were adherent and required division. The flexion gap was decided by resecting the posterior femoral condyles and posterior capsulotomy.

To correct valgus deformity, the lateral capsule, lateral ligament, popliteus tendon, and part of the lateral origin of the gastrocnemius were divided at their origin. But the use of instruments for making an extension gap was still impossible due to limited extension of the knee. We decided to resect part of the distal femur. In order to check the soft tissue balance and decide the exact amount of distal femoral resection using instruments, we temporarily resected part of the distal femur. The knee was then fully extended, but the space was still too narrow to insert the tensor. Positioning of the tensor after distraction of the joint revealed soft tissue imbalance. To correct the soft tissue imbalance and obtain more space (otherwise resection of the distal

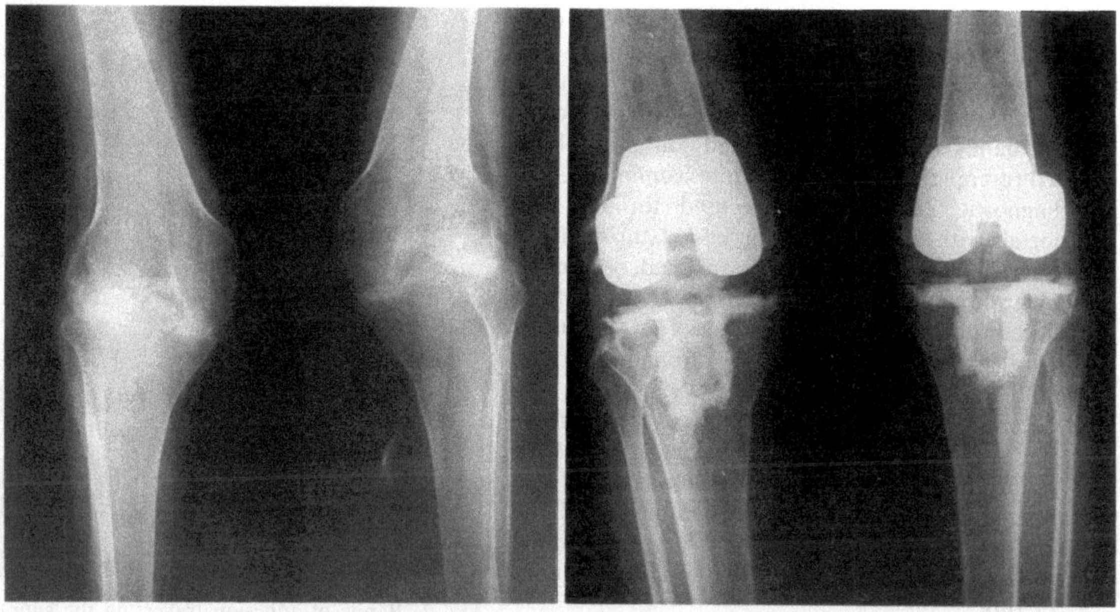

a b

**Fig. 1a, b.** Case 1. 47-year-old female patient with rheumatoid arthritis in both knees. Postoperative roentgenographic finding shows satisfactory alignment of the prostheses

femur would have violated the site of collateral ligament insertion), release was performed by stripping the soft tissues progressively from the medial upper tibia. The deep portion of the medial ligament was divided at the margin of the bone. An accurate extension gap was created by resecting the distal femur to the same amount as the flexion gap. The flexion gap was markedly increased with the lateral and medial soft tissue release. So, further resection of the distal femur was necessary for the thickness of the spacer chosen to fill the flexion gap.

The correct tightness in flexion was difficult to obtain after an extensive ligament release for the correction of severe deformity because of the limitation in distal femoral resection. It was necessary to check the flexion and extension gap frequently while performing total knee replacement in a patient with severe flexion contracture because of marked soft tissue contractures all around the knee joint, especially if bone cuts were needed before soft tissue release.

Post-operative X-rays showed a satisfactory position of each prosthesis with good alignment (Fig. 1).

**Case 2**

The patient was a 50-year-old woman with a history of rheumatoid arthritis. She had been non-ambulatory for 6 months due to severe knee pain. On examination, both knees revealed flexion contractures—about 20° on the right and 15° on the left. The right knee had further flexion to 120°, and left knee to 90°. One-stage bilateral total knee replacements were performed using a posterior stabilized condylar knee. The postoperative course was uneventful with marked improvement of pain and motion. Six months after surgery, the right knee had 130° of flexion but the left knee had a 20° flexion contracture and further flexion to only 25°.

The patient was treated by the percutaneous release of adhesion under arthroscopic visualization. The procedure was performed in an operating room under general anesthesia. After sterile preparation of the leg, the knee was manipulated without improvement of flexion. The knee joint was distended with normal saline, and the volume accepted was about 40 cm³. The sleeve for the diagnostic arthroscope and a blunt obturator were passed through an initial incision, which was lateral to the patellar tendon and a thumb's breadth above the tibial plateau, and brought beneath the patella and into the suprapatellar pouch. An attempt was made to move the sleeve and obturator across the suprapatellar pouch, into the gutters, and into both medial and lateral joint spaces, thereby rupturing some of the restrictive adhesions [13]

The diagnostic arthroscope was introduced, and the joint was inspected using a routine method.

After diagnostic evaluation, several methods were used to excise percutaneously or transect the bands of adhesions (Fig. 2). A pair of curved surgical scissors was used in a sweeping fashion to clear the bands from the pouch and gutters without arthroscopic visualization. More commonly, the diagnostic arthroscope was used through one portal, with a hook knife or basket through another, and the bands were transected or excised under direct vision. In addition, one of a variety of mechanized shaving devices was often helpful in removing debris and loose ends of bands from the joint.

Repeat manipulation followed the intra-articular debridement and the amount of passive flexion obtained under anesthesia was 125°. The interval between arthroscopic treatment and the final follow-up evaluation was 2 years. The final active knee flexion was 120° without flexion contracture.

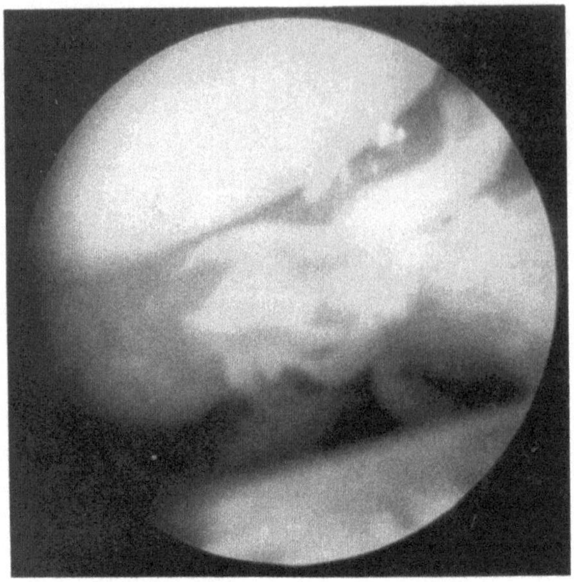

**Fig. 2.** Bands of adhesion traversing the suprapatellar pouch between the femoral and patellar components

### Case 3

The patient was a 66-year-old man with a history of syphilis and regarded as having a classical Charcot joint. The right knee joint in this patient revealed gross deformity and instability, with crepitus and effusion. On neurological examination, varying degrees of pain and proprioceptive dysfunction were noted. Laboratory evaluations such as serology tests were compatible with the neuropathic arthropathy caused by syphilis. An Insall-Burstein constrained condylar prosthesis was used due to marked collateral instability. Bone deficiency was tibial and, after making the tibial cut, a sloping defect was present in the medial tibia. The defect was corrected by a bone graft taken from the posterior femoral condyle (Fig. 3).

Histologically, hyperplastic synovium with bone and cartilage detritus was observed. Severe disorganization of the articular cartilage with invasion by a fibrous pannus was also seen. Significant amounts of hemosiderin-laden macrophages were noted in the synovium. Chronic inflammatory synovitis with patchy lymphocytic infiltrates was noted. The underlying joint capsule showed organizing fibrosis with a chronic inflammatory process and impacted bone chips.

Postoperatively, the result was excellent. The knee motion was 0°–135°. Walking was possible without support. Eighteen months after total knee replacement, an acute septic arthritis of the right knee developed. The deep infection followed a streptococcal sore throat. Subsequently, this organism was isolated from the joint. This was successfully treated by debridement, suction drains, and systemic antibiotics without removal of the prosthesis. The knee was immobilized with a cylinder cast for 8 weeks. Intravenous antibiotics were used for 4 weeks and oral antibiotics for another 3 months. After 8 weeks' immobilization, walking was gradually permitted using a cane.

Five months later, the patient came to the outpatient clinic with dislocation of the right knee (Fig. 4). The dislocation occurred while the patient was sitting cross-legged to do a new year's greeting that was a Korean traditional custom. Manual reduction was done immediately in the outpatient clinic without difficulty and the result was confirmed radiographically. A functional brace for controlling knee flexion was used to prevent dislocation with too much flexion. Ten months was insufficient to assess whether the infection was completely controlled. But during this period the patient had no signs of recurrent infection and could bend the right knee more than 90°.

## Results

In the 43 knees, the average preoperative score was 39.5 points and the average postoperative score was 87 points. Twenty-nine knees (67%) were rated excellent, 12 (28%) good, one (2.5%) fair, and one (2.5%) poor.

Prior to operation, there were eight nonambulatory patients. These patients currently walk

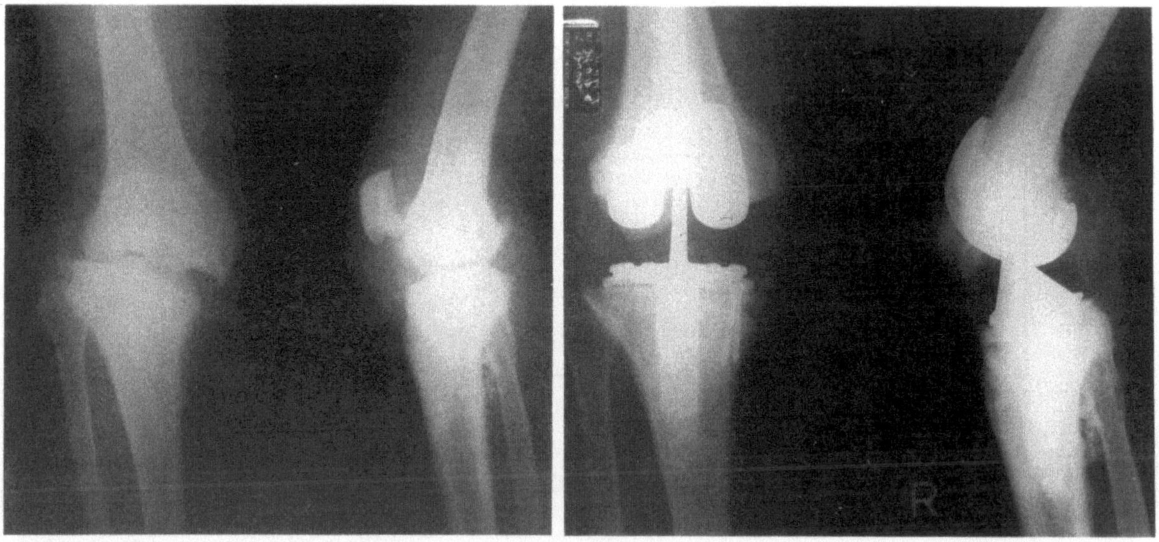

**Fig. 3a, b.** Gross deformity in Charcot knee joint secondary to ligamentous laxity and bone loss. Insall-Burstein constrained condylar prosthesis was used and the defect was filled with a graft obtained from the posterior femoral condyle

without support. Preoperatively, support was needed by ten patients and consisted of a cane in eight and crutches in two. These patients also could walk without support. Intensive postoperative rehabilitation programs were followed for one patient (case 1). Standing and walking were started when the patient was able to do straight leg raising. She was first allowed to walk using parallel bars with assistance and then gradually walked aided by walkers and crutches. At the follow-up, both knees had no flexion contractures. As to the range of motion, both knees revealed flexion to 95°. The results showed a significant improvement in function and rating was excellent. The patient was ambulatory and could walk an unlimited distance without support on final follow-up.

The average preoperative range of motion was 91° and the average postoperative range of motion was 110.2° (Fig. 5). The minimum flexion angle was 70° and the greatest flexion recorded was 140°. The improvement of flexion contracture was significant. Preoperatively, 32 knees (74%) had a flexion contracture. Postoperatively, only nine (knees 21%) had a flexion contracture. The average postoperative flexion contracture was 1.7° compared with a preoperative average of 20.1°. In the patient treated by percutaneous release of adhesion under arthroscopic control (case 2), the flexion had increased from 45° to 120° at the final evaluation, a 75° increase. There was no flexion contracture. The interval between the total knee replacement and arthroscopic adhesiolysis was 6 months. The follow-up interval was 2 years. There was no morbidity or complication, and the duration of hospitalization was brief.

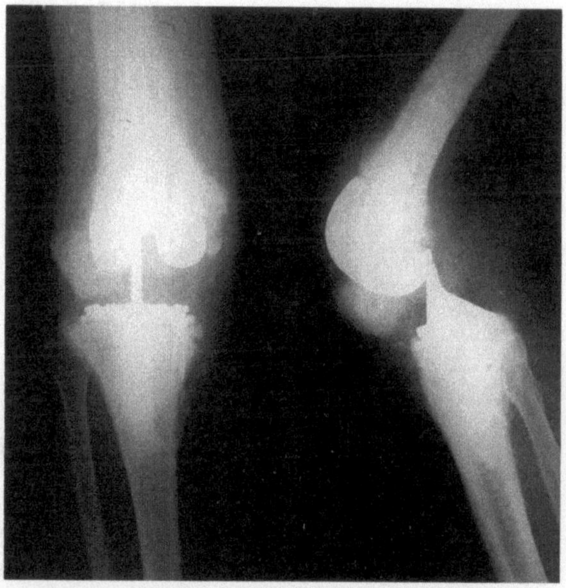

**Fig. 4.** Dislocation of the prosthesis occurred in this neuropathic patient after deep hematogenous infection

There was no case of confirmed or suspected loosening of a femoral or tibial component. Roentgenographically, an incomplete radiolucency was seen around the tibial component in two knees. The radiolucency was hairline or less than 1 mm at its widest point. In one knee with deep infection,

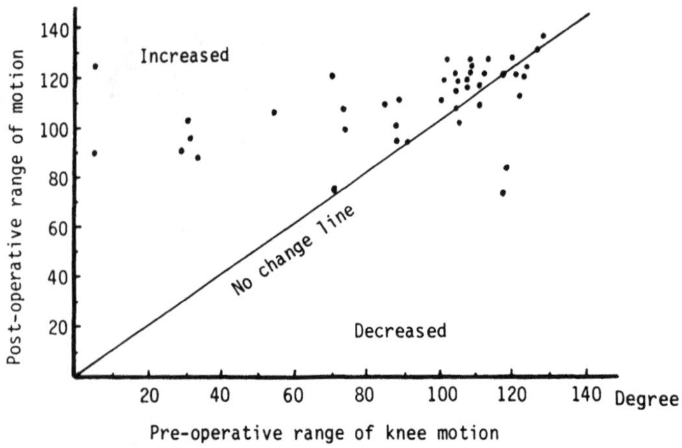


**Fig. 5.** Comparision of preoperative and postoperative range of knee motion

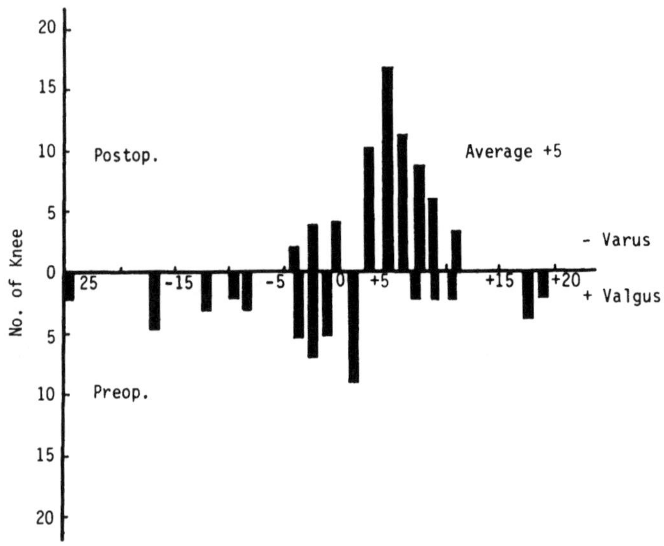


**Fig. 6.** Comparision of preoperative and postoperative tibio-femoral angle

an incomplete radiolucency around the tibial component measured 3 mm at its widest point.

Correction of varus or valgus deformity was attempted at operation. Preoperatively, the tibiofemoral angle was distributed between 25° varus and 18° valgus. Postoperatively, the tibiofemoral angle was in the range of 4° varus and 12° valgus and the average was 5° valgus (Fig. 6).

## Complications

There were three wound complications. Two knees had a spontaneously resolving wound hematoma. One knee had marginal skin necrosis with superficial inflammation. Physiotherapy was delayed until wound healing was complete in this case.

There was one deep infection which was diagnosed 18 months postoperatively. The organism that was isolated on culture was group G *Streptococcus*. Immediate joint debridement, leaving the prosthesis in situ, was performed with copious irrigation. After debridement, the wound was closed over suction drains. The range of motion and functional activity gradually increased until dislocation of the knee developed. A knee brace was applied to prevent redislocation of the prosthesis.

Peroneal nerve palsies occurred in one patient (case 1) and were associated with correction of fixed valgus deformities in both knees. The left knee showed recovery on the 3rd postoperative day, and the right knee at 6 months follow-up. The peroneal nerve should have been isolated and protected during the procedure in both knees.

## Discussion

The posterior stabilized condylar prosthesis was designed to permit excision of the cruciate ligaments and their excision affords easier correction of fixed deformities [8]. This prosthesis was initially used routinely for all types of knees at our hospital. Later, the PCA knee was employed to replace knees with lesser deformity. When using the PCA knee, we performed a 3° varus tibial cut to reproduce the mechanical axis. Hungerford believes that a prosthetic tilt will be present during standing and walking if a 3° varus is not cut into the tibia. Freeman, Insall, Ranawat, and others believe that the knee can be parallel to the floor in walking with a 90° axial cut. The mechanical axis has been shown to have a 3° varus angulation rather than be in a straight line [5]. The PCA knee system advocates the use of a 3° varus tilt cut to keep the joint parallel to the ground during stance. We tried to cut the tibia at 90° to the axis of the bone for all knee systems except the PCA.

There was a marked improvement in postoperative function when compared with preoperative knee rating scales. The average range of motion of the knees was 19.2° greater than the average preoperative knee motion. Femoral or tibial component loosening was not observed and radiolucencies, all incomplete, were observed only in two knees. Two knees required reoperation—one for infection and one for marked postoperative limitation of knee motion.

All patients were allowed to regain flexion without manipulation under anesthesia during the postoperative period [1]. We started flexion on the 2nd postoperative day if the wound was clear. At this time, we used to bend the knee once beyond 90° with active assistive or gentle passive flexion. We tried again on the 4th postoperative day if we could not bend the knee beyond 90°.

One patient who had severe knee range of motion restriction following total knee replacement was treated by the percutaneous release of adhesions under arthroscopic visualization. Restricted knee motion is a recognized complication of total knee replacement. It can usually result from intraarticular adhesion formation. When performed soon after the onset of motion limitation, vigorous physical therapy and, occasionally, manipulation of the knee with anesthesia may improve results [11]. When performed later, however, these have proven less useful. Furthermore, closed manipulation or vigorous passive attempts to gain motion may cause avulsion of the patellar tendon or fracture. The open procedure is extensive, carries considerable morbidity, and often requires initial immobilization followed by recurrent limitation of motion due to adhesion formation [10]. Using percutaneous arthroscopic means, the duration of hospitalization is brief and the morbidity is low. No immobilization is required and immediate range of motion exercises can be instituted.

In a patient with severe flexion contracture with valgus deformity, excessive ligament release was needed to overcome contracture and angular deformity. In addition, excessive tibial or distal femoral bone might be sacrificed during balance of the flexion and extension space. For optimal function with preservation of the posterior cruciate ligament, maintenance of the length of the medial collateral ligament and the posterior cruciate ligament to the anatomical joint line is critical [3]. Therefore, bone removal from the distal and posterior femoral condyles must not be much more than that replaced by the component. So, excessive tibial bone may be sacrificed with the potential for loosening of the prosthesis. For this reason, many surgeons believe this cut to be inviolate. Furthermore, femoral bone is twice as strong as tibial bone [2], so that one sacrifices less strength of bone when using the femur as the adjustment cut. In this patient, more distal femoral bone was removed than was replaced with metal, thus elevating the joint line. Elevation of the joint line by 1 cm or more is not detrimental if the cruciate is sacrificed [4].

If severe flexion contracture is present, a deeper cut will be required to allow the tibia to be brought to full extension. We made this cut on the distal femur rather than tibia. So we prefer to use a posterior cruciate-sacrificing design in a patient with severe flexion contracture or angular deformity.

Neuropathic knees can be treated by total joint arthroplasty if severe bone loss is corrected by either bone grafting or a custom-augmented prosthesis and if ligamentous balancing is adequately secured [12]. The orthopedic surgeon is usually confronted with this problem in its late stages, when preventive measures, such as bracing and protective weight-bearing, would not prove useful. In our case, the patient demonstrated severe knee instability secondary to ligamentous laxity and bone loss. Both cruciate ligaments were absent and collateral ligaments were markedly destroyed. Therefore, we used a constrained condylar knee and established bony alignment by resecting an adequate amount of bone and augmenting the remaining bony defects with bone grafts. The deep infection developed in this patient was treated by debridement, suction drains, and antibiotics because the patient did not agree to removal of the prosthesis. The result was suppression of the infection. The usual treatment of late deep infection is thorough debridement of the involved tissues and removal of the prosthetic components along with the acrylic cement [7]. The surgical salvage of an infected cemented knee arthroplasty presents a choice between arthrodesis and two-stage replacement arthroplasty. Long-term antibiotics very rarely eradicate deep infection in a cemented prosthesis; they may suppress symptoms and reduce discharge [9]. In our case, 10 months was insufficient to determine whether the infection had been controlled.

## References

1. Bae DK, Guhl JF, Keane SP (1983) Unicompartmental knee arthroplasty for single compartment disease. Clin Orthop 176: 233–238
2. Behrens JC, Walker PS, Shoji H (1974) Variations in strength and structures of cancellous bone at the knee. J Biomech 7: 201–207
3. Dorr LD, Boiardo RA (1986) Technical considerations in total knee arthroplasty. Clin Orthop 205: 5–11
4. Dorr LD, Yee L (1985) Preservation of the joint line in total knee arthroplasty. In: Dorr LD (ed) The knee. Papers of the First Scientific Meeting of the Knee Society. University Park Press, Baltimore, pp 75–82
5. Hungerford D, Krackow R, Kenna R (1983) Total knee arthroplasty: A comprehensive approach. Williams and Wilkins, New York
6. Insall JN (1981) Technique in total knee replacement. In: Instructional Course Lectures: The American Academy of Orthopedic Surgeons. Mosby, St Louis, pp 324–334
7. Insall JN (1984) Surgery of the knee. Churchill Livingstone, New York
8. Insall JN, Lachiewicz PF, Burstein AH (1982) The posterior stabilized condylar prosthesis: A modification of the total condylar design. J Bone Joint Surg 64-A: 1317–1323
9. Johnson DP, Bannister GC (1986) The outcome of infected arthroplasty of the knee. J Bone Joint Surg 68-B: 289–291
10. O'Connor RL (1977) Arthroscopy. Lippincott, Philadelphia, pp 14–22
11. O'Donoghue DH (1976) Treatment of injuries to athletes, 3rd edn. Saunders, Philadelphia
12. Soudry M, Binazzi R, Johanson NA, Bullough PG, Insall JN (1986) Total knee arthroplasty in Charcot and Charcot-like joints. Clin Orthop 208: 199–204
13. Sprague NF, O'Connor RL, Fox JM (1982) Arthroscopic treatment of postoperative knee fibroarthrosis. Clin Orthop 166: 165–172

## *Discussion*

*Koshino* (Yokohama City University): Of the many different types of total knee replacement, what is the type that you most prefer?

*Bae* (Kyung Hee University Hospital): As I said in conclusion, there is no one prosthesis that is suitable for all types of knees. Many factors are involved here.

*Koshino*: For flexion contracture in rheumatoid arthritis, do you carry out traction and casting before surgery? From your slide, it seemed that there was severe flexion contracture in surgery.

*Bae*: In severe flexion contracture of more than 40°–50°, usually the duration of contracture is important. If the contracture has persisted for many years, cast correction or traction is not helpful. In surgery, we have to release a lot of soft tissue contracture, otherwise it is difficult to straighten the knee.

*Bontemps* (Fabricius-Klinik Remscheid): Do you do any manipulations under anesthesia in the first 2–3 weeks after surgery so as to avoid subsequent arthroscopic management?

*Bae*: Immediately after surgery, I did not carry out any manipulations under anesthesia. The arthrolysis done in this patient was the only one in all my cases. I applied this technique to other knees with a limited range of motion, which showed greater firmness around the joint, or limited knee flexion contracture as a result of synovectomy or other causes.

*Yamamoto* (Matsuyama Red Cross Hospital): In dealing with rheumatoid arthritis, we have to avoid muscle release as much as possible and so preoperative management of flexion contracture of the knee joint is very important. So with a case of flexion contracture in 40° of flexion, we usually apply traction for 1 month continuously or use physiotherapy in combination with very slight anesthesia.

*Bae*: I think flexion contracture is best managed by preoperative skeletal traction or physiotherapy. However, more important is, I feel, motivating the patient toward rehabilitation and here preoperative training plays a big role.

*Ranawat* (Cornell University Medical College): We have done 12–15 total knee replacements with Charcot joints. We thought initially that the results were quite good, and they are good in at least half the cases at 5-year follow-up. We are reviewing this at present and will soon publish a report. However, a large number of patients do have problems with loosening and disengagement; sepsis has not been a problem in our experience with this device any more than with other devices. Unless there are better alternatives, I feel that this device should be approached with caution. I think that preoperatively the patient must understand the position with total knee replacement and be aware of the risk of loosening and other mechanical problems; he needs to be aware that a long leg brace should be used to maintain alignment and stability to the insensitive joint. If the patient is not in agreement with this, I do not think that we should undertake the replacement.

With respect to tuberculosis, if the disease has been treated and controlled for at least 18 months to 2 years, it is reasonable to consider such an option for replacing the joint. Following these criteria, I have done total knee replacements in two patients who had tuberculosis; the follow-up has been 2 and 5 years and both patients have remained symptom-free with respect to recurrence of the disease. There is also a report in the literature about cup-arthroplasty of the hip from a group in Iowa and they used similar indications.

# Ten-Year Follow-Up Results of St. Georg Knee Prosthesis Systems 2400 Sledges and Hinges

K. HEINERT and E. ENGELBRECHT[1]

**Summary.** A retrospective study of the St. Georg knee prosthesis systems was completed at the end of 1986. A total of 2467 knee implants inserted from 1970 to 1979 were reviewed at a minimum of 8 years and a maximum of 16 years after operation. The St. Georg prosthesis systems comprise two different types of knee replacement, a nonconstrained surface replacement and a total hinge prosthesis of the first and second generation type. Using actuarial methods, the probability of the prosthesis remaining in situ was calculated for 547 medial compartmental, 98 lateral, and 648 bicompartmental knee replacements. The results with the sledge prosthesis were compared with those of 254 St. Georg first generation hinge prostheses and 910 St. Georg second generation hinge prostheses.

Serious complications such as infection, loosening, and fracture of the components were regarded as significant determinants for the evaluation of the durability of partial and total knee replacements. The highest and lowest incidence of typical long-term complications was recorded and analyzed with respect to age, diagnosis, and the surgeon's personal experience with the method. Significant differences in the indication for a sledge or a total hinge were determined by group assessment (log-rank test).

Unlike the general trend to use semiconstrained knee replacements, the results of this clinical trial induced us to improve our hitherto used hinged knee model rather than to develop a new surface replacement. The new total knee replacement, ENDO-model, a rotating hinge, has been used since 1980 in more than one thousand cases and the results are presented.

**Keywords:** Knee joint replacement—Sledges—Hinges—Follow-up—Complications

## Introduction

It is well known among surgeons that Walldius in Sweden [21] carried out the first knee arthroplasty in 1951. Shiers in England [18] used an uncemented stainless steel hinge in 1953 [7].

Charnley's idea of low friction arthroplasty was followed by the Canadians Gunston and McKenzie [9] in 1968, who developed a cemented knee arthroplasty with polyethylene and metal bearings.

One year later in 1969, Buchholz and Engelbrecht started at the St. Georg Hospital in Hamburg, Germany a large homogeneous series of total hinge replacement based on the "low-friction" principles. Parallel to this, Engelbrecht [2] developed in 1969 the resurfacing system well known as the sledge endoprosthesis St. Georg.

The aim of knee replacement is the relief of pain, restoration of stability, and improvement of functional movement, in most cases with correction of deformity. Our present problem is to ensure that these advantages remain permanent throughout the entire postoperative period. Some hundred modifications of knee arthroplasties now in use worldwide have been classified according to their main constructional principles, degree of freedom, and type of joint stabilization [4, 5]: (a) Unconstrained surface replacements with minimal built-in restraint; (b) partially constrained surface replacements with different incongruency of the articulating surfaces; (c) total hinge systems with axial rotation; (d) total hinge systems only allowing flexion and extension.

In the order given above, the degree of freedom decreases as the extent of joint stability increases. The major requirements of construction are widest imitation of physiological kinematics, tribology, and the safety of the construction. Just as in orthopedic surgery, the true value of operative treatment only becomes apparent under normal weight-bearing conditions revealing technical and operative errors only after a long postoperative interval.

The implantation of hinge prostheses has been considered with special reservation, particularly by the Anglo-American orthopedic community, as it has been believed that the functional results of hinges are unsatisfactory and that failures are more likely to occur than with resurfacing systems. We know from hip replacement that the evaluation period for artificial joints should be at least 10 years for the number of failures to be assessed cor-

[1] Endo-Klinik, Hamburg, Federal Republic of Germany

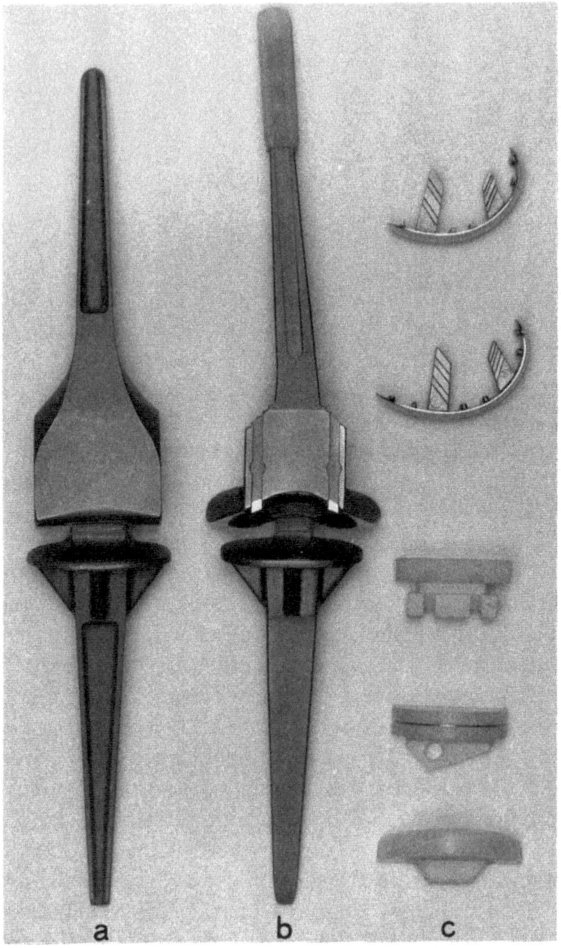


**Fig. 1a–c.** Georg knee prosthesis sytems. **a** First generation hinge. **b** Second generation hinge. **c** Sledge

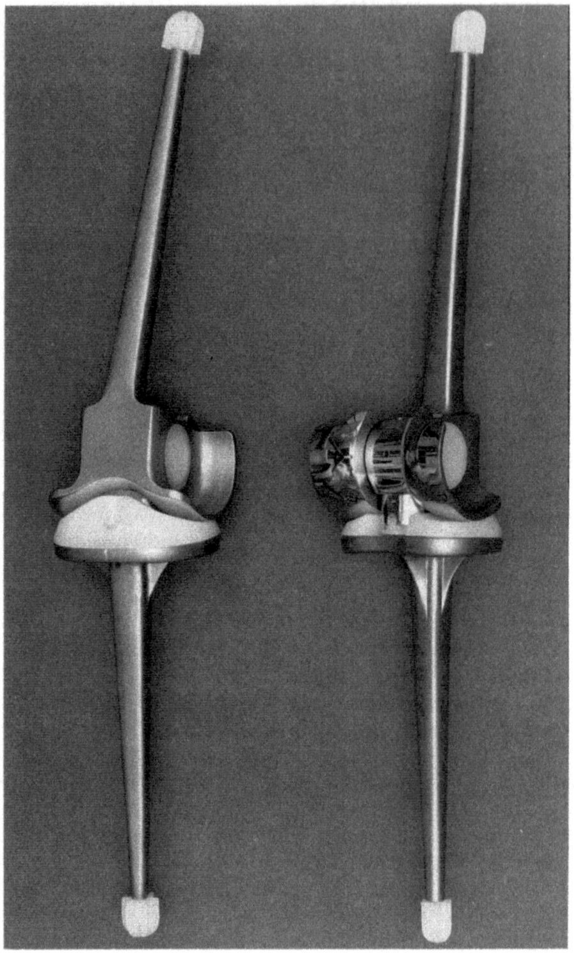

**Fig. 2.** Hinge with tibial rotation-ENDO model

rectly. Only now at the beginning of the third decade of artificial joint surgery are we confronted with unsuccessful cases resulting from inadequate operative experience and inappropriate hip prostheses from the early years [12]. For this reason, we must clearly divide technical possibilities from intuitive belief in order to avoid over-hasty judgements.

The main problems of knee prostheses are somewhat different from those of hip prostheses. Whereas with hip prostheses the dynamics of a ball joint are easier to imitate and the problem of forces is the primary issue, the knee prosthesis must imitate the complicated kinematics of the joint in a limited space. Moreover, at the present time, the only materials available have inadequate strength characteristics. The St. Georg sledge model is the system with the largest number of degrees of freedom. The capsular ligamentous system and the muscles are responsible exclusively for joint stabilization (Fig. 1).

In contrast to this, the St. Georg hinge model has just one degree of freedom, only allowing extension and flexion, but the design guarantees immediate joint stabilization (Fig. 1). (The manufacturer of the prostheses is Fa. Waldemar Link, Hamburg, Federal Republic of Germany.) According to the quoted classification criteria and characteristics, these two systems represent extremes and it is particulary interesting to note how these constructions have fared over a period of time.

The purpose of the present report is to provide a more valid and predictive analysis of our long-term follow-up data by using survivorship analysis and patient-time diagrams after 10 years in daily use. Our experience and confrontation with complications led to the development of a new system called the rotatory hinge "ENDO" (Fig. 2). This is also the name of our specialist clinic in Hamburg.

## Material and Methods

A total of 2446 consecutive St. Georg knee prostheses were inserted between 1970 and 1979 at the St. Georg Hospital and since 1976 at the Endo-Klinik in Hamburg. There were 548 medial sledges, 97 lateral sledges, and 649 bicondylar sledges. Parallel to this, 236 St. Georg total hinges of the first generation and 916 total hinges of the second generation were also implanted. After completion of follow-up in December 1986, there was no further contact after operation in 210 cases. The remaining 2236 knees were available for clinical and radiographic evaluation in 47% being sledges and 53% being total hinges.

Of the patients receiving a total hinge prosthesis, 62% suffered from osteoarthritis, 30% from rheumatoid arthritis, and 6% from post-traumatic diseases, and 2% from other causes. In the sledge group, 68% had osteoarthritis, 18% rheumatoid arthritis, and 13% post-traumatic disease, while 1% were afflicted with another disease. The patients were aged between 19 and 91 years at the time of operation, the median was 67 years (Fig. 3). The techniques used for implantation have been published [2, 3]. All the prostheses were fixed with gentamicin Palacos, which is an antibiotic-loaded acrylic cement. The same guidelines for operative techniques were followed by a small group of surgeons without significant staff changes. Thus, these series may be considered as homogeneous with respect to operative technique, the prosthesis system, and experience with implantation. Until 1979 the design of the sledge was less changed in the tibial compartment (Fig. 1). Since 1981, the second generation of sledges called the "ENDO" system has been under clinical trial.

The first generation St. Georg hinge was changed in 1975. The intracondylar part was narrowed in the second generation. The stems were given a valgus shape with lateral supporting wings. Since 1981, the Endo model, an intramedullary system with tibial rotation, has been in clinical use,—to date in approximately 1200 cases.

We think that the results of the patient assessment, such as the ability to walk, flexion arc deformity, and ability to climb stairs and get out of a chair, are preoperative parameters for the indication for operation. These clinical parameters can only be compared immediately after the operation with the preoperative situation. This type of evaluation, with the so-called knee scores, is only useful in describing the postoperative success for one patient in comparison to his individual later evaluation, perhaps with his other knee. We would now like to discuss long-term problems and possible system-related failures which come to light after long-term daily use. Therefore, we think that clinical signs should not be mixed with X-ray findings in a long-term result statement in one score system.

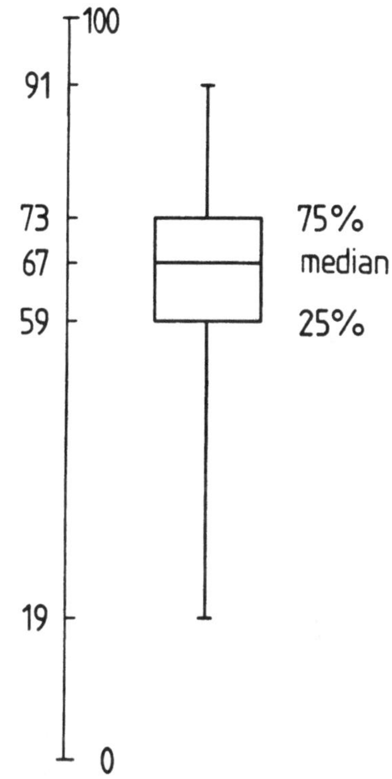


**Fig. 3.** Age of patients (all knees); box plot

For our long-term analysis, the prostheses were considered to have failed only when the implants were removed or scheduled to be removed at the next following opportunity. Patients with asymptomatic failures, so far as known, were treated as pending failures (1%–2%). Systematically and analogous to the definition of failure after total hip arthroplasty [12], we used the definition failure when the decision was made to intervene surgically. The main causes of revision after resurfacing prostheses were: *deep infection, aseptic loosening of the tibial and/or femoral component, fracture of the metal runner, tibial subluxation because of ligamentous deficiency*, and, if these are excluded, *persistent residual pain* because of malposition, multiple or unknown causes.

In arthroplasty analysis, the prognostic factor "time" must be included for final assessment. Since 1979, we have generally used the Kaplan-Meier or Cutler-Ederer estimates [11, 22] as statistical methods, taking such effects into account.

Those actuarial methods, graphically plotted as survival curves [17], are increasingly reported by orthopedic authors in cooperation with a statistics specialist. The date of the latest review was recorded together with the definition of failure or success in relation to the date of surgery. Thus, the length of follow-up for each arthroplasty was determined by the end of survey, the patient's death, or when he was lost to follow-up or the date of revision. The cumulative survival rate was estimated by successive multiplication of the annual values. It is important to realise that survival curves give a realistic picture when a large number of cases is available with approximately 10%–20% rate of failure and a minimum follow-up of 10 years. In smaller series with a shorter follow-up period, the results are misleading with a worse contribution of failure due to the evaluation criteria. At the beginning of a special series, there will in most instances be a smaller number of cases. Ten years later these "beginners" will be reduced by death and patients lost to follow-up, and very often by typical beginner's failures. So, sometimes failures were estimated more pessimistically and the recorded failure rates remain unrealistic. Further, it should be considered that it is not the primary aim of a clinical trial to specify a particular failure rate. A better aim is to identify risk groups by comparing different groups of subjects treated by the same method. In total joint arthroplasty, the surgeon is often successful when parameters such as diagnosis, age, and surgical experience are measured using one prosthetic system. Alternatively, different prosthetic principles can be compared within the same group of diagnosis, age, and the surgeon's personal experience.

With the survival techniques and life tables, the effects which are to be measured can be clearly seen in certain groups. Overlapping effects can easily be identified by regression analysis, e.g., using the method of Cox [1]. For example, it is important that an age effect exists independently of a diagnosis effect if a younger age-group is represented with certain basic illnesses (dysplasia in younger patients). All other estimates suffer from overlapping effects and no final conclusions can be drawn. In many studies, often multicentre evaluations, the result of all the efforts was that only the number of implantations performed could be reported. So, in real terms, this means that the method of follow-up was investigated and not the prosthesis with its problems.

## Results

Here, the failure rates which occurred over a 10-year period are presented comparing our different constructions of the St. Georg sledge and hinge knee prostheses with survival curves (Tables 1, 2). The patient-time diagrams (Figs. 4–7) show in detail the different types of failure for each system. This type of presentation is the first step to understanding survival curves because each failure can be seen in the year when it occurred.

In the right-angled triangle (Fig. 7) with two equal sides, the year of implantation is given on the hypotenuse. On the bottom, the year of failure is given. The vertical side shows the postoperative years. Thus, the date can be marked exactly when failure after implantation occurred. For example, if implantation was in July 1977, the midpoint of 1977 should be located at the hypotenuse and a horizontal line down through it. The revision, for example, was in March 1985, so a vertical line is drawn through a point one quarter of the way along the space for the year 1985. From the point where these two lines meet a diagonal line, parallel to the hypotenuse, is drawn upwards to cross the right axis shows that revision was performed 8 years after surgery. So we can see at the marked points at which time postoperatively how many revisions or failures had occurred and which would be the typical "failure times."

### Lateral Sledge

A total of 97 cases were implanted from 1970 to 1979. There was follow-up information from 88 prostheses. Deep infection occurred in one case (0.88%) and there was loosening, mostly of the tibial component in five cases (5.7%). Half of the loosenings occurred within 3 years postoperation; only one occurred 10 years later. Subluxation with ligamentous deficiency and persistent residual pain predominantly occurred during the first 5 years. One metal runner fractured 8 years later. In nine cases (10%), arthrosis of the medial condyles led to further operation. This was not regarded as a complication in our estimates: Four cases occurred within the first 4 years. Altogether, 13 cases of aseptic failure were found in 88 cases.

### Medial Sledge

A total of 547 medial sledges were implanted from 1970 to 1979; follow-up information from at least 505 sledges was available in 1986 (Table 1). No deep infection was observed, aseptic loosening

**Table 1.** Aspetic failures after St. Georg sledge replacement (1970–1979); end of follow up 1986

| Sledge | *n* | Mechanical loosening | | Lig. deficiency with tibial subluxation | | Fracture of fem. runner | | Persist. resid. pain and/or malposition | | *n* | Percent |
|---|---|---|---|---|---|---|---|---|---|---|---|
| | | *n* | Percent | *n* | Percent | *n* | Percent | *n* | Percent | | |
| Medial | 505 | 21 | 4.2 | 21 | 4.2 | 10 | 1.9 | 10 | 1.9 | 62 | 12.3 |
| Lateral | 88 | 5 | 5.7 | 5 | 5.7 | 1 | 1.2 | 2 | 2.3 | 13 | 14.8 |
| Bi-condylar | 612 | 20 | 3.3 | 35 | 5.7 | 9 | 1.5 | 20 | 3.3 | 84 | 13.7 |
| Total | 1205 | 46 | 3.8 | 61 | 5.0 | 20 | 1.7 | 32 | 2.7 | 159 | 13.2 |

**Table 2.** Aseptic failures after St. Georg total hinge (1970–1979); end of follow up 1986

| Complications | St. Georg Hinge 1st generation (*n* = 211) | St. Georg Hinge 2nd generation (*n* = 824) | Total (*n* = 1035) |
|---|---|---|---|
| Mechanical loosening | | | |
| Femoral | 6 } | 9 } | |
| Tibial | 3 } 11 (5.2%) | 1 } 17 (2.1%) | 28 (2.7%) |
| Both | 2 } | 7 } | |
| Fracture of femur | 5 (2.4%) | 3 (0.4%) | 8 (0.7%) |
| Fracture of prosthesis | — | 2 (0.2%) | 2 (0.2%) |
| Persistent residual pain and/or malposition | 3 (1.4%) | 3 (0.4%) | 6 (0.6%) |
| | | | 44 (4.2%) |

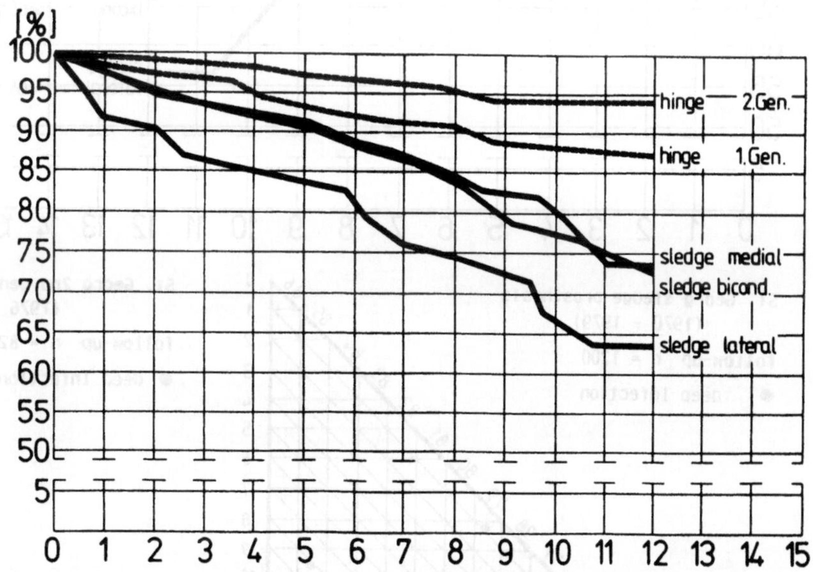


**Fig. 4.** Survival curves of St. Georg knee types (aseptic failures)

occurred 17 times in the tibial component, three times in the femoral component, both components became loose in only one case. It is obvious that in the earlier implantation years until 1975 this complication occurred at an early stage; from 1976 on, there was a longer postoperative interval.

There were ten fractures of the femoral component which occurred after the implantation years of 1975–1978. It is assumed that a special implantation technique that was previously used led to this type of failure. We do not believe that failure was due to material breakdown. Persistent residual

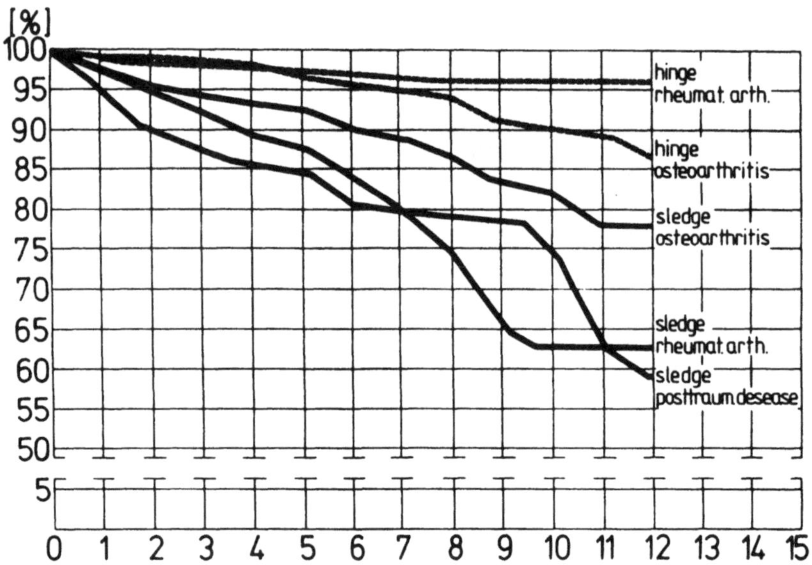


**Fig. 5.** Comparison of sledge and hinge with respect to diagnosis (aseptic failures, survival curves)

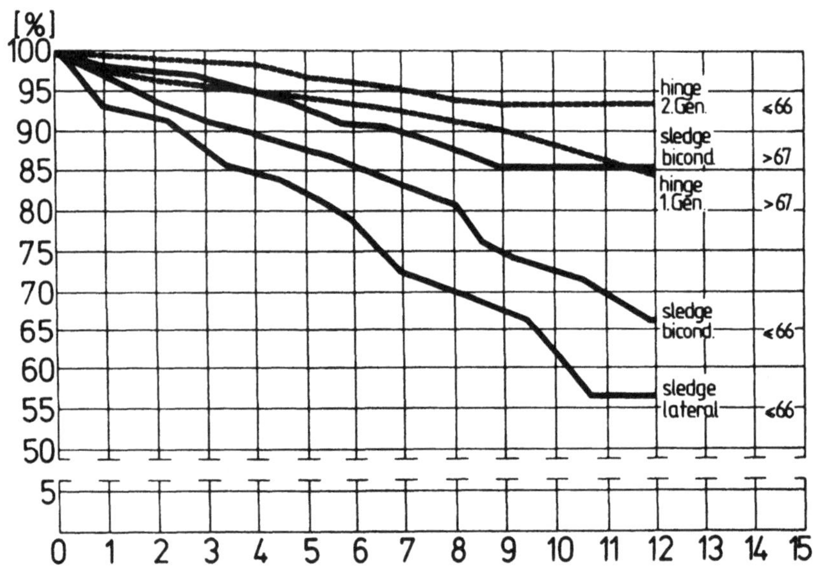


**Fig. 6.** Comparison of sledge and hinge with respect to age of patients (aseptic failures, survival curves)

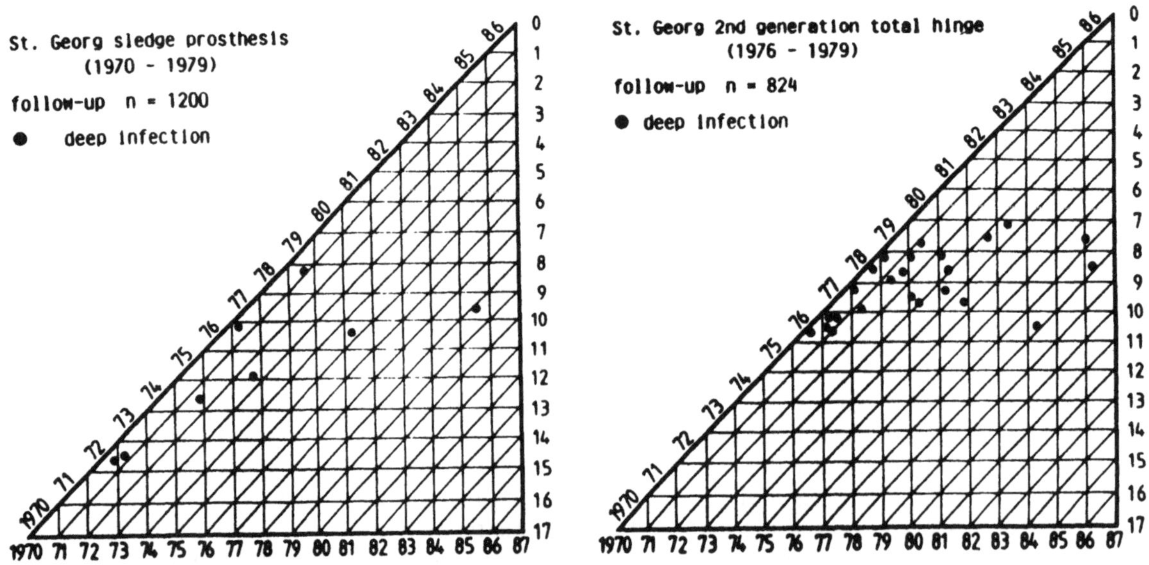


**Fig. 7.** Deep infection after sledge and hinge (patient-time diagram)

pain and/or displacement of the component was observed in ten cases, distributed over the immediate postoperative years.

Ligamentous deficiency with tibial subluxation was a major problem and occurred in 21 cases. Half of these cases occurred within 5 years after operation. Lateral arthrosis was only seen in eight cases. Altogether, 62 aseptic complications led to revision in 505 cases.

### Bicondylar Sledge

A total of 649 bicondylar sledges were implanted from 1970 to 1979. Follow-up information was calculated for 612 prostheses in 1986. We found eight deep infections, nearly all within the first 3 years after operation. Mechanical loosening of components was more frequently seen on the tibial side. This was a typical long-term complication because two-thirds of the cases occurred later than 5 years postoperation. In addition to mechanical loosening, fracture of the femoral runners was observed. Those failures were seen only during the implantation period 1975–1978, not in later years. In contrast to mechanical failure with loosening or fracture, persistent residual pain and/or malposition led to revision in 20 cases within the first 3–4 years postoperation as an example of a typical earlier complication. Ligamentous deficiency with tibial subluxation was seen during the entire follow-up period in 35 of 612 cases and is regarded as the main problem in sledge procedures.

### First Generation St. Georg Total Hinge

This type of total knee prosthesis was implanted from 1970 to 1975 in 237 cases (Table 2). Follow-up information could be used 16 years later in 1986 for 211 prostheses. Fracture at the top of the prosthetic stem occurred five times. Two revisions were required for malposition in the early years. Eleven revisions were due to loosening, mainly of the femoral component. No revision was later than 9 years postoperation, which means that with this type of prosthesis a typical mechanical long-term failure did not occur.

### Second Generation St. Georg Total Hinge

This is the most frequently used type of prosthesis and has been implanted since 1976 (Table 2). Until 1979, there were 912 prostheses implanted. Follow-up information verified 24 cases of infection at the end of the study in December 1986. This rate of 2.9% over 10 years was rather high infection. Most of those deep infections manifested within the first 3 years after surgery but were also seen even 8–9 years later. Fracture at the proximal end of the prosthesis occurred in three cases. There was malposition and/or persistent residual pain in three cases, almost all of which were revised within 2 years after first implantation. Two fractures of the condylar wings were seen 7–8 years postoperation. Mechanical loosening was seen in 17 cases, which means a very low long-term failure rate of 2.1%. In most cases, the femoral component was loose. We had only one case of isolated loosening of the tibial component.

### Prosthetic Survival with Respect to type of Prosthesis

The recorded cumulative survival rates for aseptic failure of hinges and sledges are listed for the main diagnosis and the age of the patient in Fig. 5, 6. Failure for the sledges in this analysis was defined as: (a) Ligamentous deficiency with tibial subluxation; (b) aseptic loosening of the femoral and/or tibial component; (c) fracture of the femoral runners; (d) persistent residual pain and/or malposition. Failure for the hinge model prosthesis was defined as: (a) Aseptic loosening of the femoral and/or tibial component; (b) femur or material fracture; (c) malposition with residual pain.

Within a 12-year follow-up, the postoperation survival curves are different for the hinges and sledges. Because of the small numbers, it is not appropriate to plot a period longer than 12 years (also available in the life tables within our computer lists). The log-rank and Wilcoxen-rank tests [15] show a statistical difference ($P = 0.001$). The best results were recorded for the second generation St. Georg hinge prosthesis, while the worst results were seen in the lateral sledge (Fig. 4).

### Rheumatoid Arthritis

The best results for rheumatoid arthritis were recorded when a hinged model was used (Fig. 5). In early, medium, or late follow-up intervals, a higher failure rate was seen when the patients were treated with a sledge prosthesis. The same curve refers to a group of patients with post-traumatic disease. The difference in the curves was significant ($P = 0.001$; log-rank test).

### Age

According to the median age of the patients, given by the box plot (Fig. 3), two age-groups were formed—below and above 67 years at the time of operation. The cumulative survival rates showed the best results for the older patients treated with a total hinge and the highest failure rate for the sledge model when used for the younger age-group. The difference was statistically significant ($P = 0.001$). (Fig. 6).

### Deep Infection

Comparison of the infection rate for sledges and hinges with respect to diagnosis showed the highest failure rate for rheumatoid arthritis (3.5%) and post-traumatic diseases (6.8%) (Fig. 7). This complication mainly occurred in the first 3 postoperative years but was also found some years later. In the sledge prosthesis, deep infection was only seen in patients with the preceding diagnoses, but it was never seen in the main group with idiopathic osteoarthritis.

## Discussion

The statistical model used above in the evaluation takes into account the long-term follow-up problems after total joint replacement. For a comparison of results after total hip replacement, the life-table technique or survivorship method is now established. The problem in knee arthroplasty is, which uniform definition of failure should be used. Particularly in knee arthroplasty, we have seen during the last decade that each principle, design, and construction of artificial joints produces a special type of failure at different times. Some failures occurred early, some started later, and some were equally distributed over the entire follow-up period. Nevertheless we can compare some cumulative success rates at 5 years from publications in English and German. Tew and Waugh reported 78% of the prostheses to be in situ in various knee types in 1982 [19]. Grimer et al. (1984) reported 85% good results with the Stanmore knee after 5 years [8]. Lettin et al. calculated in 1984 a 87% success rate with the Stanmore type [14]. Thacker and Fulford reported in 1986 over 95% good results with a Denham knee [20]. Knutson et al. [13] reported a nationwide study of knee arthroplasty in Sweden (1986) and found a probability of survival ranging from 65% for hinged prostheses to 90% for medial compartmental prostheses after a follow-up period of 5 years. Two- and more compartmental prostheses produced intermediate results of 87% survival. For rheumatoid arthritis, they reported significantly worse results. With the Blauth hinge a success rate of 95% was reported [10]. Our earlier results with the present series [16] gave a cumulative success rate of 80%–96% at 5 years, varying according to the type of prosthesis, diagnosis, and age of the patient.

Fortunately, the first impression after completion of this study (December 1986) was that we had fewer complications than assumed at the beginning of the knee prosthesis era. In contrast, our long-term results after total hip replacement were less satisfactory because of the rising number of aseptic loosenings, particularly of the cup in the later follow-up years (cumulative survival probability of 70% 15 years postoperation [12].

After a 10-year follow-up period, we had a low rate of deep infection (0.7%) for the sledge prosthesis. The infection rates for the total hinge were 4.3% and 2.9% for the first and second generations, respectively. The reason for this could be seen in the early implant models which had a higher amount of bone resection and exposure of the joint with restriction of nutrition, ("locus minoris resistentiae"). The number of patients with rheumatoid arthritis in the knee arthroplasty series is very much higher than in the series with hip replacement; further there was a higher number of rheumatoid arthrosis patients treated with hinge replacements than with sledges. The deep infection mainly occurred in these groups of patients and in post-traumatic diseases. It is well known that such patients form the main risk groups with respect to deep infection and the loss of bone stock in artificial joint arthroplasy.

In the resurfacing type of prosthesis, e.g., St. Georg sledge, there were three main complication groups: (a) *Mechanical loosening* sometimes with fracture of the metal runner which appeared late in the follow-up and was, therefore, regarded as a late complication. (b) *Persistent residual pain and/or malposition* which was seen much earlier within the first 2 or 3 postoperative years. Mechanical loosenings represent one third of possible failures, while persistent residual pain accounts for 20% of all failures seen in the sledge prostheses. (c) A third main group for failure of the sledge contains patients with *ligamentous deficiency with tibial subluxation*. This type of complication was found early, late, and in medium-term follow-ups. The analysis of complications has shown that the various causes are frequently mixed together and often it is difficult to demonstrate the originating cause retrospectively; thus, mechanical loosenings can be caused by technical or indication errors, for instance, and can also result in mechanical damage.

Analysis of the high number of failures of metal

runners of the femur revealed poor implantation techniques with less contact to the femoral condyle, especially within the posterior part of the runner. It is obvious that the fractured sledges were implanted within the special period from 1975 to 1978. Before and after, no biomechanical problems of the preceding type were seen. Ligamentous deficiency was predominantly found in the bicondylar sledge prosthesis. This was regarded as a typical false indication for the sledge model. Secondary deficiency by overstressing the ligaments may occur within 5 years postoperation or later. The reason for this is newly developing ligamentous deficiency due to progression of rheumatoid arthritis and increasing age of the patient; insufficient damping properties of the implant material currently used are also involved.

We saw a high number of cases of persistent residual pain and/or malposition in all three types of sledge variation. After revision with a hinge, a better success rate was obtained immediately for nearly all cases. In this group, we found avoidable failures, such as false indication and technical errors.

The first generation of the St. Georg hinge type was last implanted in 1975, i.e., more than 12 years ago. The evaluation is only of statistical and historical interest because this series was the first step in developing the larger series with the hinge type model and was, thus, the beginning of systematical development.

The second generation St. Georg hinge model has been used since 1975. Analysis of this second generation type shows that it is a very successful model because of its extremely low complication rate of 2.1% for mechanical loosening after a long-term follow-up period of more than 10 years. It should be borne in mind that these results must be seen in the light of the situation when the first steps were made in hip and knee arthroplasty. Nearly all orthopedic surgeons expected a greater number of complications with worse functional results, more than after hip arthroplasty.

Ten years later, the results were reversed: Total hip arthroplasty achieved worse results than knees with respect to mechanical problems.

## Conclusions and Tibial Rotating Knee "Endo" Model

Despite good results with hinge systems, the senior author (E.E.) started a further development of the hinge type 10 years ago. This model, like the others, derived its name from our clinic. In 1981, a larger series was started with more than 1200 operations to date. The clinical experience with both types of St. Georg model, sledge and hinge, cover an extreme sample when the degrees of freedom and joint stability are taken as the major criteria. Comprehensive tests of measurement, prospective clinical trials and analysis of failures have influenced the decision to develop more and more the total replacement of the knee with minor resection of bone and the incorporation of tibial rotation (Fig. 2). The preliminary report on the very low complication rate will be published later. There is no doubt that the fully constrained St. Georg hinge model affords predictably good results, but evaluation has shown that two serious biomechanical complications occur—mechanical failure and fracture of the femur. We conclude that the relatively high complication rate of the sledge model compared with the hinge (Fig. 8) must be attri-

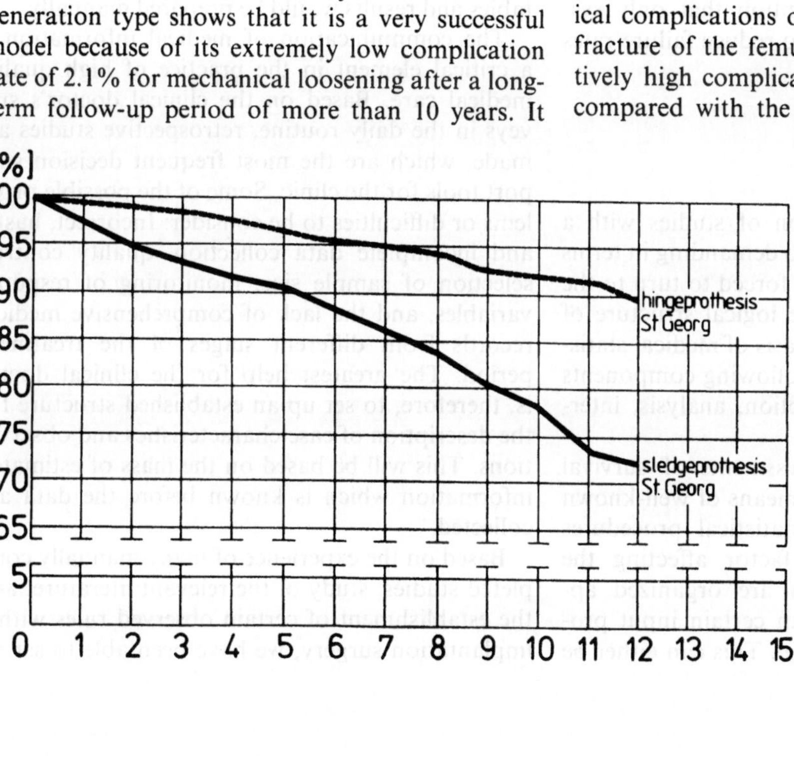


**Fig. 8.** Comprehensive survival curves of St. Georg knee endoprostheses systems after a long-term follow-up

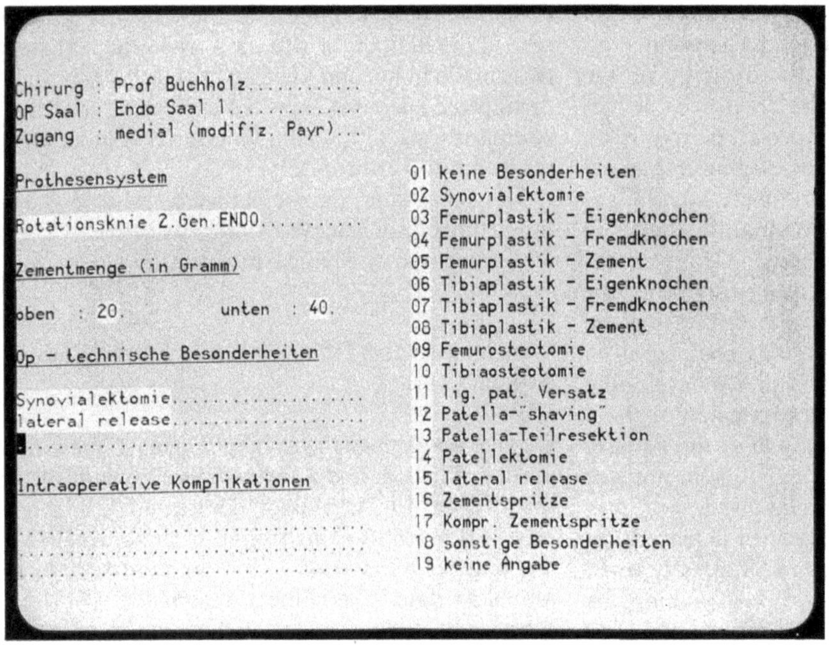


**Fig. 9.** Operation mask of the data-base KNUDS

buted to false assessment of ligaments which are changed to the same pathological extent as the resurfaced bone. The indication for sledge models has been increasingly restricted to unicompartmental lateral or medial replacements with competent ligaments in addition to a specialized and well-trained operative surgeon. With a new construction and modification of the tibial component and metal bearing, we hope that we have solved the mechanical problems of the tibial parts. We think it is important to mention that only systematic evaluation will help to reduce failure rates in the future.

## Appendix: Data Collection

The planning and completion of studies with a large number of test cases is so demanding in terms of work and time that we are forced to turn to the computer for assistance. The logical structure of all systems which forms the basis of medical statistics can be divided into the following components [12]—data collection, description, analysis, interpretation, and presentation.

The above-mentioned assessments of survival analysis were carried out by means of well-known and easy-to-use computer statistical procedures [17]. The most important factor affecting the assessment is that the data are organized appropriately, for example, with certain input programmes or basic study design. This can either be carried out by documentation assistance, working on specific computer-orientated projects or, ideally, by an internal data-collection system set up by the clinic. This would contain crucial data, often referring to cases occurring at different times and in different places, vital for conclusions which can be stored permanently in the memory and consulted at any time. Previously, these data have always had to be extracted laboriously from patients' records, following which assessment tables and results would be prepared manually.

The communication of medical information is a critical element in the practice of high quality medical care. Based on the clinical doctor's surveys in the daily routine, retrospective studies are made, which are the most frequent decision support tools for the clinic. Some of the possible problems or difficulties to be consider: Incorrect, hasty, and incomplete data collection, quality control, selection of sample size, monitoring of response variables, and the lack of comprehensive medical records from different stages of the treatment period. The greatest help for the clinical doctor is, therefore, to set up an established structure for the description of case characteristics and observations. This will be based on the mass of estimated information which is known before the data are collected.

Based on the experience of many manually completed studies, study of the relevant literature, and the establishment of certain observed rules within implantation surgery, we have been able to set up

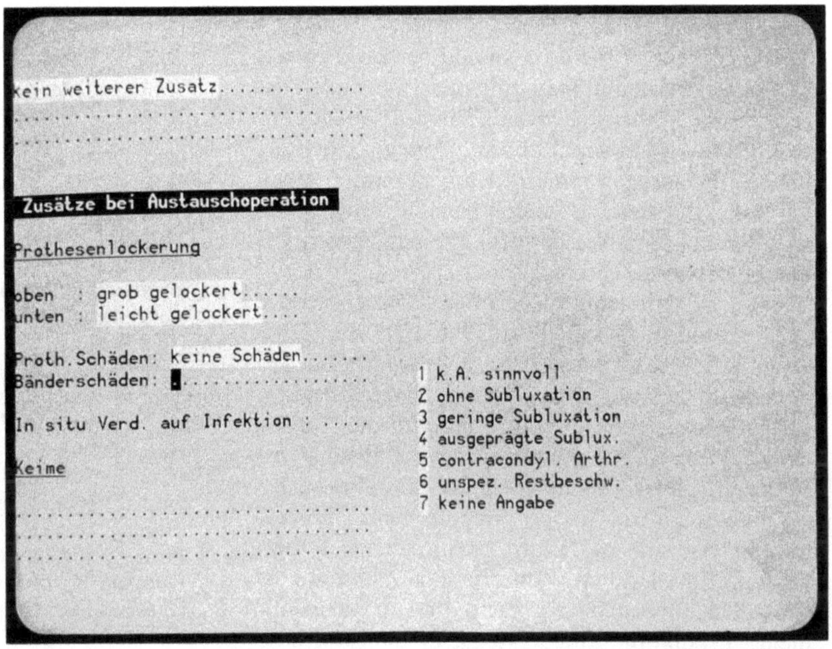


**Fig. 10.** Operation mask (revision) of the data-base KNUDS

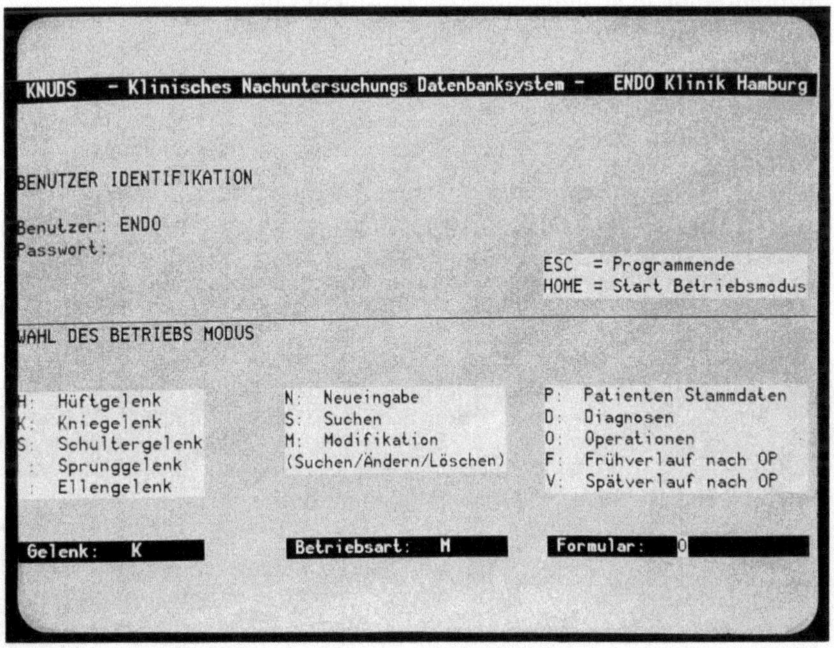


**Fig. 11.** Menu mask of the data-base KNUDS

and scale such characteristics according to size and intensity (Fig. 9).

Data management can occur in written form, whereby incomplete corrections, illegibility, and the loss of slips of paper can be significant disadvantages. Should the decision be made to move from paper to the computer terminal, the major factor to consider is to what extent the data appearing on the screen are able to describe statistical models. If these are comprehensive and disjunct, then it is simple to compose a suitable series of statistical questions for the examined data. It is also important that the data given in the user dialogue refer to the clinical location providing the information, namely the operating theatre and the examination room (Fig. 10). In this way, the disadvantages of a retrospective observation can be reduced as the data are permanently available and can be corrected or expanded at need.

The content of the data should be based on actual observation and may only in certain tested exceptions be knowledge-based. The permanent control of the system should become part of the daily task of the surgeon himself. Care should be taken to make the data as uncomplicated and "user-friendly" as possible, both for the person compiling the data-base and the user.

The base data from this examination series have been stored from 1970 to 1986 and the post-examination results added to these mean that this data-base can act as a central data collection system and be connected directly with the statistical package. Input processing and statistical results with analysis are followed via EDP (Fig. 11).

Quality control in joint replacement surgery, i.e., an estimate of failure rates, can, therefore, be reproduced at any time with a minimum of time. The time and cost factor for the development, installation, and servicing of the data base must be seen against this. As a result the degree of naturalization of an implanted joint prosthesis can be established at any time with effective use of a computer.

## References


1. Cox DR (1972) Regressions models and life tables. J Royal Statistical Society B-34: 187–220
2. Engelbrecht E (1971) Die Schlittenprothese, eine Teilprothese bei Zerstörung im Kniegelenk. Der Chirurg 42: 510
3. Engelbrecht E, Siegel A, Röttger J, Buchholz HW (1976) Statistics of total knee replacement: Partial und total knee replacement, Design St. Georg. Clin Orthop 120: 54–64
4. Engelbrecht E, Nieder E, Strickle E, Keller A (1981) Intracondyläre Kniegelenksendoprothese mit Rotationsmöglichkeit. Chirurg 42: 368–375
5. Engelbrecht E (1984) Die Rotationsendoprothese des Kniegelenks. Springer, Berlin Heidelberg New York
6. Ewald FC, Jacobs MA, Miegel RE, Walker PS, Poss R, Sledge CIB (1984) Kinematic total knee replacement. J Bone Joint Surg 66-A: 1032–1040
7. Freeman MAR, Levack B (1986) British contribution to knee arthroplasty. Clin Ortho No 210: 69–77
8. Grimer RJ, Karpinski MRK, Edwards AN (1984) The long-term results of stanmore total knee replacements. J Bone Joint Surg 66-B: 55-63
9. Gunston FH, Mackenzie RI (1976) Complications of the polycentric knee arthroplasty. Clin Orthop 11: 120
10. Hassenpflug J, Blauth W (1987) Langzeitergebnisse mit der Blauth-Knieprothese. In: Primär-und Revisionsalloarthoplastik. Springer Berlin Heidelberg New York
11. Heinert K (1982) Langzeitergebnisse von Hüftendoprothesen nach einer durchschnittlichen Verlaufszeit von mehr als 10 Jahren. Dissertation, Hamburg
12. Heinert K (1987) Computergesteuerte Langzeitauswertungen zementierter Hüftendoprothesen. In: Primär- und Revisionsalloarthroplastik. Springer Berlin Heidelberg New York, pp. 93–102
13. Knutson K, Lindstrand A, Lidgren L (1986) Survival of knee arthroplasties. J Bone Joint Surg 68-B: 795–803
14. Lettin AWF, Kavanagh TG, Craig D, Scales JT (1984) Assessment of the survival and the clinical results of tanmore total knee replacements. J Bone Joint Surg 66-B: 355–361
15. Peto R, Pike MC, Armitage P, Breslow NW, Cox DR, Howard SV, Mantel N, McPherson K, Peto J, Smith PG (1976/1977) Design and analysis of randomized clinical trials requiring prolonged observation: II. Analysis and examples. Br J Cancer 35: 1–37
16. Röttger J, Heinert K (1984) Die Knieendoprothesensysteme St. Georg (Schlitten—und Scharnierprinzip). Z Orthop 122: 818–826
17. SAS (1980) Statistical analysis. SAS Institute, North Carolina
18. Shiers GP (1954) Arthroplasty of the knee-Preliminary report of a new method. J Bone Joint Surg 36: 553
19. Tew M, Waugh W (1982) Estimating the survival time of knee replacements. J Bone Joint Surg 64-B: 579–582
20. Thacker C, Fulford P (1986) Assessment of the Denham knee replacement. J Bone Joint Surg: 600–607
21. Walldius B (1957) Arthoplasty of the knee using an endoprothesis. Acta Orthopaed Scand Suppl: 24
22. Weinstein MC, Fineberg HV (1980) Clinical decision analysis. Saunders, London

## *Discussion*

*Hashino* (Tokyo University): Current trends are now toward systems without hinges; why do you still want to use hinges? Secondly, your results with hinges are better than those with the older style hinges, e.g., GUEPAR, Shiers; why is this?

*Heinert* (Endo-Klinik): Perhaps this is due to the biomechanical construction and, above all, to the experience of the surgeon. We know from hip replacement that the experience of the surgeon is one of the most important factors in the success of arthroplasty.

*Hashino*: But, in principle, your design is a hinge. What is the difference between your design and previous designs?

*Engelbrecht* (Endo-Klinik): We know that the main problems with all-metal hinges were high infection rates, high rates of metallosis, the necessity of extensive bone resection, and bad conditions for the patellofemoral joint. We have improved this with our St. Georg design: Almost the whole prosthesis is covered by bone and most of the patellofemoral joint is preserved.

*Hoshino*: What do you think about the excessive stress?

*Engelbrecht*: We are aware of this, but you have seen the results. It is a very strong design with long stems and the forces acting on the knee can be distributed over a broad area.

# Panel Discussion

*Ranawat* (Cornell University Medical College): Dr. Iseki, could you tell us what the important advantages and disadvantages of your design are?

*Iseki* (Keio University): Our basic concept is to be as close to the normal anatomy as possible, i.e., we have to create three freedoms. We cut the anterior and posterior cruciate ligaments because in the replacement with the artificial joint these ligaments lose their function anyway. We also remove the meniscus. We keep resection of bone and cartilage to a minimum so as to maintain freedom as far as possible and have a semiconstrained knee.

The disadvantages are, as I mentioned at the end of my presentation, with regard to complications, i.e., we can change the surface but the biomechanical weak points become evident on the tibial side. Thus, we find tibial loosening, fracture of the tibia in osteoarthritic patients, loosening to a high degree in patients with rheumatoid arthritis, and infection is also seen. However, this is not limited to our joint but is common to all prostheses.

*Ranawat*: Dr. Cheng, at our center, we carry out a lot of local bone resection for bone tumors and in reply to Dr. Goldie's question we use bone resection for other bone tumor indications including osteosarcoma. Our experience is that there is a very high incidence of loosening, breakage, and fracture after 5 years and more. Perhaps your good results may be due to the fact that the patients were very light in terms of body weight. Do you have any other explanation?

*Cheng* (Taipei Medical College): What you say is correct. In the treatment of bone tumor, bioreplacement is only one possibility. Some tumors, e.g., osteogenic sarcoma, should be amputated. In less malignant tumors, such as osteogenesis of the periosteum and condylar sarcoma, if the patient does not agree to amputation, bioreplacement is an option. In benign regions of malignant tumors, if the tumor extends to the joint and the joint cannot be preserved, replacement can be performed instead of reconstruction arthrodesis.

*Ranawat*: Dr. Heinert, you presented a series today of survivorship with a hinge design. The typical problems with the hinge design were recorded by you, i.e., infection, loosening, fractures proximal to the stem. Do you think that the incidence of loosening and infection will rise with time or have we reached a plateau such that these results will not alter so much with time? Second, do you have any data on osteoarthritic patients with unilateral disease who are under 60 years of age?

*Heinert* (Endo-Klinik): I think that since we now observe the problems associated with the hinge type, we have now reached the plateau of a 94% rate after 12 years postoperation. We do not expect many more complications of a mechanical kind. We have much more experience with hip replacement and here we saw the reverse pattern: After 10 years there were many cases of loosening.

With respect to the age of the patients, I was only able to present five curves and so I took those of the older patients, but there was no statistically significant difference between patients older and younger than 67 years.

*Ranawat*: Dr. Bae, you raised the question of how to handle flexion contracture. How would Drs. Goldie and Hastings manage a patient with fixed flexion contracture of 45°?

*Goldie* (Karolinska Institute): I have gone through three phases. The first phase was only lateral release, posterior capsulotomy, and resection of the biceps tendon. Doing this combined with resection of the lateral collateral ligament, usually flexion contracture was released such that the knees could be extended to between −5° and −10°, which postoperatively was further relieved by physiotherapy. The patients were sutured only in their skin, and the soft tissues which had been sectioned were allowed to heal. The patients were put into plaster for 4 weeks and after that given physiotherapy. After 8 weeks, the patients were all stable. After 5 years, they retained their full extension, but for some reason they lost their flexion: Initially flexion was over 100°, but now it was down to 90°.

The second phase I went through was doing the same type of soft tissue release with simultaneous replacement. I then used a hinge prosthesis (Waldius). However, from the contractility of rheumatoid tissues and the stability of the joint following the healing of these tissues, I found in time that it was not necessary to have a hinge prosthesis. So there then followed the third phase, which involves the same kind of release, but in those patients in whom there is the necessity for joint replacement I use a nonconstrainted prosthesis (ICLH) and so far I have had no reason to alter this policy.

*Hastings* (Wellesley Hospital): My experience has been very much different. Faced with a rheumatoid patient with a severe knee flexion deformity, the first thing I would do would be to assess the hip flexion deformity and I would reduce this. I would agree with Dr. Yamamoto (Matsuyama Red Cross Hospital) that there is some place for physiotherapy and traction to a degree to reduce the flexion deformity. With a rheumatoid patient with a 60° flexion deformity and normal hips, it may be possible to reduce the deformity to about 30°. However, I think that the most important cause of a fixed flexion deformity, whether in rheumatoid arthritis or osteoarthritis, is probably a bony block to extension anteriorly, and there is a certain point beyond which this cannot be dealt with any further.

Removal of that bony block intraoperatively will often give an extra 20° of extension, thus reducing the extension block from 45° to 25° or 20°, which can usually be handled intraoperatively with further release of posterior capsular structures.

*Ranawat*: If posterior capsulotomy is carried out as you describe, including the posterior cruciate ligament, a disparity in stability in flexion and extension results. The knee is tighter in extension and looser in flexion. The tibia falls away from the femur. How do handle that?

*Hastings*: I am not sure that I have experienced that problem. I perform posterior release last. I do not think that removing the bony block anteriorly upsets the ligament balance in any way. Why is there any ligament imbalance in a rheumatoid patient? The problem really is bone loss and there should be relative ligament laxity. So it should be possible to distend the ligaments without causing this imbalance in flexion and extension.

*Goldie*: Yes I would agree with that, except I would say that any patient who has acquired a flexion contracture of 45° is beyond physiotherapy. If flexion contracture of the knee joint has led to flexion contracture of the hip, I would prefer doing the knee first to avoid difficulties in postoperative mobilization. Though there is much controversy here.

*Krackow* (John Hopkins University): Flexion contraction is one of the most difficult problems to deal with. With severe flexion contracture, we favor first physiotherapy and serial casting; this may not help some patients at all and some patients may be helped by 10°, 20°, or 30°, and so we feel it is worth trying. At that point, if we are still left with a flexion contracture of 35°–50°, I will perform a posterior soft tissue release done through two separate longitudinal posteromedial and posterolateral incisions so that there is no difficulty closing the skin, there is access to the hamstring tendons on both side, there is easy access to the posterior capsule and to the gastrocnemius heads, there is no worry about the popliteal vessels, and protection is provided to the peroneal nerve. It may even be necessary to enter the front of the knee joint to remove soft tissue and synovium, trim bone, and permit the tibia to come around forward on the femur, as I believe Dr. Hastings referred to. I would follow all of this again with serial casting. Similarly, I think that in most of these cases the femoral attachments of the ligaments should be such that with capsular, muscular, and tendinous release, one should still be able to obtain a ligament position so that the knee has reasonable stability in flexion versus extension. When all has been accomplished, the final management at surgery frequently represents a compromise by removing a small piece of additional bone from the distal aspect of the femur, which permits the tibia to come toward full extension; theoretically, this would invite laxity in flexion, but in fact this laxity is not so problematic because of the maintenance of the posterior femoral condyles.

*Goodfellow* (Oxford University): I have found that it is almost never necessary to perform a posterior capsulotomy in rheumatoid disease. Nor is it ever wise, I believe, to apply traction or serial casting prior to the operation because if you do you are trying to straighten out a joint whose articular surfaces do not move properly and the result is ruptures of the posterior capsule and other ligaments as well. My practice has been with deformities of up to 40°, and sometimes more, simply to perform appropriate replacement of the articular surfaces in the most physiological way I can. It is then acceptable to allow the patient to leave the operating table with 45° of flexion deformity, because traction can then be applied postoperatively, having rid the knee of the causes of the flexion deformity. The posterior capsule will stretch. The posterior capsule can shorten and lengthen in a very remarkable way. So with a flexion deformity of up to 45° that is due to rheumatoid disease and has not been present for several years, it will straighten out very fast if the corrective forces are applied after the arthroplasty and not before.

*Ranawat*: I do not use traction or serial casts. I carry out alteration at the time of surgery and I do it from the inside-out, not from the outside-in. I will release the posterior capsule and I can expose the posterior femur about 2 in from the inside. If at that time I do not do a full correction I will cut more femur. If there still remains slight flexion contracture I accept this. I then make two longitudinal incisions and do a tenotomy of both sides, thereby removing the deforming force to the knee and creating more extension. The posterior capsule is then in continuity with the periosteum to some degree. I have corrected up to 45°–50° using this method and there is a disparity in extension and flexion, at least in my hands, which I correct by Total Condylar III or some surgeons would use a Posterior Stabilizer.

Until such time as there is concensus as to the best way to handle this problem, each individual surgeon has to choose the method that suits him best.

We heard from Dr. Bae that he treated one case with suppressive antibiotics. How many of the panelists believe that they can suppress infection indefinitely by intravenous or oral antibiotics?

*Heinert* (Endo-Klinik): There are three possibilities for deep infection I think: There is antibiotic-loaded acrylic cement (4–5 g in each 20-g powder pack), postoperative treatment for several weeks, and strong perioperative treatment.

I think that suppression is possible in a big hematoma, but if it reaches the prosthesis the latter must be removed.

*Bae* (Kyung Hee University Hospital): In the case of late deep infection, I do not think that treatment with debridement and antibiotics is definitely curative; only temporary suppression can be achieved. However, in acute deep infections, antibiotic suppression may succeed in some cases.

*Cheng*: The rate of infection usually increases with the time in the hinge knee prosthesis. The success in my series may be due to the fact that the patients are careful to protect their knee joints from minor traumas.

*Iseki*: There are more cases of infection in rheumatoid arthritis than in osteoarthritis. Five or six years after implantation, there are often infections. Loosening can result from these infections; if the condition becomes severe, the prosthesis should be removed. In particular, if the hinge is quite large, a large defect can result. We try to minimize surgery, but if we detect a late infection we have to remove it for the irrigation. After this, we can consider antibiotic treatment.

*Ranawat*: I personally do not think we can eliminate or suppress an infection indefinitely if it has reached the interface. If it is only in the joint, which is hard to assess, there is a very small chance of success. But, by and large, suppression of the established infection at the interface is a failure in the long run. The treatment of choice is, therefore, removal, control of sepsis, then reimplantation with or without cement antibiotics and intravenous drugs.

# Part 3
# Cementless Total Knee Replacement I

# Arthrodesis of the Knee as a Salvage Procedure for Failed Total Knee Replacement

M. Kurosaka,[1] K. Hirohata,[1] and A.H. Wilde[2]

**Summary.** From 1973 to 1982, 30 patients underwent arthrodesis following failed total knee replacement at the Cleveland Clinic Foundation and Kobe University Hospital. The indication for arthrodesis was infection in 27, severe instability due to trauma in one, aseptic loosening of the prosthesis in one, and breakage of the prosthesis in one. Fusion was successful in 21 knees (70%). Analysis of the factors which may influence the result of arthrodesis indicated that hinge prostheses, postoperative infection, obesity, and previous skeletal surgery on the same knee increased the risk of nonunion. Although the surgical methods of fusion did not seem to influence the fusion rate in our study, adequate surgical technique with rigid fixation is essential in obtaining successful fusion.

**Keywords:** Arthrodesis—Total knee replacement—Hinge prosthesis

## Introduction

Improved design and instrumentation of total knee replacement have decreased the failure rate and increased the indications for this type of surgery. However, despite the success of total knee replacement, certain problems persist such as infection, loosening, instability, and breakage of the components. Although many failed procedures can be salvaged by the revision of a total replacement, in irrecoverably failed total knee replacement, arthrodesis may represent the best solution. In this report, we describe briefly our current approach toward the failed total knee replacement and discuss the results of arthrodesis following failed total knee replacement. We will analyze the predominant factors which have influenced the results of arthrodesis.

[1] Department of Orthopaedic Surgery, Kobe University School of Medicine, Kobe, Japan
[2] Department of Orthopaedic Surgery, The Cleveland Clinic Foundation, Cleveland, USA

## Management of Failed Total Knee Replacement

With regard to the failure of total knee replacement, mechanical causes of failure due to poor prosthetic design and poor alignment are becoming less frequent with the current generation of prostheses and improved instrumentation. In the majority of such cases, reimplantation surgery is possible. The major complication independent of prosthesis design and patient selection is infection, which occurs in 1%–2% of the knees [14]. In acutely infected total knee arthroplasty, with the exception of patients having an inadequate systemic and local defense mechanism, the success rate of early surgical debridement is reported to be reasonably high [14]; our approach is, therefore, early debridement with extensive administration of intravenous antibiotics and retention of the prosthesis. In the case of Gram-positive chronic, indolent infection, surgical debridement alone is not likely to succeed in salvaging a prosthesis in the majority of cases. Our current approach is prosthetic removal with extensive debridement followed by intravenous antibiotics. As to the timing of reimplantation, we prefer to reinsert a prosthesis once evidence of sepsis has resolved rather than proceed to immediate reimplantation. Gram-negative infections are more difficult to control and require high doses of toxic antibiotics. In such a case, reimplantation of a new prosthesis still appears to be a viable technique in the carefully selected patient; however, if a patient cannot tolerate the medication or the organism does not respond to antibiotics, primary arthrodesis is the treatment of choice (Fig. 1). In the case of a failed total knee replacement, the orthopedic surgeon must make a decision as to whether to proceed with a relatively safe arthrodesis or to perform revision arthroplasty and thereby jeopardize the chances of success of any subsequent arthrodesis.

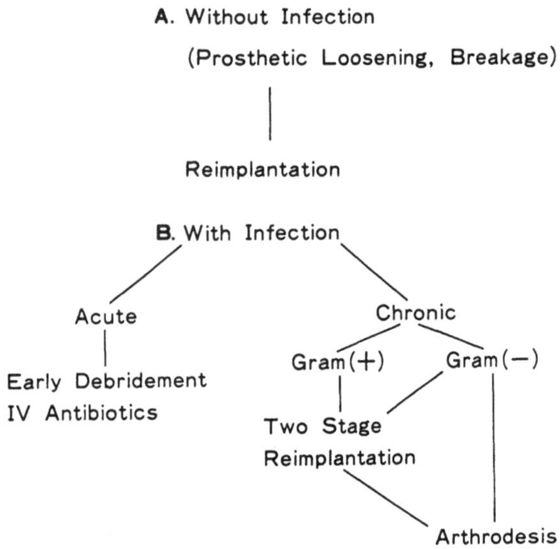


**Fig. 1.** Management of cases of failed total knee replacement

**Table 1.** Results of arthrodesis

| | Cases | Union | Nonunion |
|---|---|---|---|
| Following failed TKR | 30 | 21 (70%) | 9 |
| Without previous TKR | 28 | 26 (93%) | 2 |

*TKR*; total knee replacement

**Table 2.** Successful fusion rate in relation to primary disease

| | Cases | Union | Nonunion |
|---|---|---|---|
| Osteoarthritis | 16 | 12 (75%) | 4 |
| Rheumatoid arthritis | 13 | 9 (69%) | 4 |
| Septic arthritis | 1 | 0 | 1 |
| Total | 30 | 21 (70%) | 9 |

## Patients

During the period from 1973 to 1982, 58 patients underwent arthrodesis of the knee at the Cleveland Clinic Foundation (CCF) and Kobe University Hospital (KUH). Among these patients, 30 were treated following failed total knee replacement (27 at CCF and three at KUH), and 28 knees had arthrodesis without previous total knee replacement (16-at CCF and 12 at KUH). There is general agreement that successful fusions are much more difficult to achieve when arthrodesis is performed following failed total knee replacement than when performed as a primary procedure [3, 4, 6]. This was true in our series. The fusion rate was 70% with failed total knee replacement and 93% without previous total knee replacement (Table 1). Among the two knees which had nonunion without previous total knee replacement, one was a Charcot joint and another case showed persistent infection after post-traumatic septic arthritis.

As to the cases with previous total knee replacement, the indication for arthrodesis was infection in 27 patients, severe instability due to trauma in one, aseptic loosening of the prosthesis in one, and breakage of the prosthesis in one. The union rate was analyzed in relation to the following risk factors: age, primary disease, obesity, surgical methods, previous surgery, type of prosthesis, and postoperative infection; this was done to try to ascertain the predominant factors which have influenced the results of arthrodesis.

The mean age of patients with solid fusion was 61.2 years, which closely matched that of patients with nonunion (62.7 years). As to the primary disease, 75% of the osteoarthritic knees were successfully fused and 69% of the rheumatoid patients obtained successful fusion (Table 2). Although rheumatoid arthritis has been implicated in prosthetic infection by some authors [14, 15], the successful fusion rate in osteoarthritic and rheumatoid knees appeared to be similar in our series.

The successful fusion rate in obese patients was 44% (Table 3). Nonobese patients showed a high fusion rate compared with obese patients, and there was a statistical significance ($P \leqslant 0.02$). The heavy lower extremities of extremely obese patients may generate increased force at the fusion site or there may be a predisposing metabolic disturbance which may influence the bone-healing process.

With regard to the surgical methods, the Hoffman or Charnley external fixation device, crossed Steinmann pins with a casting technique, and internal plate fixation were utilized. Although in our series the surgical methods did not seem to influence the fusion rate (Table 4), we think it is extremely important that the procedure is performed with an adequate surgical technique [20]. If the femur and tibia have poor bone stock at the fusion site, other alternatives such as intramedullary fixation [7, 11, 12], internal fixation with plates [17], and the use of an electromagnetic field [2] should also be considered. With any type of fixation, care-

**Table 3.** Successful fusion rate in relation to obesity

| | Cases | Union | Nonunion |
|---|---|---|---|
| Men >90 kg, women >80 kg | 9 | 4 (44%) | 5 |
| Men <90 kg, women <80 kg | 21 | 17 (81%) | 4 |
| Total | 30 | 21 (70%) | 9 |

**Table 4.** Successful fusion rate in relation to surgical methods

| | Cases | Union | Nonunion |
|---|---|---|---|
| Hoffman-Vidal apparatus | 15 | 10 (67%) | 5 |
| Charnley compression device | 8 | 6 (75%) | 2 |
| Crossed Steinmann pins and casting | 6 | 4 (67%) | 2 |
| Internal fixation with plates | 1 | 1 (100%) | 0 |
| Total | 30 | 21 (70%) | 9 |

ful removal of the prosthesis and all cement, adequate debridement of the contaminated tissue, and the production of large contact surfaces are critical in obtaining successful arthrodesis.

Besides the primary total knee replacement, 21 knees underwent some kind of operation prior to the attempts of arthrodesis. The fusion rate was 78% in the nine knees which underwent primary total knee replacement only (Table 5). In 11 knees which had undergone prior soft tissue surgery alone, the fusion rate was 91%. Two knees which had revision of the patellar components and one knee which had patelloectomy were included in this group. Of the ten knees which were subjected to skeletal surgery, only four knees showed successful fusion. All of these cases except one underwent revision of the primary total knee replacement and loss of bony stock due to repeated skeletal surgery seemed to be a predisposing factor to the lower fusion rate in these cases.

The successful fusion rate with different types of prosthesis is shown in Table 6. The prostheses were classified into two groups. Of the nine patients with a hinge prosthesis, less than half the patients obtained solid fusion. The low fusion rate in the patients with hinge prostheses has been reported by many authors [3, 5, 8, 9, 13, 18, 19]; it is probably due to the fact that there is a significant amount of bone loss and extensive tissue

**Table 5.** Successful fusion rate in relation to previous surgery except primary total knee replacement

| | Cases | Union | Nonunion |
|---|---|---|---|
| None | 9 | 7 (78%) | 2 |
| Soft tissue surgery | 11 | 10 (91%) | 1 |
| Skeletal surgery | 10 | 4 (40%) | 6 |
| Total | 30 | 21 (70%) | 9 |

**Table 6.** Successful fusion rate in relation to type of prosthesis

| | Cases | Union | Nonunion |
|---|---|---|---|
| Minimally or partially constrained prosthesis | 21 | 17 (81%) | 4 |
| Hinge prosthesis | 9 | 4 (44%) | 5 |
| Total | 30 | 21 (70%) | 9 |

**Table 7.** Successful fusion rate in relation to postoperative infection

| | Cases | Union | Nonunion |
|---|---|---|---|
| No infection | 17 | 14 (82%) | 3 |
| Pin-track infection | 8 | 6 (75%) | 2 |
| Persistent infection | 4 | 0 (0%) | 4 |
| Late infection | 1 | 1 | 0 |
| Total | 30 | 21 (70%) | 9 |

damage in these cases. The reoperation rate of total knee replacement with hinge prostheses is also reported to be significantly high [1]. In addition, at the time of fusion, hinge prostheses with bulky femoral and tibial stems have an undesirably small interface at the fusion site [10]. Figure 2 depicts a patient who underwent revision surgery with a hinge prosthesis and the result was nonunion. Judging from these results, whenever revision arthroplasty is performed with the hinge prosthesis, the failure rate is significantly high and the success rate of subsequent arthrodesis is very low. Therefore, hinge prostheses should be reserved for certain limited cases and arthrodesis may be considered as an alternative to revision surgery with hinge prosthesis in some cases of failed total knee replacement.

With regard to postoperative infection, the fusion rate was 82% in those knees which did not show significant infection after arthrodesis was attempted (Table 7). Pin-track infection did not seem to influence the result of arthrodesis as long

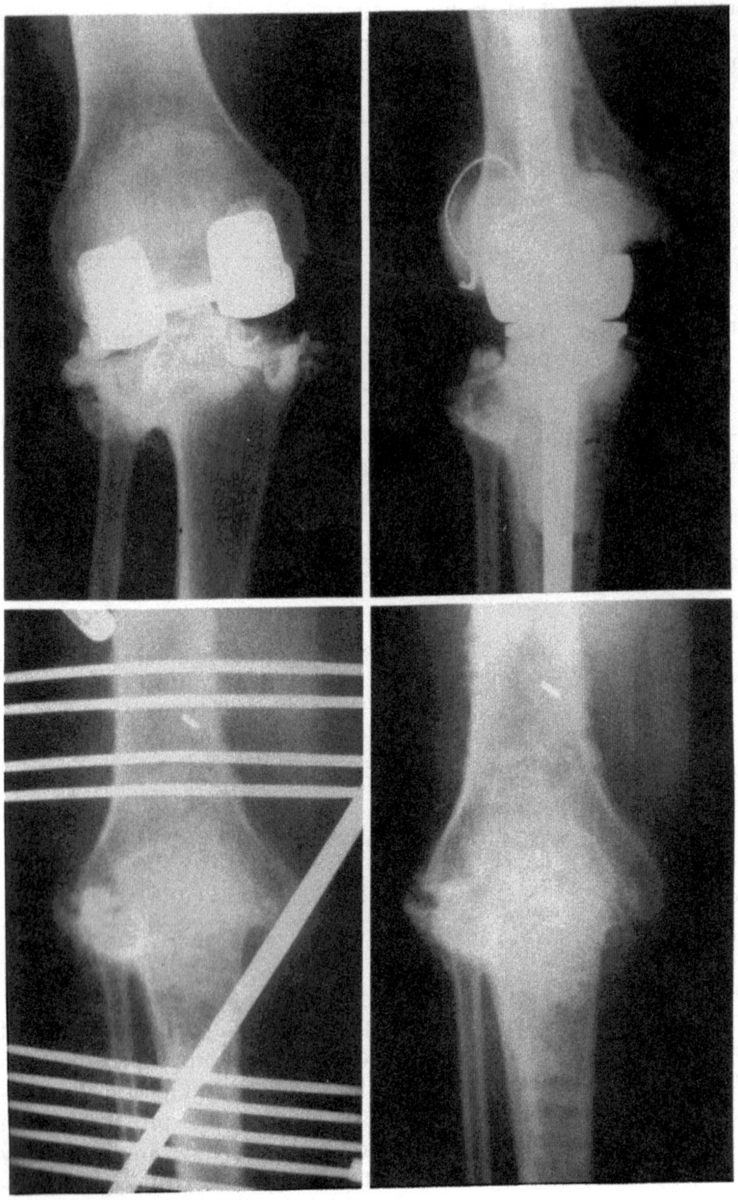

a b c d

**Fig. 2a–d.** An example of a patient who underwent revision surgery with a hinge prosthesis, resulting in nonunion. **a** Failure of primary total knee replacement. **b** Revision surgery was performed with a Guepar prosthesis. **c** Due to infection, the prosthesis was removed and arthrodesis was attempted with a Hoffman-Vidal fixation device. **d** Successful fusion was not obtained

as infection did not cause subsequent loosening of the external fixation device. On the other hand, all four knees which showed persistent infection after arthrodesis surgery resulted in nonunion despite extensive administration of antibiotics. Since arthrodesis is most frequently performed on patients who have infection following total knee replacement, all the factors which influence the control of infection such as tissue quality, virulence of organism, sensitivity to antibiotics, host defence, and general surrounding conditions should be carefully considered. Every effort should be taken to control infection, including accurate identification of the organism, appropriate antibiotic administration, extensive debridement of the contaminated tissue, and removal of foreign bodies at the time of surgery.

In summarizing all these factors, hinge prostheses and persistent postoperative infection seemed to have a great influence on the fusion rate. In fact, among the nine knees where the result was nonunion, only one had a minimally constrained prosthesis without persistent postoperative infection.

## References


1. Ahlberg A, Lunden A (1981) Secondary operations after knee joint replacement. Clin Orthop 156: 170–174
2. Bigliani LU, Rosenwasser MP, Caulo N, Schink MM, Bassett CAL (1903) The use of pulsing electromagnetic fields to achieve arthrodesis following failed total knee arthroplasty. J. Bone Joint Surg 65-A: 480–485
3. Broderson MP, Ritzgerald RH, Peterson LF, Coventry MB, Bryan RS. (1979) Arthrodesis of the knee following failed total knee arthroplasty. J Bone Joint Surg 61-A: 181–185
4. Charnley J, Lowe HG (1958) A study of the end-results of compression arthrodesis of the knee. J Bone Joint Surg 40-B: 633–635 (1958)
5. Deburge A, Guepar (1976) Guepar hinge prosthesis. Complications and results with two years' follow up. Clin Orthop 120: 47–53
6. Frymoyer JW, Hoaglund FT (1974) The role of arthrodesis in reconstruction of the knee. Clin Orthop 101: 82
7. Griend RV (1983) Arthrodesis of the knee with intramedullary fixation. Clin Orthop 181: 146–150
8. Gunn AL (1975) Arthrodesis of the knee in rheumatoid arthritis. J Bone Joint Surg 57-B: 397 (abstract)
9. Hagemann WF, Woods GW, Tullos HS (1978) Arthrodesis in failed total knee replacement. J Bone Joint Surg 60-A: 790–794
10. Hankin F, Lourie KW, Matthews LS (1981) The effect of total knee arthroplasty prostheses design on the potential for salvage arthrodesis: Measurements of volumes, length and trabecular bone contact areas. Clin Orthop 155: 52–58
11. Harris CM, Froehlich J (1985) Knee fusion with intramedullary rods for failed total knee arthroplasty. Clin Orthop 197: 209–216
12. Knutson K, Lidgren L (1982) Arthrodesis after infected knee arthroplasty using an intramedullary nail. Arch Orthop Traumat Surg 100: 49
13. Knutson K, Hovelius L, Lindstrand A, Lidgren L. (1984) Arthrodesis after failed knee arthroplasty. A nationwide multicenter investigation of 91 cases. Clin Orthop 191: 202–211
14. Petty W, Bryan RS Coventry MB, Peterson LF. (1975) Infection after total knee arthroplasty. Orthop Clin North Am 6: 1005
15. Rand JA, Bryan RS, Morrey BF, Westholm F. (1986) Management of infected total knee arthroplasty. Clin Orthop,. 205: 75–85
16. Rand JA, Bryan RS (1986) The outcome of failed knee arthrodesis following total knee arthroplasty. Clin Orthop 205: 86–92
17. Stulberg SD (1982) Arthrodesis in failed total knee replacement. Orthop Clin North Am 13: 213
18. Thornhill TS, Dalziel RW, Sledge CB (1982) Alternatives to arthrodesis for the failed total knee arthroplasty. Clin Orthop 170: 131–140
19. Vahvanen V (1979) Arthrodesis in failed knee replacement in eight patients. Ann Chir Gyn 68: 57
20. Woods GW, Lionberger DR, Tullos HS (1983) Failed total knee arthroplasty. Revision and arthrodesis for infection and noninfectious complications. Clin Orthop 173: 184–190

## *Discussion*

*Ranawat* (Cornell University Medical College): Do you have any opinion on intramedullary fixation? You concluded that obesity, infection, and type of prosthesis were important prognostic fators. Did you subject the figures to statistical analysis?

*Kurosaka* (Kobe University): I think that intramedullary fixation is a very good technique unless there is infection at the side of the fusion. In chronic infections, an external fixator would probably be the treatment of choice. As to obesity, we do not know the statistical significance owing to the smaller numbers of patients. We know the statistical significance for persistent infection and the type of prosthesis. The hinge prosthesis had a significantly lower rate of fusion than the minimally constrained prosthesis.

*Iseki* (Keio University): You said there was revision in 150 cases, of which 30 were exposed to the fusion. Is this correct?

*Kurosaka*: The revision cases included realignment of the patella and procedures of the patella. About one-third had something to do with the patella. In the last division of the tibia-femur, there were only 100 or less.

*Iseki*: How many cases of total knee replacement were there?

*Kurosaka*: Less than 100 cases.

*Iseki*: What was the population size and what was the percentage of revision cases?

*Kurosaka*: We had about 2400 cases of coinstitution, however not all the revisions were conducted in those institutions, therefore the number of revision cases in the total population could be about 5%.

*Ranawat*: You indicated that two-stage exchange for an infected knee is the treatment of choice, and I agree with that. On the same slide, you showed that if you have a Gram-negative infection you would go straight to arthresis. What evidence do you have to show that this is the correct approach and that the infection is cleared at the knee joint level?

*Kurosaka*: The Gram-negative infection does not necessarily indicate that arthrosis should be directly performed. If the patient's condition is good and the bacteria are sensitive to antibiotics, I think that we should probably remove the prosthesis and treat the patient with antibiotics. If we cannot control the infection, perhaps we should proceed to the arthrodesis. But in some patients whose general condition is not that good and the bacteria are not easy to control, it is perhaps better to proceed first to arthrodesis.

# PCA Type Total Joint Arthroplasty of the Knee

N. Matsui[1], S. Tsuboguchi[1], T. Imaizumi[1], H. Ohta[1], T. Itoh[1], and T. Suguro[2]

**Summary.** During the period from July 1984 until December 1986, we performed total knee replacement (TKR) using porous coated anatomical (PCA) knee prostheses in a total of 38 cases (50 joints) at Nagoya City University and affiliated institutions. By disease, these cases comprised 24 cases (29 joints) of osteoarthritis (OA) and 14 cases (21 joints) of rheumatoid arthritis (RA). The age of the patients at the time of surgery ranged from 63 to 81 years (average 62.9 years) for OA and from 37 to 73 years (average 58.3 years) for RA. In all cases, bone cement was used for fixation of the femur and tibia as well as the patella. The tibial components used were mostly small (7 mm thick). Prior to surgery, flexion contracture above 31° was found in six joints, and a range of motion with a contracture of less than 60° was noted in eight joints. In addition, six joints required compensation for bone loss in the medial condyle of the tibia. The post-operative observation period ranged from 2 months to 2 years 8 months. In OA, the 100-point score ranged from 41.6 points before surgery to 80.6 points after surgery, and range of motion (ROM) from 116.6° pre-operatively to 89.6° post-operatively. The values for RA were 36.2–79.8 points and 77.3°–101.6°, respectively. Adequate ROM was achieved for knees with flexion contracture and knees with contracture. The results in cases involving compensation for bone loss were also satisfactory. A comparison of our results with those obtained at Chiba University where TKR using PCA without cement (resurfacing type) was carried out on 47 cases (58 joints; 18 cases, 25 joints, of OA and 22 cases, 30 joints, of RA) led us to conclude that the use of bone cement had no bearing on the clinical evaluation. The postoperative femorotibial angle was in most cases satisfactory. The setting position of both the femoral component and the tibial component showed good alignment in the frontal plane but large variations in the sagittal plane. In cases of knees with flexion contracture, the total extent of bone resection was substantial.

**Keywords.** Total knee replacement—Porous-coated anatomic total knee—With cement—Without cement—Clinical evaluation

[1] Department of Orthopaedic Surgery, School of Medicine, Nagoya City University, Nagoya, Japan
[2] Department of Orthopaedic Surgery, School of Medicine, Chiba University, Chiba, Japan

## Introduction

In recent years, various types of artificial knee joint replacement or total knee replacement (TKR) have been performed at many institutions. Several types of artificial knee joints using no bone cement have been developed, and stable results have been reported. However, no fixing material has been shown to be superior to bone cement.

In the past, we have used various types of artificial joints at our institution. Beginning with the oldest types, they included McIntosh, Gunston, and geometric prostheses, but after 1975 we mainly used University of California, Irvine, (UCI)—Waugh. Since 1984 we have performed TKR using PCA knee prosthesis (PCA) with bone cement. In the present study, we investigated the results in cases with PCA and evaluated through postoperative X-ray photography the alignment of the lower extremity, the setting position of the components, and the extent of bone resection. In addition, we carried out a comparative study on the results of TKR using PCA without bone cement (resurfacing type) performed at Chiba University.

## Materials

TKR using PCA with bone cement was performed in 38 cases (50 joints) at Nagoya City University and affiliated institutions from July 1984 until December 1986. These 38 patients included eight males and 30 females. By disease, they comprised 24 cases (29 joints) of osteoarthritis (OA) and 14 cases (21 joints) of rheumatoid arthritis (RA). The age of the patients at the time of surgery ranged from 63 to 81 (average 69.2) years in OA and from 37 to 73 (average 58.3) years in RA (Table 1). Six joints (all involving RA) exhibited flexion contracture exceeding 30° pre-operatively, while eight joints (one OA and seven RA) had a pre-operative range of motion (ROM) of less than 60°. In addi-

**Table 1.** Materials of Nagoya City University and Chiba University

| | Sex | PCA total knee replacement with cement (stem-type)[a] | | | | PCA total knee replacement without cement (resurfacing type)[b] | | | |
|---|---|---|---|---|---|---|---|---|---|
| | | Cases | Joints | Age | Mean age | Cases | Joints | Age | Mean age |
| OA | Male | 5 | 6 | 69–79 | 75.0 | 6 | 7 | 64–88 | 73.8 |
| | Female | 19 | 23 | 63–81 | 67.7 | 14 | 16 | 65–83 | 73.7 |
| Total | | 24 | 29 | 63–81 | 69.2 | 20 | 23 | 64–88 | 73.8 |
| RA | Male | 3 | 4 | 37–63 | 52.0 | 4 | 5 | 52–73 | 61.5 |
| | Female | 11 | 17 | 41–73 | 60.0 | 23 | 30 | 38–72 | 59.0 |
| Total | | 14 | 21 | 37–73 | 58.3 | 27 | 35 | 38–73 | 59.4 |

All ages in years
*OA* osteoarthritis, *RA* rheumatoid arthritis, *PCA* porous coated anatomic
[a] Nogoya City University
[b] Chiba University

tion, a high degree of bone loss was noted in six joints (four OA and two RA) in the medial condyle of the tibia, requiring a certain amount of bone compensation at this site. In all cases, bone cement was used in the replacement of the femur, tibia, and patella. Small-size components were chosen for 38 joints, and medium-size components for 11 joints. Resurfacing-type tibial components were used for one joint, and central stem-type tibial components for 49 joints. The component thickness ranged from 7mm in 39 knees, to 9 mm in seven knees, and 11 mm in three knees. The post-operative observation period ranged from 2 months to 2 years 8 months (average 14.6 months).

Meanwhile, TKR using PCA without cement (resurfacing type) was performed in 47 cases (58 joints) at Chiba University from February 1985 until December 1986 (Table 1). Clinical evaluation was carried out by comparing the post-operative results in these cases with those in our study.

## Methods

### Clinical Evaluation

Evaluation was based on the 100-point score of knee evaluation (Table 2) by combining the points total from six parameters: pain, ROM, extension lag or flexion contracture, antero-posterior deformities or femorotibial angle (FTA), walking ability, and activities of daily living (ADL).

### X-ray Evaluation

Evaluation was carried out using the following three parameters. The setting positions of the femoral component and tibial component were evaluated through anteroposterior and lateral pictures taken during the postoperative investigation (Fig. 1): femoral prosthesis angle (FPA), tibial prosthesis angle (TPA), femoral prosthesis tilting angle (FPTA), and tibial prosthesis tilting angle (TPTA).

The femorotibial angle (FTA) was checked before and after surgery.

The total extent of bone resection was calculated from X-ray pictures taken before and after surgery.

## Results

### Clinical Evaluation

**PCA group with cement.** The total on the 100-point score was on average 42.6 points preoperatively versus 80.6 points postoperatively for the OA group, and 36.2 points preoperatively versus 79.8 points postoperatively for the RA group. In the preoperative average scores, the RA group was inferior to the OA group, but postoperatively no significant difference was noted between the two groups. ROM in the OA group showed a preoperative average of 116.6° and a postoperative average of 89.6°, against a preoperative average of 77.3° and a postoperative average of 101.6° in the RA group. In the preoperative average scores, the RA group was markedly inferior to the OA group, but since ROM in the OA group worsened postoperatively and ROM in the RA group showed improvement, no significant difference between the two groups was noted (Table 3). The totals in the 100-point score for severe cases involving flexion

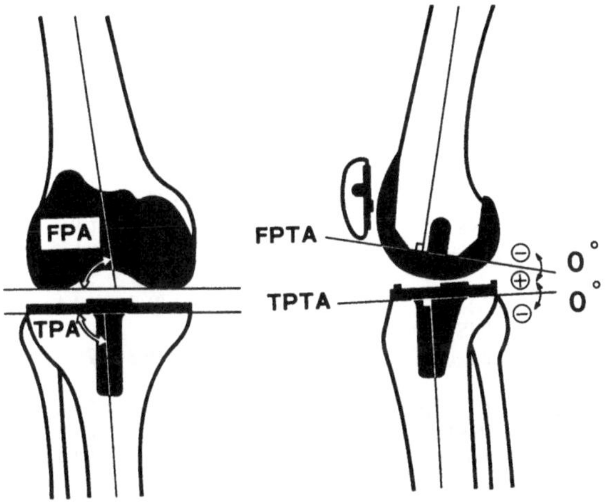


**Fig. 1.** Definition of angles used in the study of the setting conditions of the components. Ideally, in the anteroposterior view, the femoral prosthesis angle (*FPA*), i.e., the angle formed by the axis of the femoral shaft and the femoral component, should be 81°, and the tibial prosthesis angle (*TPA*), i.e., the angle formed by the axis of the tibial shaft and the tibial component, should be 93°; in the lateral view, the femoral prosthesis tilting angle (*FPTA*), formed by the perpendicular to the axis of the femoral shaft and the femoral component, and the tibial prosthesis tilting angle (*TPTA*), formed by the perpendicular to the axis of the tibial shaft and the tibial component, should both be 0°

**Table 2.** The 100-point score of knee eveluation

| | Point |
|---|---|
| Pain | |
| None | 30 |
| Mild pain with weight bearing | 25 |
| Moderate pain with weight bearing | 15 |
| Severe pain with weight bearing, mild at rest | 5 |
| Severe contiruous pain | 0 |
| ROM | |
| Over 120° | 20 |
| 90°–119° | 15 |
| 60°–89° | 10 |
| 30°–59° | 5 |
| 0°–29° | 0 |
| Walking ability (without support) | |
| Normal | 20 |
| 500–1000 m | 15 |
| Less than 500 m | 10 |
| Indoor only | 5 |
| Unable to walk | 0 |
| Extension lag or flexion contracture | |
| 0°–10° | 10 |
| 11°–30° | 5 |
| Over 31° | 0 |
| AP deformity | |
| 175° ± 5° | 10 |
| Less than 15° | 5 |
| Over 16° | 0 |
| Activity of daily living[a] | |
| Able to get out of chair | 2,1,0 |
| Able to go upstairs | 2,1,0 |
| Able to go downstairs | 2,1,0 |
| Able to stand on one leg | 2,1,0 |
| Able to run | 2,1,0 |

[a] *2* easy, *1* difficult, *0* impossible

**Table 3.** Preoperative and postoperative 100-point score and ROM in OA and RA

| | PCA total knee replacement with cement (stem type) | | | | | PCA total knee replacement without cement (resurfacing type) | | | | |
|---|---|---|---|---|---|---|---|---|---|---|
| | No. of joints | 100-point score | | ROM | | No. of joints | 100-point score | | ROM | |
| | | Preop. | Postop. | Preop. | Postop. | | Preop. | Postop. | Preop. | Postop. |
| OA | 29 | 42.6±11.0 | 80.6±5.0 (NS) | 116.6±25.7 | 89.6±15.8 (NS) | 23 | 32.3±10.7 | 82.8±5.8 (NS) | 88.6±23.8 | 103.2±12.7 (NS) |
| RA | 21 | 32.6±12.3 | 79.0±8.8 | 77.3±38.9 | 101.6±25.6 | 35 | 30.4±12.3 | 81.5±10.6 | 82.1±22.0 | 95.1±18.7 |

*ROM* range of motion in degrees, *OA* osteoarthritis, *RA* rheumatoid arthritis, *NS* not significant. $P = 0.01$

contracture, limited ROM, and bone loss were 27.2 points preoperatively versus 82.7 points postoperatively for the flexion contracture group, 22.9 versus 75.0 points for the limited ROM group, and 32.2 versus 81.7 points for the bone loss group. The ROM averages were 57.5° preoperatively versus 103.3° postoperatively for the flexion contracture group, 27.5° versus 83.8° for the limited ROM group, and 97.5° versus 100.0° for the bone loss group. Moreover, in the 100-point score and ROM evaluation, no significant difference was found between the severe cases and the corresponding cases in the control group (Table 4)

**Table 4.** Preoperative and postoperative 100-point score, ROM, and amount of bone resection in severe cases at Nagoya City University

| | Joints | 100-point score | | Extension (degrees) | | ROM (degrees) | | Amount of bone resection |
|---|---|---|---|---|---|---|---|---|
| | | Preop. | Postop. | Preop. | Postop. | Preop. | Postop. | |
| Flexion contracture (extension < −30°) | 6 | 27.2±10.9 | 82.7±6.2 (NS) | 42.5±9.4 | 4.2±2.0 (NS) | 53.5±29.5 | 103.3±10.8 (NS) | 32.3±2.3 ($P < 0.01$) |
| No flexion contracture (extension ≧ −10°) | 31 | 45.6±7.5 | 80.5±4.6 | 5.5±4.7 | 2.1±4.8 | 110.0±18.4 | 97.1±18.9 | 25.8±4.8 |
| Limited ROM (ROM < 60°) | 8 | 22.9±11.8 | 75.0±13.6 (NS) | 35.0±13.6 | 7.5±6.5 (NS) | 27.5±19.8 | 83.8±36.2 (NS) | 29.4±3.9 (NS) |
| Less ROM limitation (ROM ≧ 60°) | 42 | 43.1±8.8 | 80.8±4.3 | 9.4±8.9 | 2.2±4.4 | 107.0±18.4 | 96.7±16.8 | 26.5±4.8 |
| Excessive bone loss | 6 | 32.2±8.8 | 81.7±2.6 (NS) | 20.8±14.6 | 1.7±2.6 (NS) | 97.5±9.4 | 100.0±8.9 (NS) | 25.8±8.3 (NS) |
| No bone loss | 44 | 40.9±11.9 | 79.7±7.1 | 12.5±13.2 | 3.3±5.4 | 93.8±36.9 | 93.9±22.3 | 27.2±4.6 |

*ROM* range of motion, *NS* not significant. $P = 0.01$

**PCA group without cement.** In the 100-point score, both the OA and RA groups were significantly improved: a preoperative average of 32.3 points versus a postoperative average of 82.2 points for the OA group, and a preoperative average of 30.4 points versus a postoperative average of 81.5 points for the RA group. ROM values also showed significant postoperative improvement with a preoperative average of 88.6° versus a postoperative 103.2° for the OA group, and a preoperative average of 82.1° versus a postoperative 95.1° for the RA group.

A comparison based on the totals in the 100-point score between the PCA group with cement and the PCA group without cement showed no significant difference for either the OA or the RA group. However, a comparison of postoperative ROM values of both groups while showing no significant difference for the RA group did reveal significantly inferior results for the OA group using PCA without cement ($P < 0.05$) (Table 3).

## X-ray Evaluation

**Alignment in the A-P view (FTA).** The OA group had an average preoperative value of 186.6° versus a postoperative 177.2°, while the RA group had a preoperative average of 173.0° versus a postoperative 176.4°. Preoperatively, the OA group exhibited instances of genu varum compared with the RA group but showed good improvement postoperatively (Table 5). However, the postoperative distribution of FTA indicated inversion, i.e., a value exceeding 180°, for five joints in the OA group and two joints in the RA group (Fig. 2).

**Table 5.** Preoperative and postoperative alignment of the cases where cement was used

| | No. of joints | FTA | |
|---|---|---|---|
| | | Preop. | Postop. |
| OA | 29 | 186.6 ± 10.7 ($P < 0.01$) | 177.2 ± 3.9 (NS) |
| RA | 21 | 173.0 ± 11.5 | 176.4 ± 3.4 |

*OA* osteoarthritis, *RA* rheumatoid arthritis, *FTA* femorotibial angle

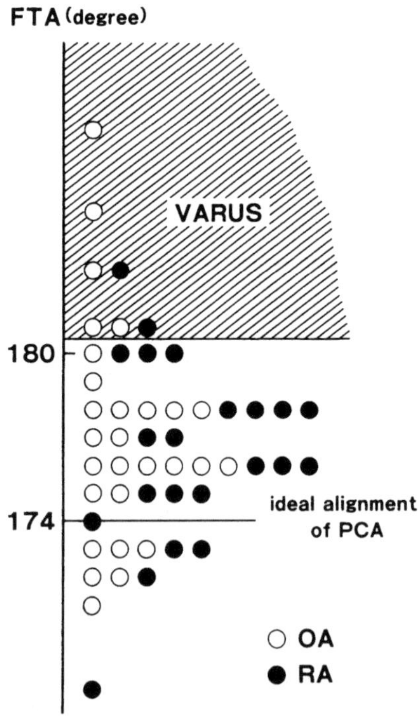


**Fig. 2.** Postoperative alignment in the anteroposterior view. Ideal alignment is 174°; cases that exceed 180° are regarded as varus malalignment

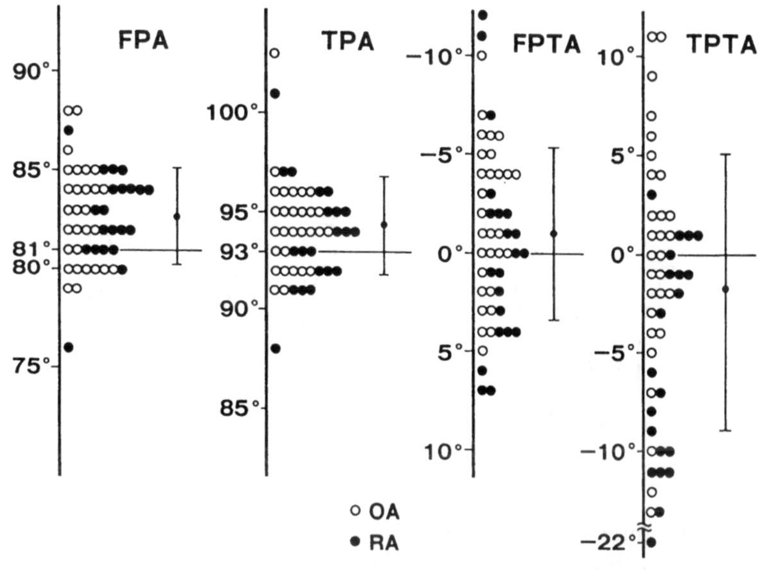


Fig. 3. Setting angles of components (see Fig. 1). In the anteroposterior view, FPA and TPA are seen to be close to the ideal values; but in the lateral view, FPTA and TPTA show a large variation, indicating that accurate bone resection and component setting is difficult. The various angles are: FPA 82.7° ± 2.4°, TPA 94.2° ± 2.5°, FPTA − 1.9 ± 6.9°, and TPTA − 1.0 ± 4.4°

**Setting angle for the components.** The FPA (Fig. 1) had an average value of 82.7° (76°–88°), the TPA an average of 94.2° (88°–103°). By contrast, both the FPTA with an average of −1.0° (−12°–+7°) and TPTA with an average of −1.9° (−22°–+11°) showed a high degree of variation (Fig. 3).

**Extent of bone resection.** A comparison of the extent of bone resection between the group with more than −10° and the group with less than −30° of preoperative extension showed extensive bone resection for the group with less than −30°, which amounted to a significant difference ($P < 0.01$). Postoperatively, none of the cases requiring extensive bone resection showed any extension insufficiency (Table 4).

## Surgical techniques

Originally, we used the PCA cutting jig system [5], but since Japanese have a small physique, jigs can be accurately fitted in only a few cases even when using small components. As a result of excessive bone resection from the posterior condyle of the femur, the femoral component can easily set in the anterior position. In cases of extensive deformation of the tibial joint surface, we experienced difficulty in determining the line for bone resection. Accordingly, we independently devised our own jig system and the corresponding instrumentation as shown in Fig 4 and Fig 5.

**Femoral side.** We determined a reference point (P) for bone resection from the transverse distal femur

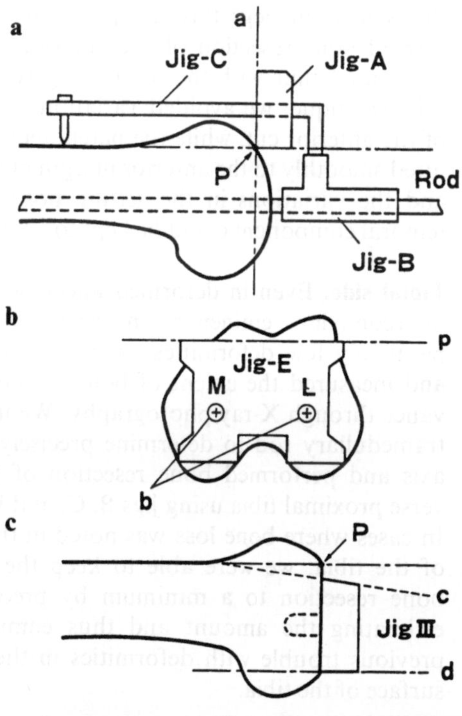


**Fig. 4. a** *Jig-A*, *Jig-B*, and *Jig-C* are attached to the *Rod* embedded in the bone marrow cavity, and point *P* is determined as the point where the elongated line of the anterior margin of the femur intersects the femoral condyle. Bone resection of the transverse distal femur is performed at *plane a* (the whole frontal plane is at 9° valgus with regard to the femoral shaft). **b** Holes are bored to accommodate the femoral prosthesis fixation pegs by matching *Jig-E* with the line where *plane p* intersects the femoral condyle. **c** Bone resection of the anterior femur and the posterior femur is performed with the original *Jig III*

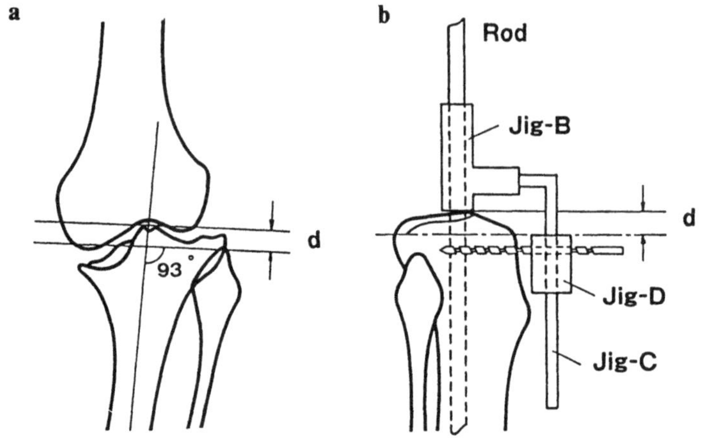


**Fig. 5.** **a** The width (*d*) of bone resection is determined in advance by taking the intercondylar eminence in the anteroposterior view located through preoperative X-ray as the reference point. **b** *Jig-B*, *Jig-C*, and *Jig-D* are attached the *Rod* embedded in the bone marrow, and bome resection of the transverse proximal tibia is performed at the destance (*d*) distally from the intercondylar eminence

and the anterior femur through jig A, jig B, and jig C fixed with an intramedullary rod. At a line passing point P, we carried out bone resection from the distal femur at 9° valgus from the femoral axis and bored holes to accommodate the femoral prosthesis fixation pegs through jig E. We then performed bone resection of the anterior femur and posterior femur with the original jig III. Through this technique, we avoided variations of the level of the anterior cut, while the patellofemoral flange fitted smoothly to the anterior margin of the femur, and the variations in the setting position of the femoral component could be kept to a minimum.

**Tibial side.** Even in deformed knees, we took the intercondylar eminence in cases with comparatively few deformities as the reference point and measured the extent of bone resection in advance through X-ray photography. We used an intramedullary rod to determine precisely the bone axis and performed bone resection of the transverse proximal tibia using jigs B, C, and D (Fig. 5). In cases where bone loss was noted in the condyle of the tibia, we were able to keep the extent of bone resection to a minimum by preoperatively estimating the amount and thus eliminated the previous trouble with deformities in the articular surface of the tibia.

## Complications

We experienced one case of rupture of the patellar ligament that occurred as a result of knee bending during walking. We treated this case by attaching the patellar ligaments by wire to the tibial tubercle and reinforcing the patellar ligaments by inverting the iliotibial band with a pedicle.

## Cases

**Cases 1** (female, 72, OA). Since about 1972, when the patient experienced bilateral gonarthralgia, conservative treatment was employed; but when the pain in the right knee joint worsened around March 1986, a right TKR was performed on September 9, 1986. The preoperative 100-point score for the right knee was 49, with ROM from 10° to 130°, and FTA 189°. At the time of examination these values had changed to 86 points, 5°–100°, and 178°, respectively (Fig. 6).

**Case 2** (female, 68, classical RA, stage 4, class III). The onset of the disease was about 1970. Since about 1982, when the patient experienced bilateral gonarthralgia, conservative treatment was employed; but when the pain in the left knee worsened, a left TKR was performed on July 2, 1985. The preoperative 100-point score for the left knee was 25, with ROM from 30° to 70°, and FTA 182°. At the time of examination these values had changed to 79 points, 5°–120°, and 178°, respectively (Fig. 7).

**Case 3** (female, 64, OA). Since about 1977 when the patient experienced bilateral gonarthralgia, conservative treatment was employed, but in March 1985 the bilateral gonarthralgia worsened and inversion deformities were reinforced.

Left TKR was carried out on November 28, and right TKR on December 17. Bone resection of the tibia was kept to an absolute minimum; bone loss was replaced with a bone graft and fixed with a ceramic screw of monocrystalline $Al_2O_3$. The preoperative 100-point score was 26, with ROM from 20° to 110°, and FTA 211°. At the time of examination these values had changed to 80 points,

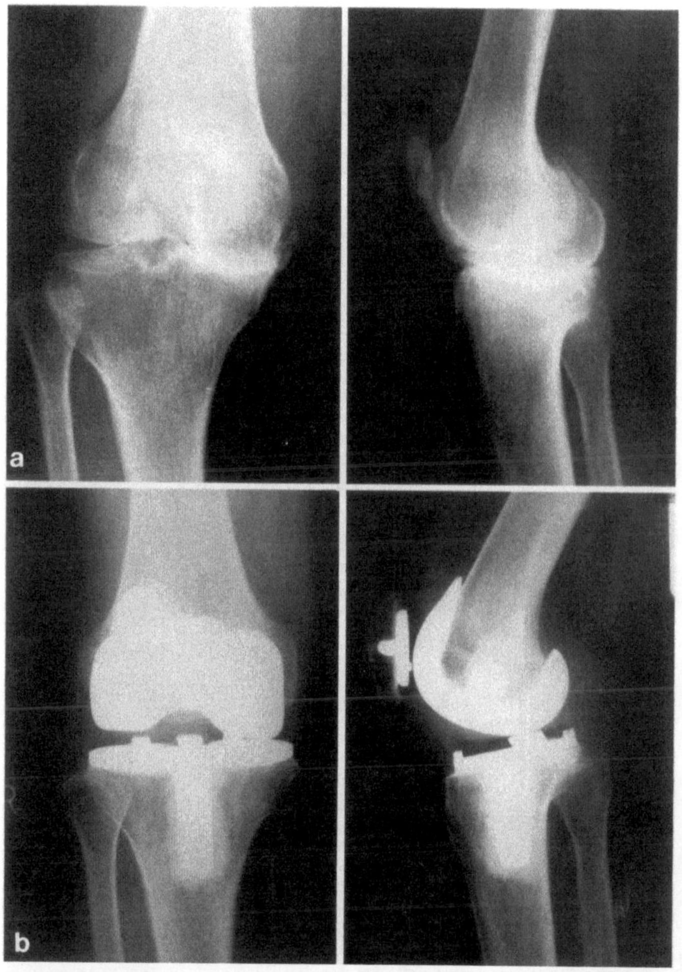


**Fig. 6a, b.** Radiographs of the right knee of a 72-year-old woman with OA. **a** Preoperative radiographic view. **b** Six months after TKR using PCA with cement

0°–90°, and 176°, respectively. Meanwhile, the preoperative 100-point score for the right knee was 31, with ROM from 15° to 130°, and FTA 215°. At the time of examination these values had changed to 80 points, 0°–100°, and 178°, respectively (Fig. 8).

## Discussion

The PCA knee system developed by Hungerford et al. is an artificial joint system designed to accomplish tricompartment replacement either with or without the use of cement. Its characteristics are a porous coating on the metal surface in order to strengthen adhesion between metal and bone as well as between metal and bone cement; it also incorporates a shape for each component that closely resembles the anatomical structure of a normal knee [2–4]. We carried out TKR using PCA with bone cement for several reasons.

Despite dynamic problems involving the bone-bone cement interface and despite extensive bone loss in the case of repeated replacement, there is at present no material superior to bone cement for fixing artificial joints, and by continuing rehabilitation therapy during the early postoperative period full load can be placed on the joint during that period.

The increased adhesion between bone cement and the artificial joint is an important advantage.

Stress on the interface between the artificial joint and bone is reduced if physiological movement of the knee can be properly simulated.

Walker et al. [9] regard the metal tray type with one or two attached pegs as suitable for the tibia, while Lewis et al. [7] consider the metal tray type with one stem adequate. The central stem type tibial component of the PCA system can also be regarded as adequate in this respect.

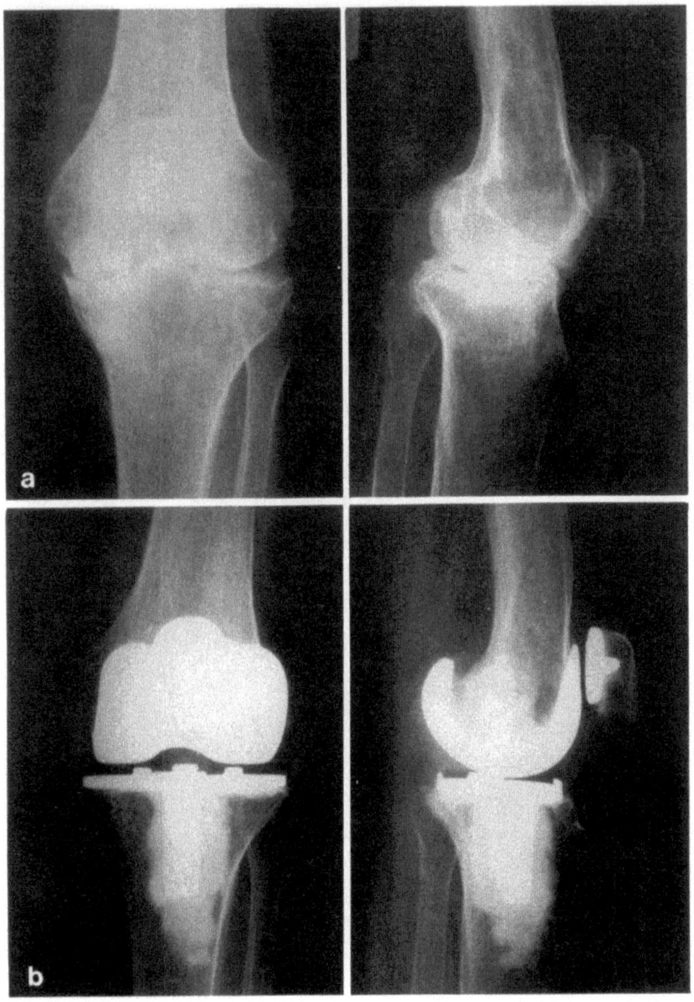


**Fig. 7a, b.** Radiographs of the left knee of a 68-year-old woman with RA. **a** Preoperative radiographic view. **b** Twenty months after TKR using PCA with cement

## Clinical Evaluation

Both OA and RA groups showed good results in the 100-point scores of knee evaluation with no difference between the two. Our present data include only short-term follow-up observations, but the use of bone cement had no bearing on the clinical evaluation. Consequently, it is considered important, particularly with older people and RA patients, to use PCA with bone cement, because sufficient fixation can be achieved during the early postoperative period, and the period of no load on the knee can be shortened. In OA cases where bone cement was used, a worsening of ROM was noted, but a clear cause-effect correlation with the use of bone cement could not be established. However, suitability and surgical technique in two cases with insufficient flexion of only 55° require reconsideration. In joints restricted by handicaps such as flexion contracture and ROM limit (contracture), ROM after TKR improved remarkably, leading to good results. With regard to bone loss in the tibia, tibial bone resection was kept to a minimum, and bone grafting was performed with subsequent anchoring by ceramic screws. The good postoperative results indicate that this approach constitutes a suitable method (Fig. 8). We have reached the conclusion that application of this technique to such cases should be expanded.

## X-ray Evaluation

To prevent loosening and instability of the prosthesis, proper alignment of the lower extremity and correct position of each component is essential [6, 8]. Bargren et al. [1] have reported that the success rate in long-term follow-up of cases where FTA exceeded 180° is no higher than 14%. However, in seven joints treated at our institution where the postoperative FTA exceeded 180° we

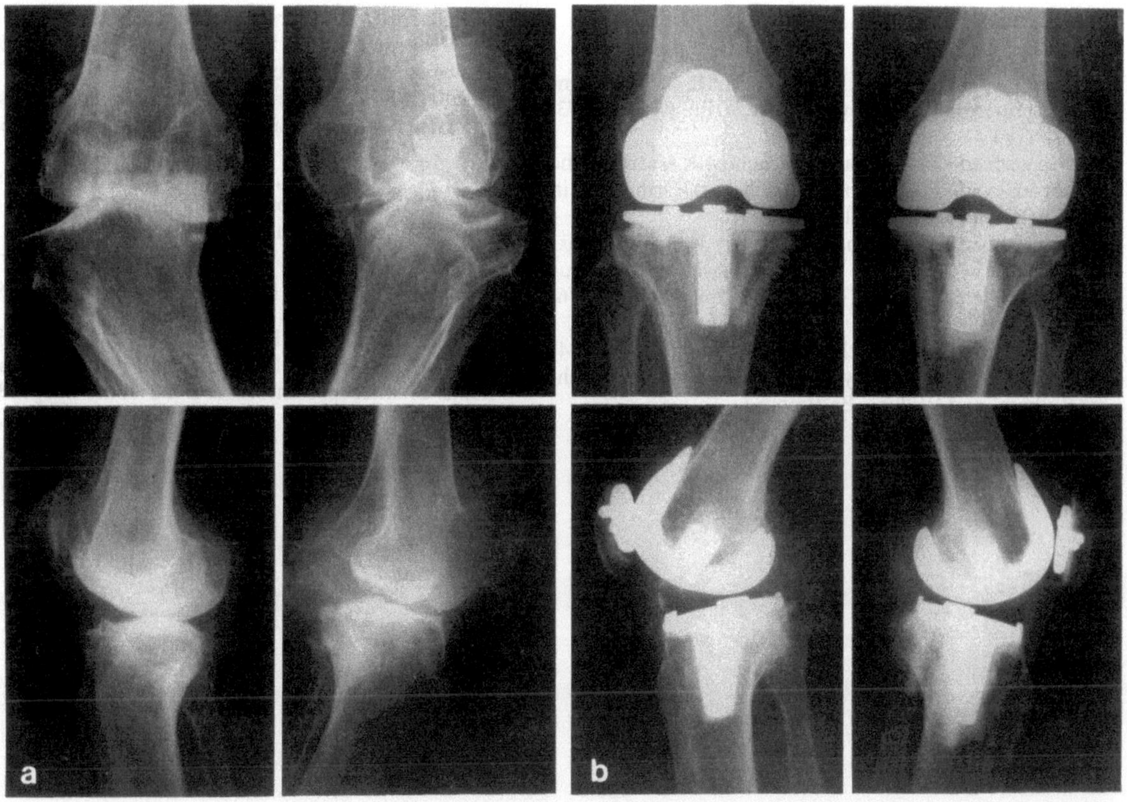


**Fig. 8a, b.** Radiographs of the knees of a 64-year-old woman with OA. **a** Preoperatively bilateral knees had severe varus angulation and marked bone loss in each medial tibial condyle. **b** Fourteen months after right TKR and 15 months after left TKR. Bone graft was performed and anchored with ceramic screws

have so far experienced no loosening or instability of the prosthesis, though further strict observation is required. In some cases there were large variations in the setting position of each component in the sagittal plane with marked deviations from the ideal setting angle (Fig. 3), indicating difficulty in achieving perpendicular bone resection with regard to the bone axis and correctly setting each component. Remedying this situation requires further improvement in the jigs when performing bone resection. In order to cope with flexion contracture, the extent of bone resection was increased, and since no extension insufficiency occurred, it is assumed that flexion contracture of about 40° can be handled by adjusting the extent of bone resection.

## Conclusion

We carried out a comparative clinical evaluation based on 100-point scores between TKR performed on 38 cases (50 joints) using PCA with cement at out institution and TKR using PCA without cement (resurfacing type) performed on 47 cases with 58 joints at Chiba University. In addition, we examined by X-ray photography FTA the setting angle of femoral and tibial components and the total amount of bone resection in the cases treated at our institution.

The short-term follow-up concerning postoperative evaluation of TKR using PCA revealed no difference between the OA and RA groups for PCA with cement versus PCA without cement.

In virtually all cases, alignment remained within an FTA of less than 180°, with a correct setting position noted for each component in the frontal plane. However, in addition to cases with genu varum, variations in the setting angle viewed from the sagittal plane were also noted. This point requires further study.

Flexion contracture can be handled by increasing the extent of bone resection.

In cases of bone loss in the condyles of the tibia, bone grafting and subsequent anchoring with ceramic screws is considered useful.

## References

1. Bargren JH, Blaha JD, Freeman MAR (1983) Alignment in total knee arthroplasty. Clin Orthop 173: 178–183
2. Hungerford DS, Kenna RV Krackow KA (1982) The porous-coated anatomic total knee. Orthop Clin North Am 13 (1): 103–122
3. Hungerford DS, Kenna RV (1983) Preliminary experience with a total knee prosthesis with porous coating used without cement. Clin Orthop 176: 95–107
4. Hungerford DS, Krackow KA, Kenna RV (1984) Total knee arthroplasty: A comprehensive approach. Williams and Wilkins, Baltimore
5. Hungerford DS, Krackow KA, Kenna RV: The PCA™ primary total knee system: Surgical technique Howmedica, Rutherford, NJ. USA
6. Insall (1984) Total knee replacement *in* Surgery of the knee. Churchill Livingstone, New York, pp 587–696
7. Lewis JL, Askew MJ, Jaycox DS (1982) A comparative evaluation of tibial component designs of total knee prosthesis. J Bone Joint Surg 64-A: 129–135
8. Lotke PA, Ecken ML (1977) Influence of positioning of prosthesis in total knee replacement. J Bone Joint Surg 59-A: 77
9. Walker PS, Greene D, Reilly D, Thatcher J, Ben-Dov M, Ewald FC (1981) Fixation of tibial components of knee prosthesis. J Bone Joint Surg 63-A: 258–267

## *Discussion*

*Bae* (Kyung Hee University Hospital): In your latter cases, you did more bone resection in patients with flexion contracture, what part of the bone did you remove—the tibial or femoral part?

*Matsui* (Nagoya City University): Mainly, the femoral side.

Bae: The PCA knee is an anatomical prosthesis, so if you remove more bone from the femoral part the joint line will be elevated and the tension in the posterior cruciate ligament and major collateral ligament will be altered. What do you think about this?

*Matsui*: If there is to be a great deal of bone removal, we take more bone from the side of the tibial plateau.

*Ryu* (Nihon University): You seem to use small prostheses, but in my experience with Japanese patients the anterior of the femoral component was too big. Do you think this type of prosthesis can be adapted to smaller patients?

*Matsui*: In a small number of cases, we did experience a problem with the size. In the posterior of the condyle, we may have had to cut a great deal of bone and so in these cases we had to suit the individual patient.

*Watanabe* (Hokkaido University): What is the difference in pain during the first weight bearing between cemented and cementless prostheses with the PCA? At our center, we use the Total Condylar and we found that there was more pain in the cementless than in the cemented cases upon weight bearing.

*Matsui*: Yes our experience has been the same as yours. Without cement at the beginning, there is more pain and this persists for the first 3 months. Dr. Suguro of Chiba University Hospital my co-author, is scheduled to discuss this point tomorrow afternoon. Isotope tests indicate that during the first 3 months, the prosthesis is not quite settled and clinical pain improves after this initial settling period.

# Results of Uncemented Total Knee Replacement

K. Ogata, M. Naito, Y. Sasaki, and Y. Sugioka[1]

**Summary.** From 1982 to 1986, we performed 71 uncemented total knee replacements (TKRs) on 48 patients with osteoarthritis and 11 patients with rheumatoid arthritis. Four different types of total knee prosthesis were used: 15 Ceramic (KOM-1), 6 Whiteside OrthoLoc, 48 PCA, and two Miller/Galante total knee systems. Instrumentation of the OrthoLoc system was simple and excellent in precise and reproducible cuts while that of the PCA system was overly complicated with many components. Bone cement had to be used for three tibial components of the PCA system due to poor initial fixation. Postoperative management of uncemented TKRs was more difficult than that of cemented TKRs. An early range of motion was occasionally deferred due to bleeding and pain, and full weight bearing was not allowed for 2 months. One Ceramic patellar component fractured at 3 months postoperatively, requiring later revision. All Ceramic Knees developed radiolucencies at the implant-bone interface, however no symptomatic loosening was noted at an average follow-up of 3.5 years. Symptomatic loosening of the tibial component occurred in one PCA knee at 10 months postoperatively, and revision surgery was performed. Significant subsidence of tibial components occurred in three PCA knees and one Ceramic knee. There was no case of infection. No significant difference was found in range of knee motion between the types of total knee system with a mean flexion of 95°–110°. Pain relief has been excellent with all types of uncemented total knee replacement.

Although the uncemented total knee replacements implanted into well-vascularized and mechanically sound bone will produce a stable and painless interface, it is still necessary to develop optimum press-fit fixation and strength to allow early rehabilitation and a new surface design to give a near-anatomical range of motion.

**Keywords:** TKR—Cementless fixation—Ceramic—Clinical trial

There are certain disadvantages to using cement in the total joint replacement. It has been well documented that the bone-cement junction is always separated by a layer of fibrous tissue which may lead to prosthetic loosening with increasing time and stress. Acrylic debris may hasten wear on the polyethylene component. The amount of bone stock is reduced by the mass of cement, and the chance of infection may be increased with the use of cement [2]. Recently many types of total knee prosthesis have been developed for implantation without cement.

In this paper we report our experience with the use of four different types of cementless total knee prosthesis and analyze the instrumentation, postoperative management, complications and prognoses on these total knee systems.

## Materials and Methods

From 1982 to 1986, we performed 71 uncemented total knee replacements on 48 patients with osteoarthritis and 11 patients with rheumatoid arthritis. Fifty patients were female and nine were male, and their age at the time of operation ranged from 48 to 81 years (average, 69 years). Nine patients underwent two-stage and three patients underwent one-stage bilateral total knee replacements. Three patients had contralateral cemented knee prostheses and four patients had contralateral high tibial osteotomies.

Our requirements for cementless implantation were: (a) The patient could tolerate 2 months of postoperative partial weight bearing, and (b) the bone was well vascularized and mechanically sound. However, if the mechanical stability of a component of the prosthesis was not obtained at the termination of the procedure, that component was reinserted with cement.

Four different types of total knee prostheses were used: 15 Ceramic (KOM-1, Kyocera), 6 Whiteside OrthoLoc (Dow Corning Wright), 48 porous-coated anatomical (PCA, Howmedica), and 2 Miller/Galante (Zimmer) total knee systems. Ceramic knees were used between 1982 and 1983, the PCA knees from 1983, the OrthoLoc knee from 1984, and the Miller/Galante knee in 1986. The patella was not replaced in 12 of the 48 PCA

[1]Department of Orthopedic Surgery, Kyushu University Hospital, Fukuoka, Japan

knees.

Postoperative management of uncemented total knee replacements was more limited than that of cemented ones. Suction drainage was discontinued at 24–48 h. Range of knee motion was started at 2–5 days postoperatively with or without the continuous passive motion (CPM) machine and partial weight bearing ambulation at 5–7 days. Full weight bearing without brace or aids was allowed at 2–3 months.

## Results

### Instrumentation and Prosthesis Design

The ceramic knee instrumentation system was simple but required too much eyeball judgment in making the bone cuts. Initial press-fit fixation of the prostheses was not always optimum. The instrumentation of the OrthoLoc system was simple and excellent in precise and reproducible cuts for the insertion of prostheses. Excellent initial stability was accomplished with the tibial components. The PCA knee instrumentation was overly complicated with many jigs; some eyeball judgment was required for femoral bone cuts. Although the instrumentation of the Miller/Galante system was also complicated, this system appeared to be better in the reproducibility of cuts than the PCA system.

Bone cement had to be used for one tibial component of the Ceramic knee, three tibial components of the PCA knee, and one femoral component of the OrthoLoc knee due to poor initial fixation. Initial stability of the tibial component could be best accomplished with the Miller/Galante system. The fixation screw of the tibial component of the PCA system did not appear to add further stability.

A limited range of prosthesis size was a problem with the OrthoLoc and PCA systems. A small size was not available with the OrthoLoc system and only the standard size was used in all six patients. With the PCA system, a small size was used in 40 knees and a medium size in eight knees. A wider range of prosthesis size was necessary, especially a smaller size, for Japanese patients.

Post-operative management of uncemented total knee replacement was more difficult than for cemented replacements. Early range of knee motion was occasionally deferred due to pain. A more cautious approach was required with range of motion exercises and ambulation due to a biomechanical concern about the bone-implant interface. Although full weight bearing was not allowed for 2 months, several patients did not follow the advice and apparently started full weight bearing ambulation as early as 1 week postoperatively.

### Complications

There were no cases of superficial or deep infection. Although we did not use any form of prophylactic anticoagulant therapy, none of our patients developed thromboembolic diseases.

One Ceramic patellar component fractured at 3 months postoperatively, requiring later revision (Fig. 1).

Symptomatic loosening of the tibial component occurred in one PCA knee approximately 10 months postoperatively, and revision surgery was

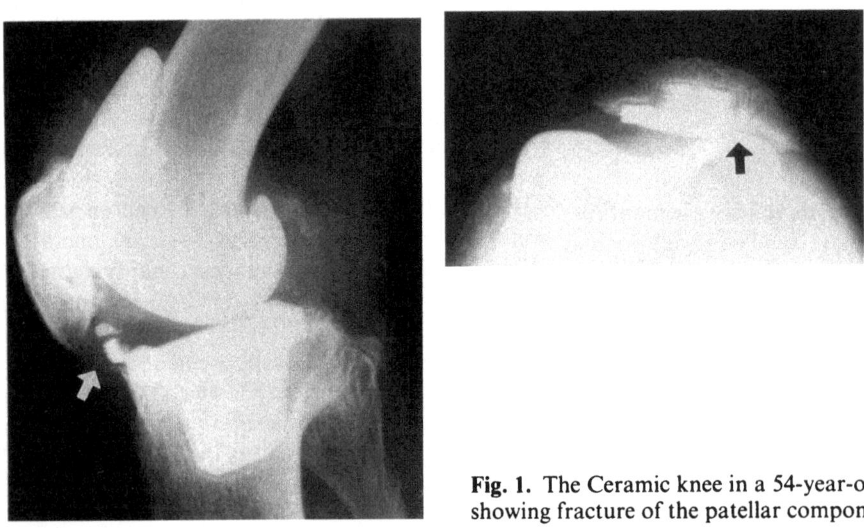

**Fig. 1.** The Ceramic knee in a 54-year-old male with osteoarthritis showing fracture of the patellar component (*arrows*)

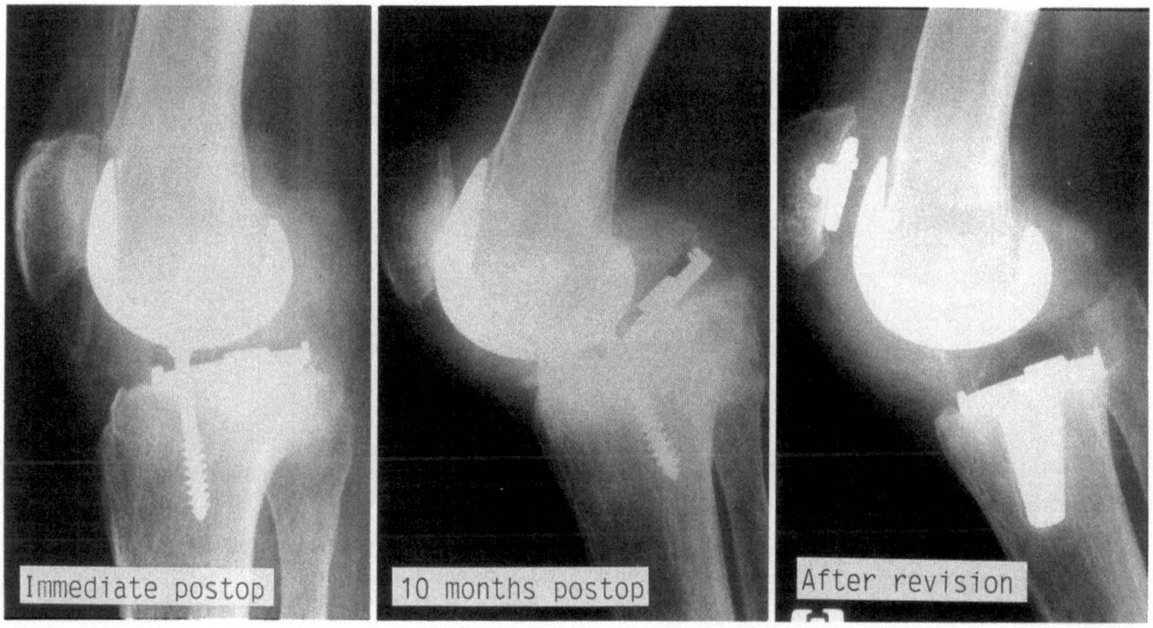


**Fig. 2.** Symptomatic loosening of the tibial component, which occurred in one PCA knee in a 60-year-old female with rheumatoid arthritis

performed using the stem-type tibial component without cement (Fig. 2). The patient was a 60-year-old female with rheumatoid arthritis. It was speculated that the loosening in this case was caused by two factors: inadequate size of the prosthesis, which did not entirely cover the cortical bone of the tibial cut surface, and osteoporosis, which would have induced progression of sinking. Although the femoral component was clinically stable without evidence of a radiolucency for 1 year, that component was easily removed and only small fragments of bone were attached to the porous coating surface. The patellar articular surface, which was not replaced at the initial surgery, showed progression of degenerative changes and, therefore, the patella was replaced at the time of revision.

All Ceramic knees developed radiolucencies at the implant-bone interface which could be noted as early as 3 months postoperatively. Although symptomatic loosening was not noted at an average follow-up of 3.5 years, use of the Ceramic knee was abandoned for fear that radiolucencies would progress to symptomatic loosening (Fig. 3). One PCA knee showed a radiolucency at the patellar bone-implant interface. This patient occasionally complained of mild discomfort about the anterior aspect of the knee, which may have been related to possible loosening of the patellar component. No significant radiolucency has been observed in the OrthoLoc and the Miller/Galante Knees.

Significant subsidence of the tibial components occurred in three PCA knees and one Ceramic knee. All of these knees were asymptomatic and clinical results were excellent. One PCA knee in a 73-year-old female has shown slowly progressive subsidence and has been kept under careful observation (Fig. 4).

Separation of the porous coating beads was noted on postoperative roentgenograms from nine tibial, six patellar, and five femoral components of the PCA knees. This was already observed on the immediate postoperative films, suggesting that the beads were detached from the substrate at the time of insertion of the prosthesis.

Patellar problems were seen in four knees, including one dislocation in the Ceramic knee and three subluxations in the PCA knees, which were mainly related to operative technique. In none of these knees was a lateral release performed at the initial surgery. Incorrect bone cut was noted in two patellae of these knees: resection of the medial facet was not sufficient. A lateral release was performed 3 years postoperatively on one knee with patellar subluxation which showed poor range of knee motion.

For poor range of knee motion, manipulation under anesthesia was performed on four PCA knees and one Miller/Galante knee at 4–6 weeks post-operatively.

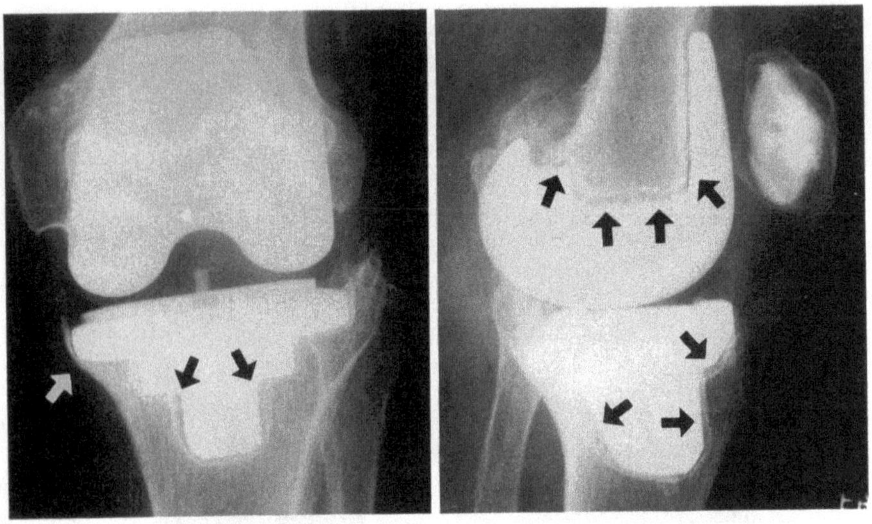

**Fig. 3.** Five years postoperative roentgenograms of the Ceramic knee showing significant radiolucencies at the bone-implant interfaces (*black arrows*). Note subsidence of the tibial component in the medial tibial condyle (*white arrow*)

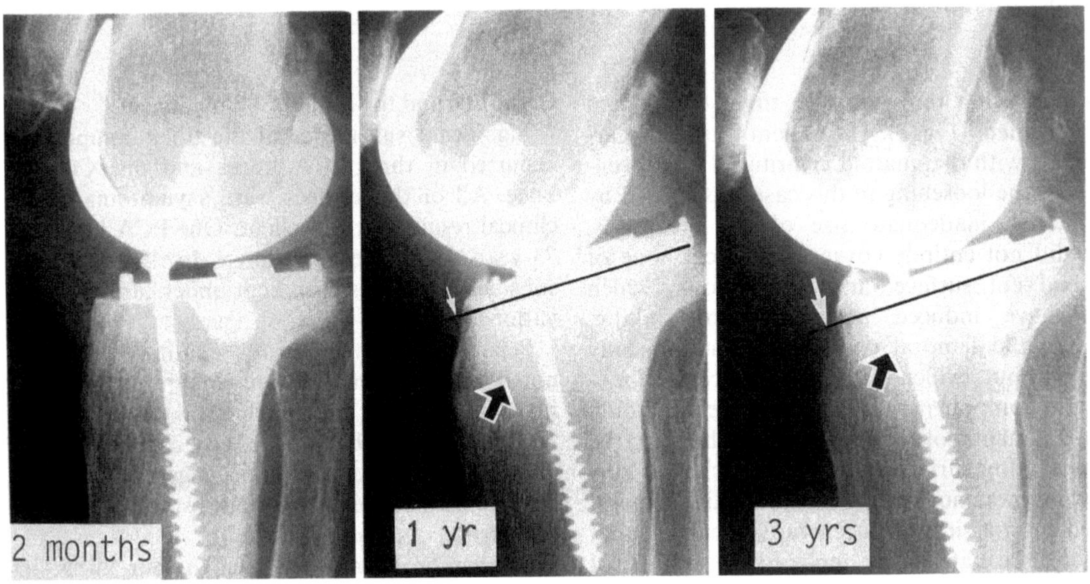


**Fig. 4.** The PCA knee in a 73-year-old female with osteoarthritis, showing slowly progressive subsidence of the tibial component (*white arrow*). Note sclerotic change of bone underneath the anterior portion of the tibial component, suggesting stress concentration (*black arrows*)

## Clinical Results of Primary Cementless Total Knee Replacements

Clinical results were evaluated at the average follow-up period of 42 months for 15 Ceramic knees, 27 months for six OrthoLoc knees, 21 months for 48 PCA knees and 4 months for two Miller/Galante knees.

No significant differences were found in the range of knee motion between the four types of total knee system with mean flexion 95°–110°. The best range of motion was noted in a PCA knee with 140° of flexion. On the other hand the poorest range of motion was 50° in a PCA knee which underwent arthrotomy for release of adhesion. Although the continuous passive motion (CPM machine) was introduced in the postoperative management of these patients in 1985, no significant improvement was noted in the attained range of knee motion with the use of the CPM machine.

Overall results were evaluated with the Insall knee score system [3]. Scores of more than 85 were estimated as excellent, between 70 and 84 as good, between 60 and 69 as fair and less than 60 as poor. Eighty percent of the Ceramic knees, 83% of the OrthoLoc knees, and 90% of the PCA knees were rated as excellent or good. Although the follow-up period was short, two Miller/Galante knees were rated as excellent. Among the knees with good results, two Ceramic, one OrthoLoc, and two PCA knees showed occasional discomfort. Poor results were seen in two Ceramic knees, one with a fracture of the patellar component and the other with patellar dislocation, and in two PCA knees, one with loosening of the tibial component and the other without patellar resurfacing which showed retropatellar pain.

## Discussion

Although the uncemented total knee replacement is a fascinating alternative to a more conventional cemented procedure, careful selection of patients and advanced surgical technique are essential. We think that osteoporosis and inappropriate size of the prosthesis are two major risk factors in loosening. Great attention should be paid to initial stability of the prostheses at the time of surgery. It is of supreme importance that the tibial component be placed entirely over the cortical bone of the tibial cut surface to avoid subsidence of the prosthesis. In our experience, optimum initial stability of the tibial component was not always achieved with the Ceramic, the OrthoLoc and the PCA systems, suggesting the need for better press-fit fixation of prostheses.

Our results suggest that bone ingrowth at the bone-implant interface does not always occur with the materials presently available. In particular, the ceramic prosthesis appeared to be separated from bone by fibrous tissue. It was surprising to find that the femoral component of the PCA knee was easily removed at the time of revision surgery for the loosened tibial component. Although the femoral component was clinically stable in this case without evidence of radiolucency for one year, only small fragments of bone were attached to the porous coating surface of the extracted prosthesis. Similar findings have been recently reported by several authors [1, 5]. Whether or not the lack of bone ingrowth leads to symptomatic loosening is a question that awaits longer experience in cementless porous-coated knee arthroplasty.

Separation of the porous-coating beads from the substrate in PCA knees has been observed by several authors. Rosenqvist et al. [6] have drawn attention to and expressed concern over the phenomenon of loose beads following implantation of the PCA prosthesis in a group of patients with rheumatoid arthritis. Ranawat et al. [5] suggested poor integrity of the metal beads to the solid metal substrate.

Most of our patellar problems were related to surgical technique. It is important that both medial and lateral facets be equally resected and the patellar tracking be balanced to avoid subluxation or dislocation. We have paid special attention to the effect of surgical dissection on the patellar blood flow because we think that adequate bone blood flow is necessary for biological fixation of the patellar component. Experimental study has shown that patellar blood flow is significantly decreased if fat pad removal and lateral release are combined [4]. Therefore, it is important that the fat pad be preserved as much as possible or lateral superior genicular vessels be preserved when a lateral release is performed. In fear of patellar complications, the patella was not replaced in 12 of 48 PCA knees. Of these 12 knees, only one knee has shown retropatellar pain. We do not know the long-term outcome of nonresurfaced patellae, however it is possible that they will develop further degeneration, resulting in a painful patella.

Postoperative management of uncemented total knee replacements was more difficult than that of cemented ones due to greater blood loss and a biomechanical concern related to strength of initial fixation of prostheses and bone ingrowth. Although the CPM machine is a convenient tool for the range of motion exercise, it should be kept in mind that muscle power is not strengthened by this machine and that there is no significant difference in the attained range of motion between knees with and without CPM exercises. The average range of knee motion in our patients was 95° at follow-up. This may not be satisfactory for elderly Japanese patients because they are used to sitting on the floor with the knees fully flexed. We speculate that one of the causes of a poor range of motion is related to the surface design of the prostheses.

## Conclusions

Although uncemented total knee replacements implanted into well-vascularized and mechanically sound bone will produce a stable and painless interface, it is still necessary to develop optimum press-fit fixation and strength to allow early rehabilitation and a new surface design to give a near-anatomical range of knee motion.

The interpretation of the eventual nature of the biological fixation of the bone-implant interface requires longer clinical experience and further basic research.

## References

1. Cook SD, Scheller AD, Anderson RC, Haddad RJ (1986) Histologic and microradiographic analysis of a revised porous-coated anatomic (PCA) patellar component. A case report. Clin Orthop 202: 147–151
2. Hungerford DS, Kenna RV (1983) Preliminary experience with a total knee prosthesis with porous coating used without cement. Clin Orthop 176: 95–107
3. Insall JN, Ranawat CS, Aglietti P, Shine J (1979) A comparison of four models of total knee-replacement prostheses. J Bone Joint Surg 58-A: 754–765
4. Ogata K, Shively RA, Shoenecker PL, Chang S-L (1987) Effects of standard surgical procedures on the patellar blood flow in monkeys. Clin Orthop 215: 254–259
5. Ranawat CS, Johanson NA, Rimnac CM et al. (1986) Retrieval analysis of porous-coated components for total knee arthroplasty. Clin Orthop 209: 244–248
6. Rosenqvist R, Bylander B, Knutson K, et al. (1986) Loosening of the porous coating of bicompartmental prostheses in patients with rheumatoid arthritis. J Bone Joint Surg 68-A: 538–542

## *Discussion*

*Miller* (McGill University): You showed a PCA knee which had sunk anteriorly. Was that an osteoarthritic or rheumatoid case?

*Ogata* (Kyushu University Hospital): The patient was a 73-year-old women with osteoarthritis. She had very severe varus deformity preoperatively. The patient was rather small for the femoral component, but she had quite a big tibial cut surface for the small tibial components. We had to insert a small component on the tibial side. That is the main reason for the sinking.

*Miller*: We have seen in rheumatoid patients what we consider a different mechanism for loosening, one which we distinguished from the situation where there is progressive increase in the size of a radiolucent line. We have observed acute loosenings which we believe to be due to cancellous bone failure and while we have seen these in osteoarthritics they are more common in rheumatoid patients.

# Clinical Experience with the Cementless Application of the PCA Knee and Bone Remodeling by Computerized X-ray Analysis

G. Bontemps[1] and J. Mockenhaupt[2]

**Summary.** The calculated forces on the knee joint with an implanted Porous Coated Anatomic (PCA) prosthesis and the resultant stresses on the bone anchorage are reviewed. The analysis reveals considerable loading at the tibia and patella, which can exceed the load-carrying capacity of the bone. Two tibial and three patellar loosenings confirmed this risk during a 4-year follow-up of 89 cementless PCA knee prostheses. An evaluation of these complications shows that the basic failure is breakage of the bone overloaded from eccentric force application. At the tibia, slight overcorrection of the preexisting frontal deformity is advised to compensate for muscular insufficiencies and to strive for neutral dynamic alignment. At the patella the design should minimize excentric loading in extreme flexion without compromising wear. The densitometric analysis showed remodeling at the tibia for about one year. Stable interfaces had only minor changes at a later stage.

**Keywords:** Bone ingrowth—Cementless fixation—Porous cobalt-chrome—Interface stress—Bone remodeling

## Reasons and Rationale for the Cementless Implantation Technique

Late aseptic loosening still represents the main problem in alloarthroplasty. Fixation of endoprostheses with bone-cement is quite satisfactory for short-and medium-term ranges, however over longer periods of observation the shortcomings become evident. These are primarily due to low tear and shear strength, the low fatigue strength and brittleness and—most importantly—resting macro-phages are often found at the interface and must be regarded as biologically unstable [5].

The danger of infection is another important matter. Germs can spread unhindered on the surface of the poly-methylmethacrylate as the nonvascularized tissue keeps them beyond the reach of cellular defence mechanisms. The addition of antibiotics to the cement introduced by Buchholz and Engelbrecht [4] is an attempt to meet this problem and shows good intermediate results. However in the long run we still have to cope with the danger of infection.

Improved cementing techniques with low-viscosity cement—pulsatile lavage and cement pressurization—have also been unable to avoid these handicaps. In the case of revision, owing to greater depth of cement penetration, more bone stock has to be sacrificed. It is also to be noted that the fatigue strength of these cements is even lower.

Efforts toward improving the quality of the cement as well as its application were made simultaneously with tests on direct anchorage of the prosthesis to the bone. Although the latter lead back to the beginnings of artificial joint replacement in general, it was expected that the shortcomings of the former systems might be avoided by a more advanced prosthesis design. Yamamoto et al. [24] and Freeman et al. [10] were the first to use the press-fit techniques in combination with new design features for knee prostheses. They put priority on minimizing the interface stresses under the following criteria:

- Unlinked, semiconstrained surface replacement
- Stability provided by balanced capsuloligamentous complex
- Large prosthesis/bone surface area and intimate prosthesis/bone contact
- Correct leg alignment
- Exact component positioning

Special instruments were developed to achieve precise and reproducible implantation and to assist deformity correction as well as soft-tissue adjustment.

Subsequently, numerous attempts were made to improve the cementless integration of the prostheses. Along with screws, pegs, etc., microstructured surfaces have been developed to allow bone or tissue ingrowth in order to ensure "biological" fixation. The results of studies with porous surfaces of sintered cobalt-chrome beads by Pilliar et al. [18] and Robertson et al. [21] were employed in the design of the PCA prosthesis. Hungerford et

[1] Fabricius-Klinik Remscheid, Remscheid, Federal Republic of Germany
[2] Anatomisches Institut der Universitaet Koeln, Federal Republic of Germany

al. [14] have described the features and rationale of this three-compartmental semiconstrained surface replacement extensively.

In the following, some of the features which are especially important for the cementless application are presented. All fixation interfaces of the PCA knee are coated with a double layer of cobalt-chrome beads, which form a three-dimensional porous surface. The mean pore size is 425 μm with a porosity of 35%. This large pore size was chosen to allow tissue ingrowth despite the relative movements between the prosthesis and bone, which are inevitable even in a perfect stable fit.

The inducible displacement of the prosthesis on the tibia condyle, where it is most evident with eccentric loading, was registered at 100–300 μm (Pauly 1986, personal communication). Ryd [22] even reported a mean displacement of 700 μm for the cementless PCA, but these patients were treated postoperatively with immediate full weight bearing. The cemented components also had inducible displacements ranging from 200–1000 μm. With perfect stability, tissue and bone ingrowth in such porous surfaces has been found in several animal studies and in the meantime also has been confirmed by explanted prostheses from humans [8, 12].

The advantage of such a porous structure over nonporous material is that once tissue ingrowth has taken place the interface becomes able to transmit shear and tensile forces. The resistance of this compound against shear forces ranges, according to animal studies, from 7.0 to 17 $MN/m^2$ [2, 21]. These values would be satisfactory to withstand the expected shear forces.

The sagittal shear forces along the X-axis have to be calculated at twice the body weight (Fig. 1), which comes to approximately 1500 N [23]. These shear forces are less important on the femoral component because of its inherent three-sided stability. However, in the tibial component the interface mechanism must be able to withstand these significant shear forces. They are, of course, variable depending on the constraint of the prosthesis. According to studies by Postak et al. [19], the anterior stability of the PCA prosthesis was 600 N and the posterior stability 1000 N before he registered failure through dislocation or gross polyethylene deformation. For a rough calculation of the stresses at the interface we divide these values by 2000 $mm^2$ of the bone/prosthesis contact area. The resulting interface shear strength is below 1 $N/mm^2$. This level can be reached by most porous materials and is well under the above-mentioned range of 7–17 $N/mm^2$. The shear forces in the

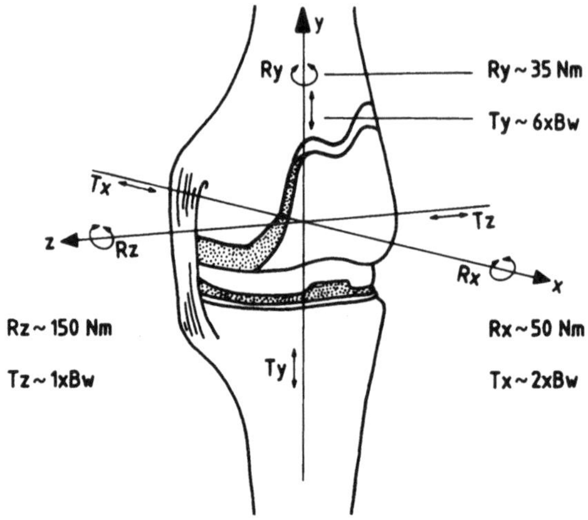


**Fig. 1.** Forces and moments at the knee

medial-lateral direction are lower—500 N for the PCA [19].

For the rotational torque, the following values were reported. Internal and external rotation around the Y-axis was up to 35 N. m [17]. In the design of the PCA prosthesis special attention was paid to the imitation of the torque rotation pattern in the normal knee. Therefore, the resulting shear stresses at the fixation interface are in the safe region [19].

The varus-valgus angulation around the x-axis has moment values of up to 50 N. m, mostly as the so-called functional genu varum [7]. Angular deformities or misalignment, of course, increase this value considerably. The flexion-extension moment around the z-axis has reported moment values of up to approximately 150 N. m [16, 23].

The latter two loads are absorbed by tensile forces in the capsulo-ligamentous system and muscles and transformed mainly into compressive forces at the joint. For compressive forces in the vertical direction, the values reported go up to six times body-weight, i.e., approximately 5000 N [15–17]. This level implies that with a supporting area of 2000 $mm^2$, loadings on an area of about 2.5 $N/mm^2$ are attained if the stress is uniformly distributed. This is the mean value of area forces permissible on cancellous bone of the tibia, which has a compressive strength of 1–6 $N/mm^2$ [1, 9, 13].

Because the strength of the proximal tibia decreases with the depth below the subchondral plate, the level of bone resection should be as proximal as possible. To reduce the stresses on the area, the prosthesis should also rest upon the whole surface of the top of the tibia including the cortices. The PCA comes in four sizes to ensure these possibilities in most cases. As the bone at the femoral condyles is usually stronger than at the tibia, the margin of safety is larger here [6].

The forces in the patellofemoral joint are reported to be up to four times body-weight for climbing stairs [20, 23]. Because the bone/prosthesis contact areas are smaller, about 400 $mm^2$, the calculated interface stresses can exceed the upper level of the permissible stresses in the cancellous bone. In flexed activity patterns, this anchorage is thus highly stressed. The risk might even increase because of the difficulty in calculating shear forces and tilting moments with eccentric proximal or distal loading in different flexion positions (Fig. 2).

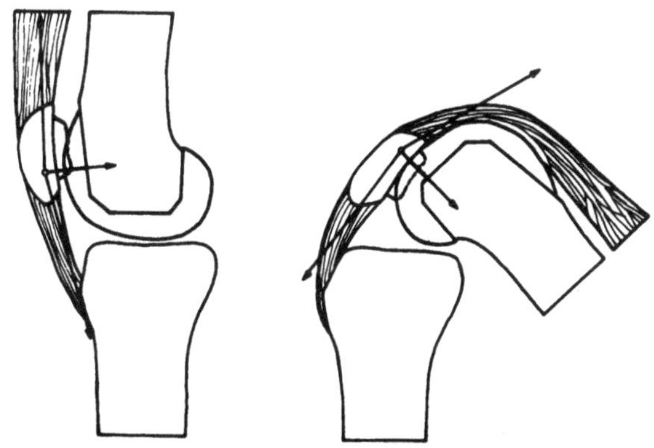

**Fig. 2.** Peripheral force application to the patellar component with flexion beyond 90°

## Prerequisite for Biological Fixation

The deciding factors for the application of the cementless implantation technique are the quality of the bone and the quality of the fit. In our experience, 70% of the supporting bone surface should be vital enough to allow for potential ingrowth. This process resembles fracture healing. Any local and systemic factors which impair fracture healing will also affect the ingrowth of bone into a porous surface. Furthermore, the bone must have sufficient strength to provide rigid initial fixation and a good press-fit. No tilting should occur when putting the prosthesis through the full range of movement. Primary stability and the achievement of intimate bone/prosthesis contact are imperative conditions for bone ingrowth.

Smaller bone cysts are filled with cancellous chips and should not impair the biological fixation process considerably. Larger bone defects of up to one-third of the supporting surface can be compensated with corticocancellous grafts. These are usually gained from the femoral condyles and/or the other tibial plateau.

Extensive bone destruction, usually in connection with extreme deformities (>30°), is a contraindication to the application of the cementless PCA system.

Concerning the postoperative management, a partial weight-bearing period of 2–4 months is judged essential for bone adaptation and remodeling. Patients who have larger bone grafts should be protected for an even longer period.

## Materials and Methods

From April 1983 until September 1986, 95 PCA prostheses in 87 patients were implanted cementless in at least two components. In seven cases, the tibia was cemented, in two the femur, and in nine the patella. In ten cases, the patella was not replaced. Two patients died from unrelated causes and three patients with four prostheses were lost to follow-up, leaving 89 cases for detailed review. Roughly 60% of them had osteo-arthritis, the rest inflammatory diseases. The follow-up ranged from 9 months to 4 years with an average of 2.3 years. The age distribution showed the greatest number of patients to be between 60 and 80 years. The youngest was 28 years, the oldest 86. The average age was 66 years, 72 years for osteoarthritis (OA) and 59 for rheumatoid arthritis (RA).

The follow-up evaluation was done according to a slightly modified British Orthopaedic Association (BOA) system, first after a 3-month, later after a 6-month interval.

## Results

Cases of OA and RA are analyzed together because they did not show much difference in most respects.

The leading symptom for undergoing surgery was *pain*. It was almost completely eliminated in 27 cases and completely eliminated in 59 cases (together 97%) by this procedure. Only three patients complained of moderate pain; the reason was algodystrophy in one case, a loosened patellar component in another, and patellar subluxation in the third.

The postoperative analysis showed that 85% could *walk* for more than 30 min. Here, the OA patients did slightly better than the RA patients who were handicapped by other diseased joints. In three RA cases, this was also the reason for the limitation of the walking ability to 10 min. Eighteen patients (mostly RA) used walking aids.

The *range of movement* is demonstrated in Fig. 3. The mean flexion ability beyond 100° is important for rising from a chair, and nearly complete extension is important for economical walking.

Long AP X-rays revealed correct *leg alignment*. In 93% of cases, we found physiological conditions with a femorotibial valgus of 2°–10°. Four cases were in varus and two in valgus. In all of these cases the original deformity was not totally corrected. Analysis of each component showed that malpositioning of the tibial prosthesis was responsible for the varus deviation and that of the femoral component for the valgus. These faults happened initially when using the first set of instruments without the intramedullary femoral rod.

Checking the X-rays, we found *loose beads* under the tibial prosthesis in 31 cases; this was less frequent (12 cases) at the femur and five cases at the patella. This is in our opinion due to micromotion at the interface, if beads are knocked off during implantation. This cannot be avoided totally during the fixation process when the prosthesis settles, especially on the tibial side. As long as the number of loose beads does not exceed five and does not increase we consider the phenomenon harmless, as in the case of Fig. 4, which shows an excellent clinical result after 3 years.

*Radiolucent* lines of more than 1 mm were registered at the bone/prosthesis border in 22 cases, mainly at the outer medial and lateral areas of the tibial condyles (Fig. 5). We saw a dorsal narrow demarcation line in three cases at the femur, and in five cases at the patella. These signs usually appeared in the first year and did not subsequently show significant progression, except of course in cases of loosening.

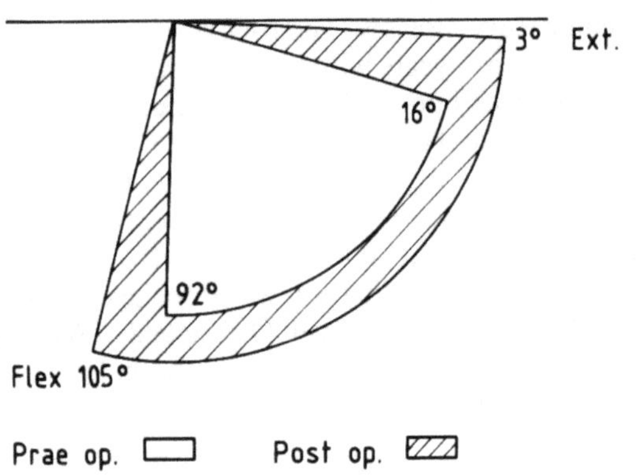

**Fig. 3.** Pre- and postoperative range of motion

## Computerized Densitometric X-Ray Evaluation

The anteroposterior (AD) radiographs were analyzed with an image-analyzing system (IBAS II, Kontron, Eching, Federal Republic of Germany). The radiographs were scanned with a K30 videocamera (Siemens, Berlin, Federal Republic of Germany) through an S-Orthoplaner macro-lens (Zeiss, Oberkochen, Federal Republic of Germany) by transmitting illumination. The IBAS II is equipped for conversion of analog brightness to digital grey-values. By the application of several functions, it is able to evaluate the X-ray images. Image pixels are stored in an array with a size of 512 × 512 points. The grey values are 0–255 for each pixel.

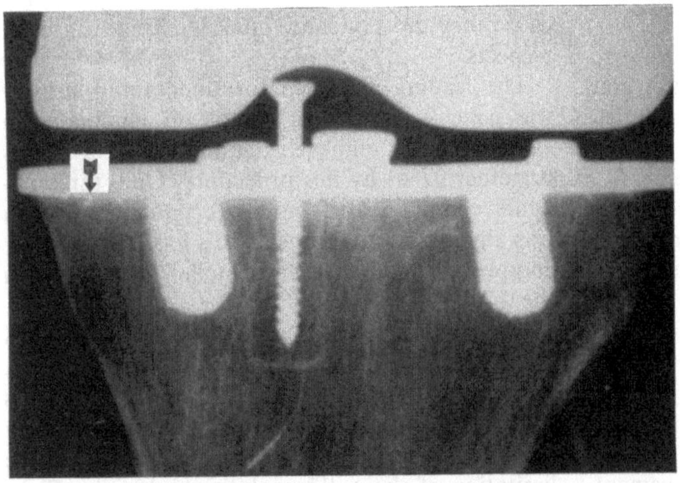

**Fig. 4.** Anteroposterior radiograph to show beads separated from tibial tray with stable interface 3 years after implantation

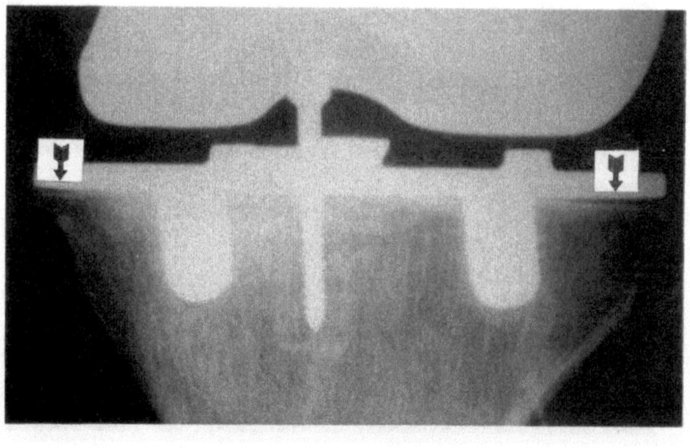

**Fig. 5.** Anteroposterior radiograph to show non-progressive radiolucency underbeneath the borders of the metal tray 3 years postoperatively

The first instruction in the measuring program was an average function to reduce camera noise. The image is improved by shading correction, followed by median filtering at a size 5 × 5 and a rank of 13.

The grey values were arranged and attributed to pseudo-colors: Dark-blue symbolizes lower density; light-blue, green, and yellow mark higher densities; red marks the greatest density. Radiographs offer no reference scales of density. Therefore, the grey-levels of the images could not be standardized, for example, in comparison to an aluminium wedge. Hence, the measuring procedure allowed an analysis of density distribution only in the same image. Precise evaluation concerning changes in density in several images was not possible.

The process described is recommended for observing special zones of radiographs with respect to their relative densities. The analysis showed areas of osteolysis at the tibia beneath the outer medial and lateral borders of the metal tray, running distally beside the pegs. These areas of osteolysis were not found beneath the central part of the metal tray. Here we noticed, usually more on the medial side, a zone of X-ray density growing weaker distally. This zone reached the density of the compacta directly beneath the metal tray and grew weaker distally where it ran down from the pegs to link with the diaphysial corticalis.

The osteolyses at the borders were judged to be the result of lack of stress on the bone. The bone beneath the central part of the metal tray has to take more stress after the implantation of the prosthesis and therefore starts to reinforce itself. This is evident in the increased bone density. In natural joints, it is mainly the tibial condyles that are stressed.

After a period of adaptation of approximately 1 year, we found only a few changes in the distribution of bone density in the series surveyed, showing that resorption as well as restructuring of the bone were equal. This might indicate stabilization and acceptance of the prosthesis.

## Complications

The complications are listed in Table 1.

The two cases of loosening of the *tibial component* occurred in very active and overweight women. The primary diagnosis for both was osteoarthritis. It is note-worthy that 6 months postoperatively these patients still complained of pain during weight bearing. At that time, X-rays did not show any striking irregularities at the inter-

**Table 1.** Complications

| Complication | Number of cases | Treatment | Result |
|---|---|---|---|
| Tibial component loosening | 2 | Revision | OK |
| Patellar component loosening | 3 | Revision (2 cases) | OK |
| Patellar component maltracking | 2 | Distal realignment, | OK |
| | | proximal realignment | Recurrence |
| Patellar fracture | 1 | Revision | OK |
| Instability | 1 | Revision | OK |
| Delayed Healing | 1 | | OK |
| Thrombosis | 2 | | OK |

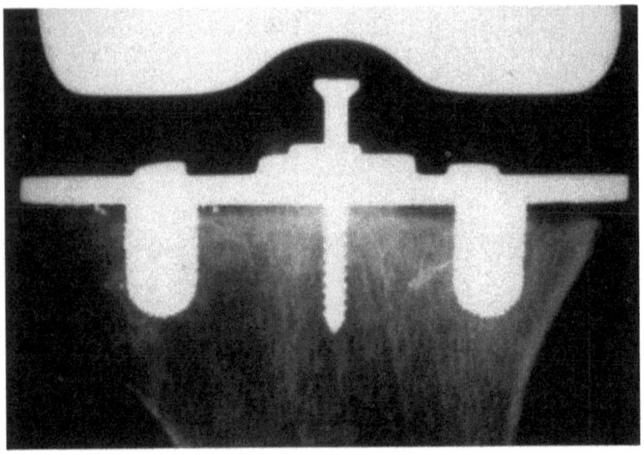

**Fig. 6.** Postoperative X-ray at 10 months shows a loosened tibial component with slight varus displacement

face. However, in one of the cases, we found broad osteolysis under the tibial plateau (Fig. 6) with a slight varus displacement 10 months postoperatively. Basic mistakes in implantation were not evident. The original alignment was correct. During revision operation, osteonecrotic changes were evident in the central area of the tibial condyle. Therefore, we assume the failure to have been caused by overstraining the bone of this 102-kg patient with too early an introduction of full weight bearing 10 weeks postoperatively.

In the second case, a slight varus tilt of the tibial component (95°) might have caused the loosening. Radiolucency and separated beads under the medial part of the metal tray became obvious at 9 months follow-up. With time, these signs increased together with the complaints so that revision had to be performed 1 1/2 years after implantation.

In both cases, histological examination of the tissue attached to the porous coating revealed connective tissue with vascularity and some chondroid cell units.

These findings were different in one case in which the tibial component was exchanged after 2.3 years because of varus-valgus instability. The same patient had a separated patellar prosthesis described below. The tibial component was clinically well fixed to the bone. The X-ray showed a thin radiolucent line underneath the metal tray with adjacent sclerotic bone and five loose beads. The bead on the lateral polyethylene plateau probably originated from the patella (Fig. 7a). The microradiograph demonstrates the bone layer more precisely (Fig. 7b). Direct contact to the beads at the surface was visible in some regions, but there was no considerable ingrowth in the interconnective spaces. This was also evident in the histological examination (Fig. 7c). The bone made close contact with the beaded surface, but in the pores we found mainly connective tissue.

Concerning the *patella*, the following complications were noted. Three loosenings of the patellar component occurred in very active women with flexion abilities of 115°–125°. These patients were overweight, 90–105 kg, and the basic disease in two of them was osteoarthritis. One patient had complete separation of the patellar prosthesis (as mentioned above). In the other two cases, radiolucency at the base plate and osteolysis around the pegs indicated loosening (Fig. 8). One patient is at present awaiting surgery, reoperation was carried out on the other two and a cemented component was inserted. Two patellar maltracking problems necessitated reoperation. The proximal realignment did not last very long. The distal realignment was successful. The one patellar fracture of the proximal pole healed after revision.

The overall classification was done using a slightly modified Hungerford scoring system [14]. This evaluates pain, stability, deformity, range of movement, and flexion contraction as well as quadriceps forces. Using this system we obtained 90% good and excellent results (excellent 46%, good 44%, fair 6%, poor 4%). The revision cases remained in their group as noted before reoperation, which means that the two tibial and two patellar loosenings are classified as "poor." The "fair" group includes the other revision cases—the third case of loosened patella and one patient with pain and poor motion.

## Discussion

Component loosening occurred mainly in OA not in RA patients. The latter had softer porous bone on the one hand, but usually also less weight and, in particular, fewer functional demands.

The two *tibial loosenings* show that cementless fixation of that component still presents a prob-

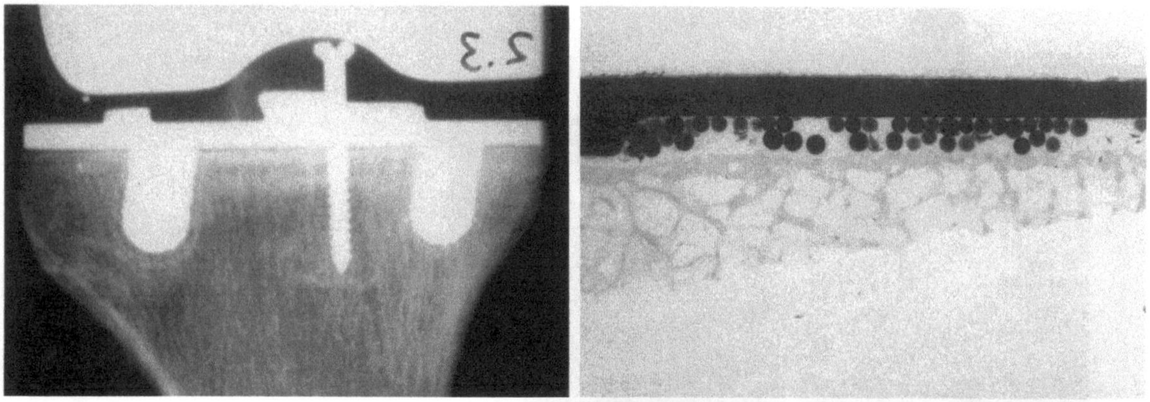

a b

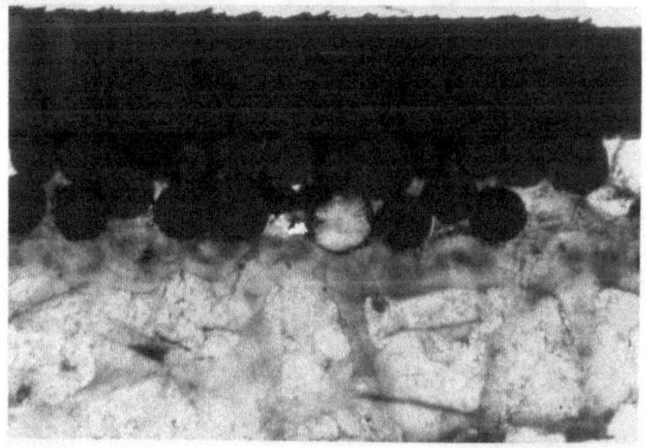

c

**Fig. 7. a** Radiograph taken 2.3 years after operation. For explanation see text. **b** Microradiograph of section through tibial component. Close contact of bone and porous surface is seen **c** Histological section of the tissue at the tibial tray. Bony apposition to the beaded surface is evident

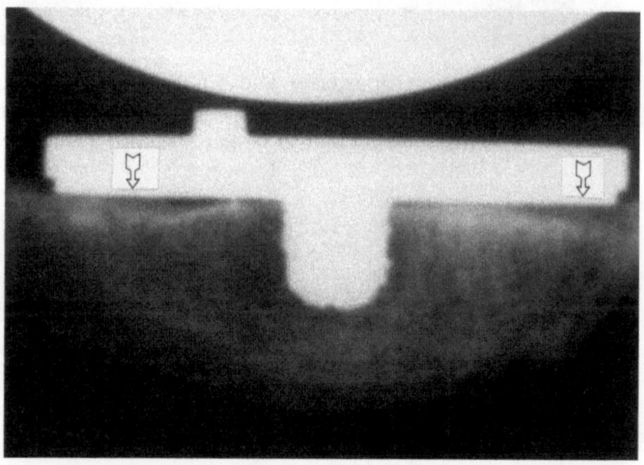

**Fig. 8.** Close-up of a lateral view showing loosened cementless PCA patellar prosthesis. Wedge-shaped radiolucency at the base plate indicating tilting due to eccentric loading

lem. Even with perfect static alignment, the dynamic forces occurring during walking are individually different and difficult to calculate. Especially problematic are the mediolateral movements of the main vertical force vector, primarily in the sense of the so-called functional genu varum [7]. This causes mediolateral tilting motions on the tibial plateau with micromovement and considerable increasing peak loads stressing the anchorage. Metal reinforcement of the polyethylene reduces high local compressive stresses to the underlying bone but also creates greater displacement with eccentric loading and higher tensile forces on the unloaded side. If the bone breaks down on the overloaded side with resulting component subsidence, the implant might lift off the bone on the unloaded side unless prevented by biological fixation (Fig. 9). Freeman et al. [10] devised a relatively long medullary stem for their tibial component to neutralize the tilting moments. We have tried to counteract the crushing of the bone on the loaded side which is responsible for the failure by reducing the forces with a slight overcorrection of the previous malalignment. In particular the varus deformity,

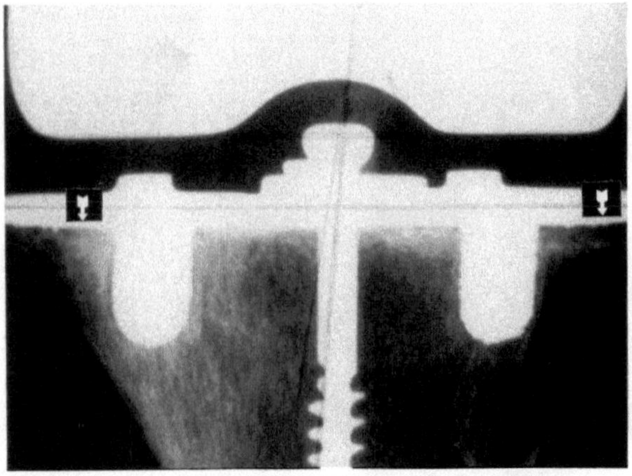

**Fig. 9.** Anteroposterior X-ray at 2.5 years shows medial component subsidence and lateral elevation despite correct static alignment

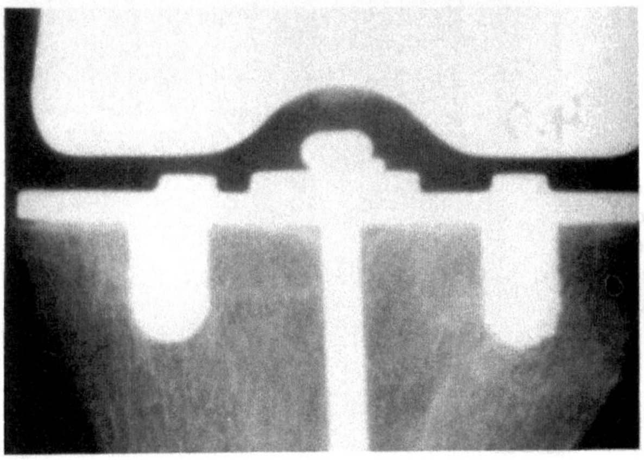

a

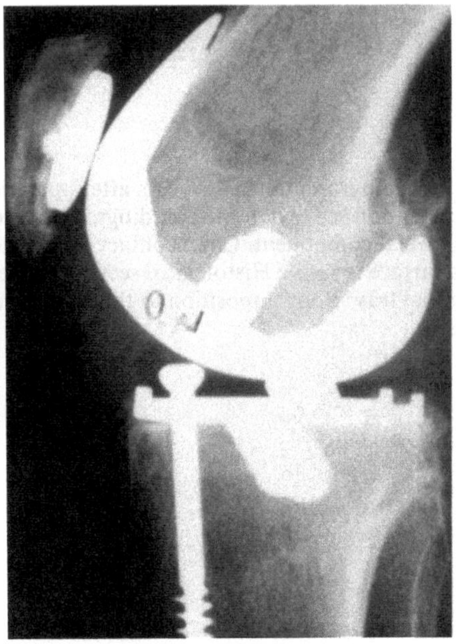

b

**Fig. 10. a** Anteroposterior and **b** lateral view of a non-cemented PCA prosthesis 4 years after implantation, showing intimate contact of bone to fixation interfaces

progression of which is at least partly due to the weakening of the dynamic stabilizers (tractus iliotibialis, biceps femoris, etc.), needs this slight (1°–2°) over-correction towards valgus [11, 15].

With regard to tibial osteotomy, our experience has been established over a long period. In our opinion, it is also valid for artificial knee replacement since here too the alignment-related decompensation usually reverts back to the initial deformity because of persistent muscular insufficiencies.

For the future, one can only hope that more sophisticated analysis of gait will provide a more precise definition of the individual force vectors. This will enable us to discard empirical measures and to strive for dynamic neutral alignment of the main walking phases on a more scientific basis. For the time being only the postoperative remodelling of the bone shows us whether we have reached our goal. The bone needs approximately 1 year for adaptation. We found that once stabilization was reached after this period there was no sign of any decompensation during the observation period of more than 4 years (Fig. 10). Theoretically, decompensation can only be expected if alterations occur in the biomechanical or biological conditions.

The anchoring of the *patellar prosthesis* is also still a problem. Primarily, we were unable in nine cases to achieve a good press-fit stability, which forced us to perform cement fixation. There was also some loosening of three cementless components. The high forces on the patellar anchoring mentioned above can exceed the load-bearing capacity of the bone. The design of the "anatomical patella" and the relatively conforming femoral groove increase both the shear forces and the tilting moments. In particular, the eccentric forces during extensive flexion can put too much strain on the anchoring as illustrated by the three failures in the overweight patients with more than average good flexion.

The newly developed "dome patella" is less constrained and exposed to peripheral force application and fits more securely with its three pegs. However, it remains to be seen if this will also minimize the risk of loosening. Increasing wear is probable because of a smaller contact area of polyethylene against the patellar groove. However, such pressure distribution exceeding the yield stress of the polyethylene is also found in many similar designs. The fact that wear problems have not been apparent in the past shows that the stresses in femoropatellar joints of these patients were lower because of the reduced flexion activity.

## Conclusion

Primary stabilization of the tibial components succeeds well in most cases, though secondary biological fixation is sensitive and can be endangered and compromised by overweight and errors in the alignment. However, bone adaptation is usually adequate and stabilizes the prosthesis satisfactorily. This was also confirmed by X-ray densitometric examinations.

Fixation of the patellar prosthesis is not yet fully satisfactory. Nine components had to be cemented since there was not enough press-fit stability. Three cementless components loosened. Whether the modified version with three pegs provides advantages remains to be seen.

Biological stabilization of the femoral component was reliable and did not cause any problems.

## References


1. Bargren JH, Day WH, Freeman MAR, Swanson SAV (1978) Mechanical tests on the tibial components of non hinged knee prostheses. J Bone Joint Surg (Br) 60: 256
2. Bobyn JD, Pilliar RM, Cameron MB, Weatherly GC, Kent GM (1980) The effect of porous surface configuration on the tensile strength of fixation of implants by bone ingrowth. Clin Orthop Rel Res 149: 291
3. Bobyn JD, Pilliar RM, Camerson HU, Weatherly CG (1980) The optimum pore size for the fixation of porous-surfaced metal implants by the ingrowth of bone. Clin Orthop Rel Res 150: 263
4. Buchholz HW, Engelbrecht H (1970) Über die Depotwirkung einiger Antibiotika bei Vermischung mit dem Kunstharz Palacos. Chirurg 41: 511–515
5. Charnley J (1979) Low friction arthroplasty of the hip: Theory and practice Springer, Berlin
6. Colley J, Cameron HU, Freeman MAR, Swanson SAV (1978) Loosening of the femoral component in surface replacement of the knee. Arch Orthop Traumat Surg 92: 31
7. Debrunner AM, Seewald K (1964) Die Belastung des Kniegelenkes in der Frontalebene. Z Orthop 98:508
8. Edmunds JO (1986) Biologic fixation of total knee—Implant retrieval studies. Third Remscheider Knee Symposium. Howmedica, Kiel, FRG
9. Evans FG (1973) Mechanical properties of bone. Thomas, Springfield
10. Freeman MAR, Samuelson KM, Bertin KC (1985) Freeman-Samuelson total arthroplasty of the knee. Clin Orthop Rel Res 192: 46
11. Grammont P (1985) Einfluss der Patella auf das Gleichgewicht des Kniegelenkes. Orthopädie 14: 193
12. Cook SD, Scheller AD, Anderson RC, Haddad RJ Jr (1986) Histologic and microradiographic analysis of noncemented retrieved PCA knee components. Clin Orthop 202: 147–151
13. Hvid I (1985) Cancelleous bone at the knee. A comparison of two methods of strength measurement Arch Orthop Trauma Surg 104: 211
14. Hungerford DS, Krackow KA, Kenna RV (1984) Total knee arthroplasty—A comprehensive approach. Williams and Wilkins, Baltimore
15. Maquet PGJ (1976) Biomechanics of the knee. Springer, Berlin Heidelberg New York
16. Morrison JB (1968) Bioengineering analysis of force actions transmitted by the knee joint. Biomed Eng 2: 164
17. Paul JP (1976) Force action transmitted in the knee of normal subjects and by prosthetic joint replacement. Total knee replacement. Institute of Mechanical Engineering, London, pp 126–131
18. Pilliar RM, Cameron HU, Macnab I (1975) Porous surfaced layered prosthetic devices. Biomed Eng 10: 126–131
19. Postak PD, Matejczyk MB, Greenwald AS (1986) Stability characteristics of total knee replacements. Mount Sinai Medical Center, University Circle, Cleveland
20. Reilly DT, Martens M (1972) Experimental analysis of the quadriceps muscle force and patello-femoral joint reaction force for various activities. Acta Orthop Scand 43: 126
21. Robertson DM, St. Pierre L, Chahal R (1976) Preliminary observations of bone ingrowth into porous materials. J Biomed Mater Res 10: 335
22. Ryd L (1985) Micromotion in knee arthroplasty. PhD Thesis, University Hospital, Lund
23. Smidt Gl (1973) Biomechanical analysis of knee flexion and extension. J Biomech 6: 79
24. Yamamoto S, Hachinota M, Yuzuki O, Miyake T (1981) The Kodama-Yamamoto knee prosthesis. Ryumachi 21: 21

## *Discussion*

*Shinmei* (National Defense Medical College): I have had similar results to yours in 80 cases of cementless implantation with PCA. Do you do anything special in surgery to improve bone ingrowth? In 90% of rheumatoid patients with osteoporosis, I carry out cementless implantation. In bone grafting, can you carry out cementless PCA?

*Bontemps* (Fabricius-Klinik): I think bone ingrowth is very important in fixation. The pore size (425 μm) may be a little small for ingrowth despite the relative movement. From several investigations, we have displacement of the prosthesis against the bone at about 200, 300, and sometimes even 400 μm, even with a perfect stable fit. Therefore, the pore size could be a little greater, especially on the tibial component; it may be sufficient on the femoral component because of its three-sided inherent stability and the resultant reduction in micromovement between prosthesis and bone.

With regard to bone grafting, all our failures and complications occurred as a result of osteoarthrosis. Of the 89 patients, about 40% of cases were rheumatoid arthritis, in about half of which we had to perform bone grafting almost immediately. I am very concerned that this should work well.

I think it is important to have a stable fit even if there are defects which have to be filled. We sometimes carried out magnetic field therapy, but I do not have a great deal of faith in this.

*Walker* (Harvard Medical School): With respect to bone ingrowth, shearing motion is often discussed, which is why I believe you wish to increase the size of the beads. However, if there is shearing motion and bone ingrowth only occurs in the areas that are not moving, the ingrowth is not doing anything useful; it is not preventing the motion. On the other hand, the up-down motion, especially on the tibia, may be important. Our group and Prof. Miller's group have demonstrated that when a tibial component is vertically loaded the gap between the metal and the bone varies, tilts, and rocks very considerably. Perhaps it is this up and down motion that retards the bony ingrowth. What do you think about this?

*Bontemps*: This was a point with eccentric loading; tensile forces occurred on the unloaded side. I think this happens with every step. It is well known that even if there is correct static alignment, when the patient moves the weight bearing goes to the medial and lateral sides. Therefore, we have this tilting movement in the medial-lateral direction and also in flexion there is the femoral roll-back in addition to compressive forces at the back and elevating forces at the front. It is thus important, I believe, to promote ingrowth so as to prevent this and take up these tensile forces.

*Onishi* (Osaka Minami National Hospital): With regard to bone growth, I have treated 70 cases with PCAs. With a hard tibia, the contact is not so good; using cancellous bone and a metal tray, the bone can be broken into chips by means of a hammer. The bone chips are then spread over the tibial surface to allow good contact. I will discuss this in my presentation tomorrow. Using a ceramic total knee and such bone chips, we are able to prevent the clear zone from appearing. What are your thoughts on this?

*Bontemps*: I think this is an important point. We use a sort of bone paste: We have a machine which makes the bone very fine; we put the machine paste over the tibia surface and using a glass plate we see whether we really have a flat surface. We aim for 100% contact over the whole area. I think it is useful to use bone chips or bone paste to fill all these defects. For sclerotic areas, it is of course important to drill the holes.

*Miller* (McGill University): Bone fails to ingrow in porous surfaces in all kinds of total joint implants. It is important for us all to be aware of our objective, which is to achieve bone ingrowth or fixation. Many authorities are tempted to say that we do not really want bone ingrowth and that fibrous tissue fixation is sufficient. I do not believe this is correct because fibrous tissue fixation will not function in shear and tension.

# Porous-Coated Anatomic Total Knee Replacement: A Clinical and Radiographic Review

M. Bushuk, D.E. Hastings, and E. Bogoch[1]

**Summary.** Between November 1983 and October 1986, 61 porous-coated anatomic (PCA) total knee replacements (TKRs) were implanted. One patient had deceased and 12 patients were unavilable for follow-up at the time of this review. Forty-eight PCA TKRs in 44 patients were personally reviewed. The mean patient age was 71 years, the range of follow-up was 6–42 months (mean 18 months). The original diagnosis was osteoarthritis in 30 knees and rheumatoid arthritis in 18 knees. Twenty-four knees were uncemented, 21 knees were cemented, and three knees had combined cemented and uncemented components. Three patients did not undergo patellar resurfacing, and one patient was symptomatic at the time of review.

Using the Hospital for Special Surgery knee evaluation scale, the mean preoperative score was 42 and the mean postoperative score 87. The average postoperative range of motion was 97°. Of 48 knees (85%), 41 were rated good to excellent (80–100 points). Seven knees (15%) were rated as fair (70–79 points), and these were carefully analyzed. Neither preoperative diagnosis nor method of component fixation greatly influenced the final result.

The most common technical error was malpositioning of the femoral component into flexion in 13 knees (27%). Two tibial components were placed in extension measuring 9° and 12°. Loose beads were observed in 20 of the 48 knees (42%). Of the knees with loose beads, 80% were uncemented. The majority (80%) of loose beads were first noted between 6 and 19 months postoperatively. Loose beads did not influence early results.

Complications included two deep vein thromboses (DVTs), two urinary tract infections (UTIs), one hematoma which resolved spontaneously, one small area of defective wound healing, and one synovial fistula requiring excision. There were no infections, pulmonary emboli, patellar dislocations, or component revisions. Two uncemented patellae and three tibial components (one cemented) showed lucent lines on X-ray. Only one of the uncemented tibial components was clinically loose.

Our study suggests that the PCA knee, both cemented and uncemented, is an effective arthroplasty for the arthritic knee and has consistently reproducible results. The exact significance of loose beads in this short-term study is unknown but requires careful observation in the long term.

[1] Wellesley Hospital, University of Toronto, Toronto, Canada

**Keywords:** Porous-coated anatomic total knee replacement —Osteoarthritis—Rheumatoid arthritis—Cemented—Uncemented—Loose beads

## Introduction

Present day total knee arthroplasty represents approximately 120 years of development in evolution of surgical technique and prosthetic design. The concept of knee arthroplasty appears to date back to 1861 when Ferguson reported on a patient who underwent a resection arthroplasty which was functioning in a satisfactory fashion 5 years postoperatively [1]. In 1863, Verneuil used the joint capsule of the knee as an interposition arthroplasty to cover the resected articular surfaces [2]. Since then, several other autogenous tissue transplants have been utilized for interposition arthroplasty, including fascia lata [3], skin [4], prepatellar bursa [5], chromicized pig bladder [6], cellophane [7], and nylon [8]. Hemiarthroplasty of the distal femur and tibial plateau eventually led to the development of total knee replacement (TKR) in the late 1950s. The first popular TKR utilized a hinge designed by Walldius.

The prototype of the modern low-friction TKR was developed in 1968 by the Canadian Gunston while working with Charnley in Wrightington, England [9]. It consisted of a metal femoral component and a high-density polyethylene tibial component, both of which were secured to bone with polymethylmethacrylate. Gunston's polycentric design was minimally constrained, required minimal bone resection, retained the cruciate and collateral ligaments, and allowed polycentric motion similar to that found in the normal human knee. The total condylar TKR developed by Insall and Burstein in 1974 was a semiconstrained unit which sacrificed the cruciate ligaments and allowed for resurfacing of the patellofemoral joint. Stability was achieved by deepening of the tibial cups and by altering the thickness of the high-density polyethylene tibial component in order to maintain the appropriate tension in the joint capsule and collateral ligaments throughout the normal arc of motion. Insall and Kelly [10] recently reported a 10-year follow-up of 40 knees with total condylar prostheses. There were five failures—one due to infection and four due to improper patient selection or technical reasons. The remaining 35 knees (87.5%) had a satisfactorily functioning arthroplasty after 10 years.

Refinement in design resulted in the development of the Kinematic TKR. This cemented semiconstrained unit had a metal-backed tibial component and allowed for retention of the posterior cruciate ligament. In addition, the Kinematic had design features which (a) allowed increased flexion, rotation, and gliding motion at the tibiofemoral articulation, and (b) decreased posterior stresses during flexion. Ewald et al. [11] reported on 124 Kinematic TKRs with 90% good to excellent results 2–4 years post-operatively (average follow-up 27 months).

Advances in prosthetic materials and design have led to the development of porous-coated implants, which allow bone ingrowth into the porous structure and thus direct osseus fixation of the prostheses to bone. The porous-coated anatomic (PCA) TKR with a porous coat made up of sintered Vitallium beads and the Miller-Galonte TKR with a sintered Titanium wire mesh porous coat are two examples of TKRs which are designed for insertion without the use of polymethylmethacrylate. Utilizing an uncemented TKR allows the patient and surgeon an alternative to the potential complications associated with the use of polymethylmethacrylate. These complications have included monomer toxicity [12–14], thermal and pressure necrosis of bone [15–17], vascular compromise [18], and aseptic loosening with marked bone resorption due to the associated histiocytic reaction [17].

A certain amount of precision is required to insert a cemented TKR, but it is absolutely critical when inserting uncemented components since initial mechanical stability must be achieved at the time of surgery in order to allow normal postoperative rehabilitation. To ensure precise and properly oriented bone cuts, one must minimize the amount of "eyeball" technique and utilize an instrumentation system which is simple, allows for alignment checks prior to making any bone cuts, and provides reproducible results.

Recently loosening of beads from the porocoat [19] have been reported following PCA TKR. The significance is as yet uncertain. Lucent lines are not infrequently seen and are a radiological sign of potential loosening and implant failure. The aims of this paper are to: (a) report our short-term experience with the PCA TKR and provide a basis for establishing a prospective study on total knee arthroplasties; (b) compare the results in specific subgroups, such as osteoarthritis and rheumatoid arthritis, cemented, uncemented, and hybrid, and patellar replacement compared with no patellar component; (c) review component position and identify common technical errors; (d) examine the problem of loose beads; and (e) analyze the significance of radiolucent lines on postoperative follow-up X-rays.

## Materials and Methods

A total of 61 PCA TKRs were inserted at the Wellesley Hospital, Toronto, Canada, between November 1983 and October 1986. One patient was deceased at the time of review and 12 patients were unavailable for follow-up. A total of 48 PCA TKRs in 44 patients were personally reviewed and evaluated according to the Hospital for Special Surgery (HSS) 100-point knee-rating system. A preoperative HSS score was obtained through review of hospital charts and consultation notes. Follow-up ranged from 6 to 42 months (mean 18 months). Forty-one knees were inserted in females with an age range of 52–89 years (mean age 72 years). Seven knees were in males with an age range of 53–79 years (mean age 67 years). The original diagnosis was osteoarthritis (OA) in 30 knees and rheumatoid arthritis (RA) in 18 knees. A total of 13 patients had prior surgery on the knee which underwent TKR. Five patients previously had a high tibial osteotomy, six patients had a MacIntosh double hemiarthroplasty, one patient had a McKeever prosthesis inserted and one patient underwent an arthrotomy for septic arthritis 7 years prior to insertion of a PCA TKR.

Twenty-four knees were uncemented (15 OA, 9 RA). A total of 21 knees were cemented (13 OA, 8 RA). Three knees were classified as hybrids: one patient with only the tibial component cemented, and two patients with the tibial and patellar components cemented. In three patients, patellar resurfacing was not carried out.

The Universal Total Knee Instrumentation system was used in all cases. This instrumentation system offers several advantages, including: (a) jigs which are sequentially numbered according to their use: (b) alignment guides which aid the surgeon in correct positioning of the jigs as well as allowing for alignment checks prior to making any bone cuts; and (c) utilization of appropriate and readily available reference points, i.e., femoral shaft, center of the knee, and the center of the ankle [20].

Radiological assessment included AP standing views of the knees, a lateral view and skyline view of the patella with the knee in 30° of flexion. Evaluation of the X-rays included: (a) analysis of the femoral and tibial component position with respect to flexion/extension and valgus/varus; (b) examination for presence of loose beads, noting time of first appearance, location, number, and evidence of migration; and (c) examination for presence of radiolucent lines, noting time of appearance, location, and evidence of propagation of the lucent line.

## Results

Using the HSS 100-point knee evaluation scale, the mean preoperative score was 42 and the mean postoperative score was 87 (Table 1). Twenty-four knees (50%) were rated as excellent (90–100 points), 17 knees (35%) as good (80–89 points), and seven knees (15%) as fair (70–79 points). Therefore, a total of 41 knees or 85% had a good to excellent postoperative result. No patient had a postoperative rating lower than their preoperative score. Neither preoperative diagnosis nor form of fixation (i.e., cemented, uncemented, or hybrid) obviously influenced the final result. All patients experienced marked pain relief following TKR.

Preoperatively, the average range of motion was 7°–101°. Postoperatively, the average range of motion was 0°–97° (Table 2). Preoperatively, 32 knees had a fixed flexion contracture of 3°–45° (average 12°). Postoperatively, seven patients had a residual flexion contracture of less than 5°. One patient, in whom we were able to achieve full extension intraoperatively, had postoperative recurrence of her 20° fixed flexion contracture. This patient was one of the fair results with a total postoperative score of 75. Preoperative diagnosis (i.e., OA or RA) and method of fixation (cemented or uncemented) did not seem to influence the final range of motion. No significant difference in the postoperative score or range of motion could be demonstrated for the hybrid group and the knees without patellar components when compared with the knees which were entirely cemented or uncemented. Examination of the three patients with no patellar component revealed that two of the patients (diagnosis OA) were asymptomatic and one patient (diagnosis RA) had moderate patellofemoral pain.

Of the seven knees which were rated as fair (70–79 points), three patients had severe generalized RA, which limited their overall functional level. One patient with RA and no patellar resurfacing and malposition of the femoral component had patellofemoral pain and recurrence of her preoperative 20° fixed flexion deformity. One patient had clinical and radiographic findings compatible with a loose tibial component (Fig. 1.). One patient with OA was taking Prednisone 5 mg/day and had a previous McKeever prosthesis. One patient on Worker's Compensation benefits had global discomfort in the knee but no obvious clinical or radiographic findings to explain the pain.

**Table 1.** Mean HSS score

| | Preoperation | | Postoperation | |
|---|---|---|---|---|
| | OA | RA | OA | RA |
| Uncemented | 45 | 47 | 87 | 88 |
| Cemented | 41 | 33 | 89 | 85 |
| Hybrids | 40 | 50[a] | 93 | 79[a] |
| No patella | 40 | 21[a] | 86 | 75[a] |
| Overall mean | 42 | | 87 | |

[a] One knee only
*OA* osteoarthritis, *RA* rheumatoid arthritis

**Table 2.** Mean range of motion

| | Preoperation (degrees) | | Postoperation (degrees) | |
|---|---|---|---|---|
| | OA | RA | OA | RA |
| Uncemented | 7–106 | 17–108 | 1–103 | 0–108 |
| Cemented | 5–102 | 12–88 | 0–92 | 2–102 |
| Hybrid | 7–85 | 30–100[a] | 0–100 | 0–90[a] |
| No patella | 4–87 | 20–80[a] | 2–100 | 20–90[a] |
| Overall mean | 7–100 | | 0–97 | |

[a] One knee only
*OA* osteoarthritis, *RA* rheumatoid arthritis

Preoperative and serial postoperative X-rays were analyzed. Femoral component positioning in the AP X-ray was felt to be satisfactory (between 6° and 12° of valgus) in 46 knees. One femoral component was in neutral and a second in 14° of valgus. In the lateral projection, 34 of 48 knees were within 5° of neutral. The most common malposition of the femoral component was flexion in 13 knees; this was 6°–10° in 12 knees and 12° in one other. One femoral component was placed in 11° of extension (Fig. 2). On the AP X-ray, 47 of the tibial components were in satisfactory alignment (3° ± 3° varus). One component was in 8° of varus. On the lateral view, 46 tibial components were in neutral and two in extension of 9° and 12°, respectively (Fig. 3). Three of the knees with component malposition scored below 80° on the HSS evaluation scale.

Loose beads were documented in 20 of the 48 knees (42%). Of the knees with loose beads, 80% were uncemented. Loose beads were noted in the a 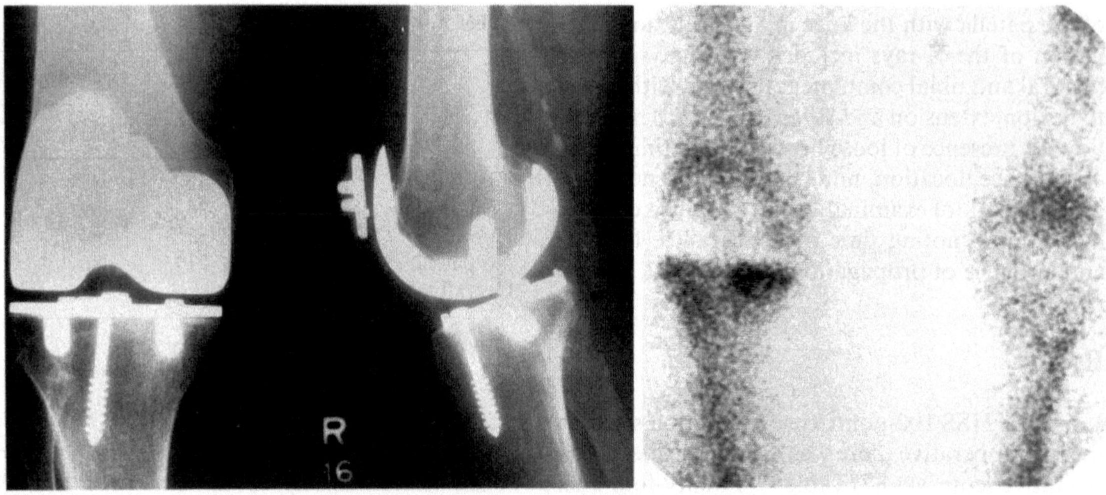 b


**Fig. 1. a** Anteroposterior standing and **b** lateral right knee demonstrating radiolucent line under medial edge of tibial component. Technetium 99 bone scan demonstrating increased uptake in medial half of tibial plateau

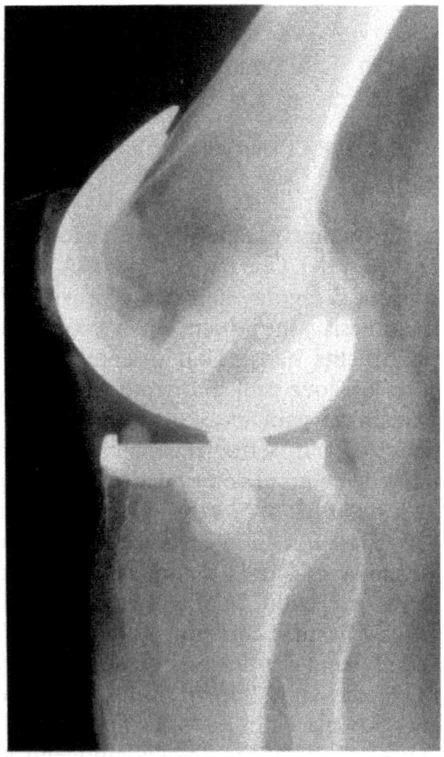

**Fig. 2.** Femoral component inserted in 11° of extension

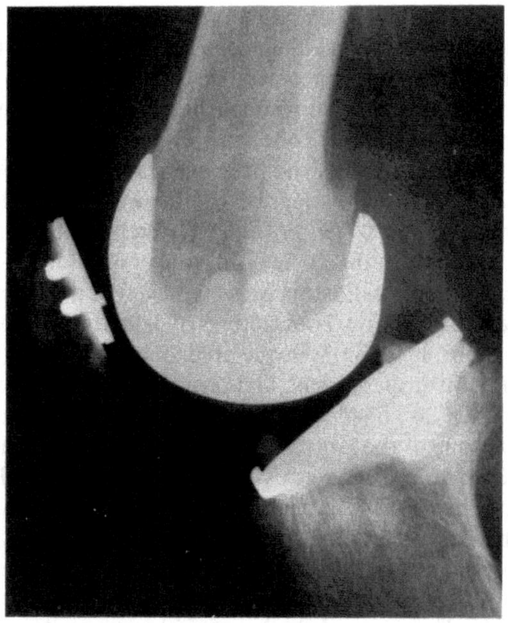

**Fig. 3.** Tibial component inserted in 12° of extension and limiting flexion to 85°

immediate postoperative film in four knees and were noted between 6 months and 19 months postoperatively in 16 knees (80%). The maximum number of loose beads in any single knee was four. Bead migration was less than 1 mm in 18 knees. Two knees had beads which had migrated 1–4 mm. No intra-articular loose beads were observed. There was no correlation between loose beads and fair results. The one patient who we thought had a loose tibial component had only one loose bead at the inferior margin of the lateral peg of the tibial component.

No lucent lines were visible around any of the

femoral components. Two uncemented patellar components had nonpropagating radiolucent lines opposite the one pole of the patella without any porous coating. There was intimate contact between the portion of the patellar component with porous coating and the bone, suggesting good bony ingrowth. Both of these patients were clinically asymptomatic. One cemented and two uncemented tibial components had evidence of lucent lines. The lucent line in the case of the cemented tibial component was in the region of the posterior lip of the component. In the case of the two uncemented tibial components, the lucent lines were in the region of the medial and lateral lips of the components (i.e., peripheral to the medial and lateral pegs). No progression of the lucent lines could be documented on serial X-rays. One of these patients had chronic pain in the region of the lucent line under the medial tibial plateau and had increased uptake in this region on a bone scan 2 years postoperatively. Based on this evidence we felt that the tibial component was loose and that the pain experienced by the patient was due to micromotion of the component. However, the patient felt that the level of pain that she was experiencing did not warrant revision of the component.

Complications included two deep vein thromboses, two urinary tract infections, one wound hematoma which resolved spontaneously, one small area of defective wound healing, and one synovial fistula. The synovial fistula was excised 7 days postoperatively and the patient's subsequent postoperative course was uncomplicated. Two patients required manipulation of their knees under a general anesthetic 14 days postoperatively as a result of stiffness. It is notable that there have been no infections, pulmonary emboli, patellar dislocations, or component revisions to date in this consecutive series of PCA TKRs.

## Discussion

Although a mean follow-up of 18 months is short in terms of studying any total joint replacement, we feel that 41 of 48 knees (85%) with good to excellent results is very encouraging. Many of these patients are enjoying vigorous, active lives and some of them are stressing their prostheses by walking several miles a day or by playing 18 holes of golf. The form of fixation, whether the components were completely cemented (21 knees), uncemented (24 knees), or a hybrid (three knees), did not seem to influence the final result. The completely uncemented TKRs were a little slower to regain function as they were kept restricted weight bearing for the initial 6 weeks, while the cemented TKRs were allowed immediate full weight bearing postoperatively. Although there were seven knees that were classified as fair results with scores of less than 80 points, it should be noted that four of these patients had severe generalized RA. All four patients experienced improved alignment of their extremity and significant pain relief from their TKR. Their scores of below 80 were largely the result of their generalized RA, which limited the overall functional level. The high proportion of patients with polyarthritis does affect the overall result to some degree in this series.

No significant difference in final results could be demonstrated when comparing uncemented to cemented techniques for insertion of the component. Nonetheless, there are several advantages to avoiding the use of methylmethacrylate, including: (a) decreased operating time, (b) no methylmethacrylate debris to hasten the wear of the high-density polyethylene tibial component, and (c) preservation of a maximum amount of bone stock in the event that the TKR has to be converted to a cemented TKR or knee fusion. In addition, methylmethacrylate is brittle, prone to fatigue fracture, and is a poor transmitter of tensile stresses, all of which are factors affecting the long-term survival of the bone-cement interface.

The primary goal of cementless fixation is to achieve long-term prosthetic stability. Bone ingrowth into the porous coating results in an interface that is responsive to the forces that are transmitted across it. Correctly aligned precision bone cuts and proper balancing of soft tissue structures around the knee are two critical factors in achieving adequate bony ingrowth into the porous coating. The universal instrumentation system did allow reliable component positioning in most cases. The most common error in component positioning was that of flexion of the femoral component in 13 knees. In chapter 4 of Instrumentation for Total Knee Arthroplasty, Greenberg et al. stated in reference to the intercondylar drill hole that "the position of this hole is not critical to the orientation of any femoral bone cut" [20]. We would tend to disagree with this statement. Ideally, the intercondylar drill hole should be centered in the intercondylar notch so that the posterior spike on the drill guide is just anterior to the femoral attachment of the posterior cruciate ligament. It is crucial that the alignment guide is centered over the shaft of the femur and is parallel to the femur. In addition, the intramedullary rod must be centered down the intramedullary shaft. If the intercondylar drill hole is not in the correct location, then the intramedullary rod will not be centered in the intramedullary canal and thus will run the risk of being deflected from its correct alignment by the normal anterolateral bow of the femur. If the hole is too posterior, jig I A and B will tend to sit in flexion. If the hole is too far anterior, the jig will tend to sit in an extended position. Therefore, it is crucial to use the built—in alignment checks to ensure that the guide pin is centered over the femoral shaft and parallel to it before any bone cuts are made. This should prevent malpositioning of the femoral component. A femur with a large anterior bow tends to place the femoral component in flexion. This variation can be recognized, and appropriate correction taken.

Proper soft tissue balancing is critical in achieving joint stability, which in turn is a major factor affecting bone ingrowth into the porous coating. Fixed flexion, varus, or valgus are the common deformities that must be dealt with when performing a total knee arthroplasty. In some cases, there may be a combination of these deformities.

Fixed flexion deformities are initially managed by resection of bony blocks to flexion such as bony ridges or large osteophytes anteriorly. As much as 20° of correction can be obtained by this simple measure. One then releases the posterior capsule and removes any posterior osteophytes or loose bodies. Occasionally, the femoral attachments of the gastrocnemius muscle have to be elevated in a subperiosteal fashion. Further resection of bone is rarely required, but should it become necessary it should be resected from the distal femur. Resection of further bone from the proximal tibia to achieve full extension of the knee results in ligamentous instability in flexion.

Management of fixed varus deformities begins with resection of osteophytes and loose bodies followed by sequential subperiosteal medial release. Fibular shortening can be done for significant residual lateral laxity. In cases where there is extensive bone loss along the medial tibial plateau, it is best to bone graft the defect in order to minimize the amount of proximal tibia to be resected. The best bone for grafting is that obtained from resection of the posterior femoral condyles (Fig. 4).

Correction of fixed valgus deformities of less than 30° can be achieved by Z-lengthening of the iliotibial band and sequential subperiosteal release of the lateral capsule, lateral collerateral ligament, popliteus tendon, and arcuate ligamentous complex. For valgus deformities of greater than 30°, one should, through a separate incision, identify, free, and protect the common peroneal nerve at the fibular neck. In addition to the releases described for valgus deformities of less than 30°, one should release or Z-lengthen the biceps femoris tendon and, rarely, the lateral gastrocnemius tendon. For residual medial collateral ligament laxity, advancement of the medial soft tissue envelope should be done (Fig. 5). Large lateral plateau defects should be bone-grafted to minimize the bone resection from the proximal tibia.

Mechanical stability must be achieved at the time of surgery in order to allow for bone ingrowth into the porous coating and to allow for normal postoperative rehabilitation. If there is any evidence of movement of the components at the time of implantation, the component should be removed and cemented into place. There is growing evidence that micromotion at the bone implant interface will inhibit bone ingrowth into the porous coating [21, 22]. The maximum limit of movement to allow bone ingrowth has not yet been determined. However, Pilliar et al. suggest that if shear displacement at the bone-prosthesis interface is greater than about 30 $\mu$m, bone ingrowth will be inhibited [23]. Greater initial implant movement could result in implant fixation by nonmineralized fibrous connective tissue. Larger relative movements would result in fibrous tissue and encapsulation only [24].

The porous coating found on the PCA TKR consists of a double layer of sintered Vitallium beads [25]. The porous layer is 1.25 mm thick and has an average pore size of 425 $\mu$m. The overall porosity has been measured at 35%. The mechanical shear strength between the sintered beads on the PCA prosthesis has been reported to be 43 MPa (7000 lb/in$^2$) [26]. Bone ingrowth into the porous coating has been estimated to be at least 50% in the femoral component, 50% in the patellar component, and 20% in the tibial component (Peter Van Syckle, Howmedica, personal communication) (Fig. 6). There have been several recent in vitro and animal studies which have demonstrated increased bone ingrowth rates attributed to thin hydroxyapatite coatings applied to the porous coating of implants [27–29]

Rosenqvist et al. recently reported on 34 PCA TKRs in 28 patients with RA [19]. In these 34 knees, 23 tibial and 15 femoral components were cemented. Nineteen knees (56%) had loose displaced beads on follow-up X-rays. In fourteen knees, the beads loosened more than 3 months postoperatively. Six knees had intra-articular beads. The number of loose beads per tibial component ranged from one to eleven (mean three), and per femoral component from one to six (mean one). Rosenqvist et al. concluded that: "the metallurgical technique for porous coating with heat sintered cobalt-chromium beads does not produce a coating that is sufficiently strong

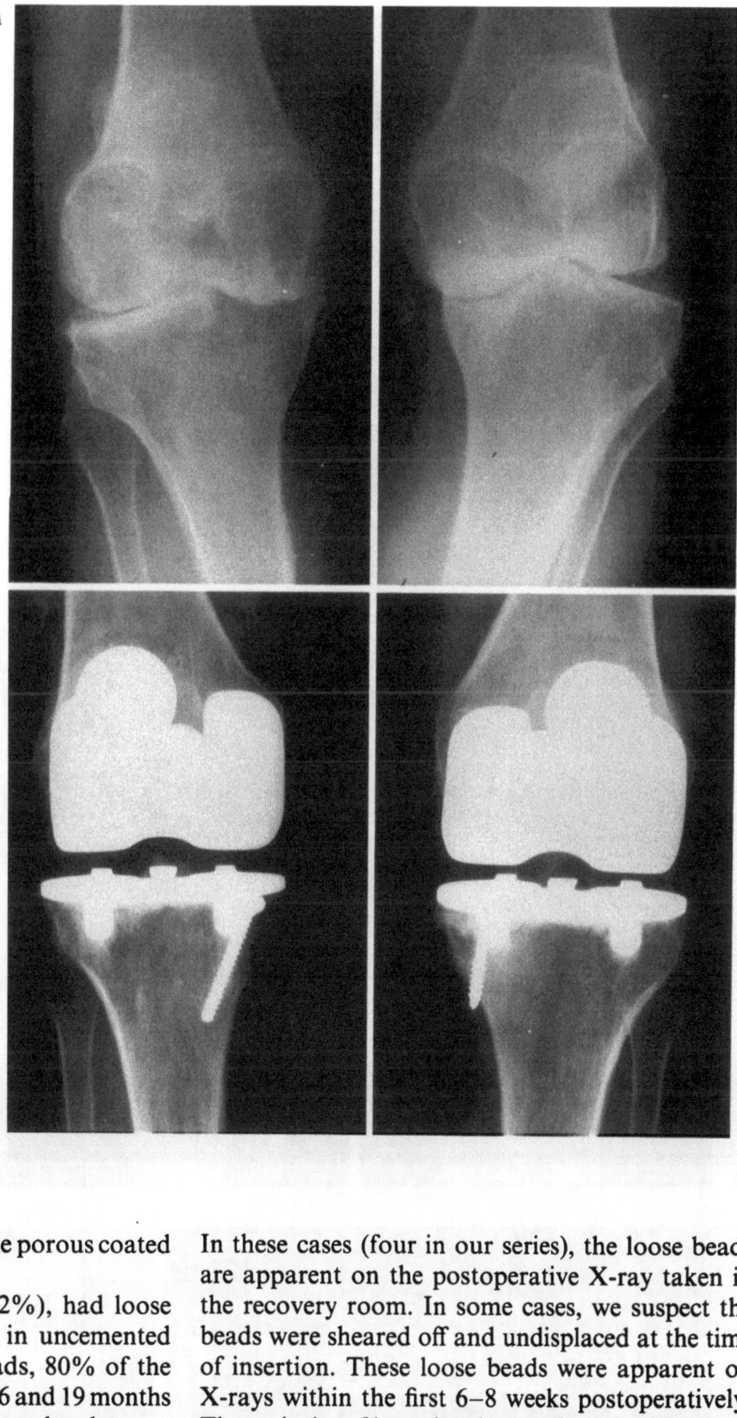

**Fig. 4.** **a** Bilateral varus deformity with bone loss. **b** Reconstruction with bone graft from posterior femoral condyle

to prevent loosening in the case of the porous coated anatomic prosthesis" [19].

In our study, 20 of 48 knees (42%), had loose beads and 80% of these occurred in uncemented TKRs. In the knees with loose beads, 80% of the loose beads were first noted between 6 and 19 months postoperatively. The majority of loose beads came from the tibial component. There were no intra-articular loose beads. The maximum number of loose beads for any single TKR was four. We could not correlate loosening of beads to any clinical failures.

The origin of loose beads seen on the postoperative X-rays is variable. In some cases, the beads are sheared off and displaced at the time of insertion. In these cases (four in our series), the loose beads are apparent on the postoperative X-ray taken in the recovery room. In some cases, we suspect the beads were sheared off and undisplaced at the time of insertion. These loose beads were apparent on X-rays within the first 6–8 weeks postoperatively. The majority of loose beads were first noted between 6 and 19 months postoperatively. One cannot rule out completely that these beads were sheared off at the time of insertion and displaced later, but we feel a more likely explanation is that the beads sheared off after implantation due to micromotion or cyclic loading with subsequent fatigue failure (Fig. 7). It is likely that some of the beads are predisposed to failure for two distinct reasons. Firstly, some of the

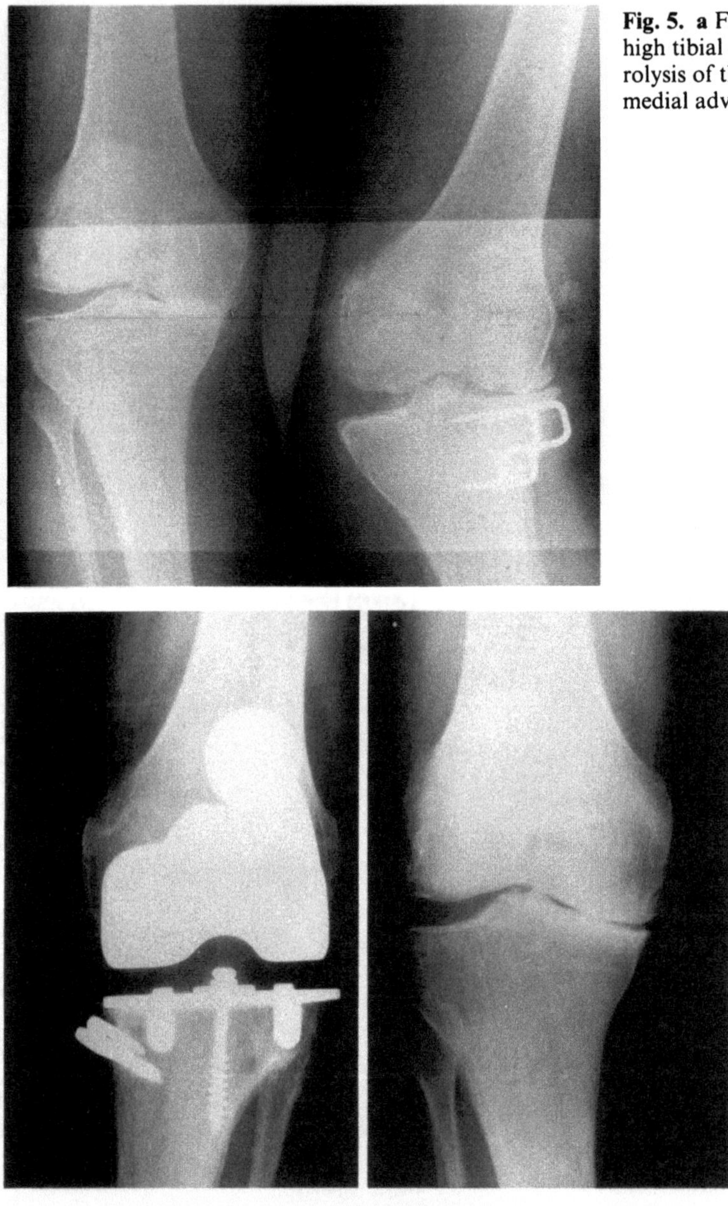

a

b

**Fig. 5.** **a** Forty degrees valgus deformity after failed high tibial osteotomy. **b** Reconstruction with neurolysis of the peroneal nerve, lateral release, and medial advancement

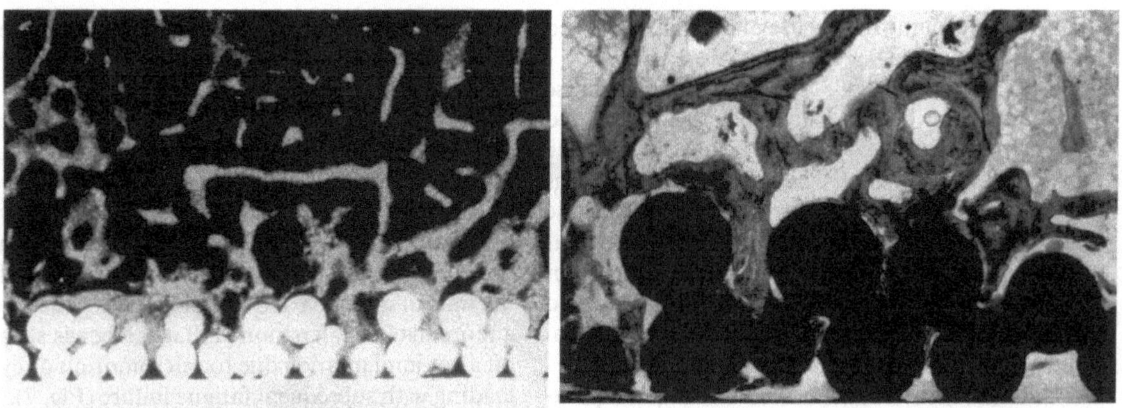

a

b

**Fig. 6.** **a** Fine-detail radiograph demonstrating bony ingrowth into porous coating. **b** Histological section demonstrating bone ingrowth

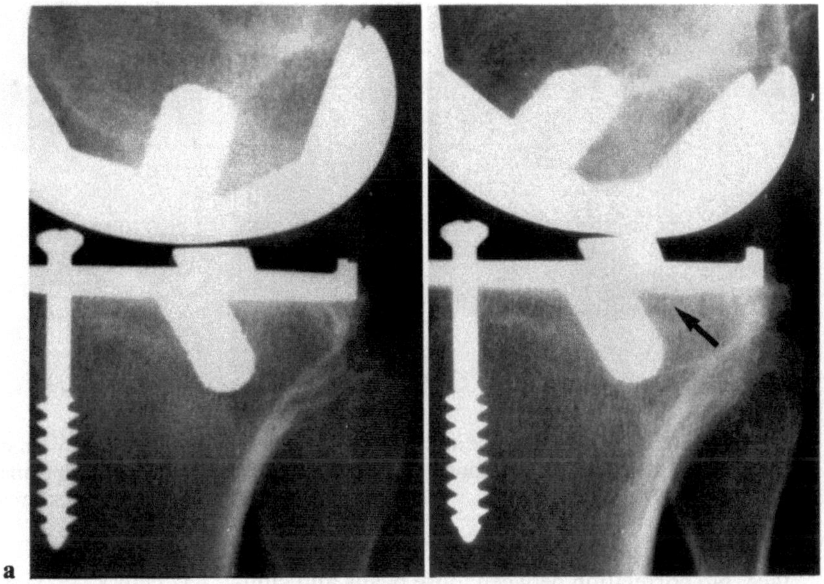

**Fig. 7.** **a** Immediate postoperative radiograph with no evidence of local loosening. **b** Comparable view 1 year later demonstrating loose bead

beads are sitting somewhat "proud" on the main layer of the beads making up the porous coating. As a result, these beads were exposed to much greater stresses. Secondly, some of the beads were predisposed to loosening as a result of a defect in the sintering process, which results in a weaker than normal bond between beads at what is referred to as the "neck" region. The exact details of the powder sintering process utilized by Howmedica to produce the porous coating on the PCA TKR and total hip replacement are protected under proprietary laws. However, the various processes involved in producing porous coating on orthopedic implants has been well described by Pilliar [30].

The bead-type porous coating is made from atomized metal alloy powders formed by a technique referred to as the "spun electrode process". Spherical alloy particles of the required size range can be made by controlling the rotation speed of a consumable electrode. Both the starting powder size range and the sintering conditions utilized determine the structure of the porous coating. The sintering procedure basically involves a high-temperature annealing process that causes the powder particles to bond to each other and to the solid metal component with only minor changes to the particle shape. Cobalt-chrome-molybdenum powders are sintered at temperatures in the range of 1300°. Particle bonding for this alloy is dependent upon, to a degree, liquid-phase sintering. The region at which the liquid phase and bonding occur is referred to as the "neck" zone. The kinetics and the strength of the bonds which form are influenced by the chemical composition of the cobalt-based alloy as well as by the sintering time and temperature. Higher carbon levels and rapid cooling during the sintering process result in the formation of chromium-carbide phases in the neck regions. These carbides are intrinsically brittle and if they are found in a continuous form along the neck regions this can result in easy particle separation from the implant. Bonding of the particles can be improved by suspending the particles in an organic binder phase, which aids in the coating of the prosthesis. A second method which could be used to improve the particle bonding involves a process by which particle bonding is achieved at a lower sintering temperature through the application of pressure during the sintering process. This process is referred to as diffusion bonding.

The microstructure of the neck region of the particle-implant and particle-particle junctions, which are found in the porous coatings of PCA TKRs, is seen in Fig. 8. The microstructure of the neck region which occurs in the porous coating on the PCA total hip replacements is shown in Fig. 9. It is interesting to note that there are large, continuous chromium-carbide phases evident in the porous coating on the total knee component, but not the total hip component. This might suggest that a slightly different sintering process is being used for the total knee components. Although some loose beads appear on post-operative X-rays in patients who have had a PCA total hip arthroplasty, they are not as prevalent as in patients with TKRs. The true significance of the loose beads in our study is not known as the length of follow-up is short (mean 18 months). The late appearance of loose beads with obvious migration does suggest that there is incomplete bone ingrowth into the porous coat and that micromotion is occurring at the bone-implant inter-

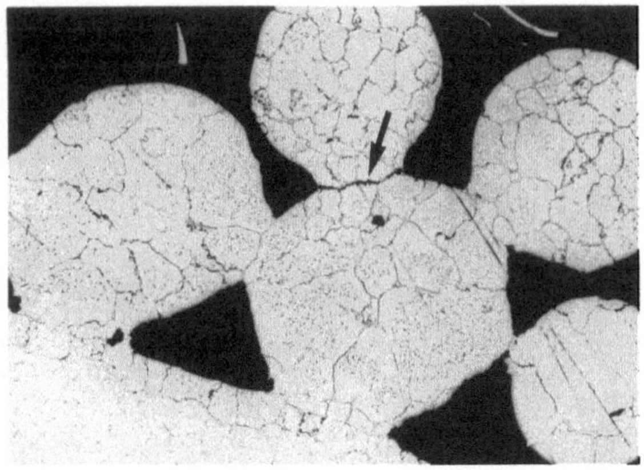

**Fig. 8.** Chromium-carbide phase in the "neck" region of a bead on a PCA tibial component. Courtesy of RM Pilliar

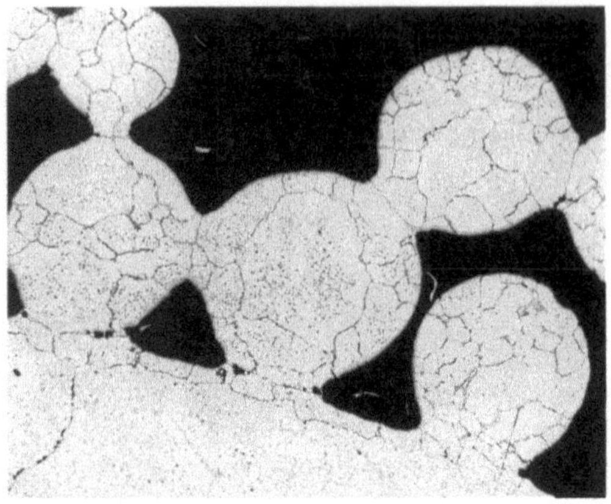

**Fig. 9.** Chromium-carbide phase in a PCA hip femoral component. The lines are finer and do not extend across the entire "neck" region. Courtesy of RM Pilliar

face. No correlation between loose beads and clinical failures could be found in this short-term study. However, we think the loose beads could potentially represent a serious problem which bears close observation in the long term.

There are two other in vivo effects of porous-coated implants which remain a concern. First, there is possible resorption of host bone due to disuse atrophy, often referred to as stress shielding. There have been several studies of uncemented porous-coated hip implants which indicate that some resorption of the medial calcar can occur as a result of stress shielding [31, 32]. No problems due to this factor were seen in the present series, but again the follow-up is relatively short. The distal femur is a potential site of stress shielding. The second problem relates to the surface areas present in porous-coated implants. Increased corrosion rates, five to ten times higher than normal, appear to be directly related to the increase in surface area of the porous-coated implants [33, 34]. There is a potential for significant metal ion migration into the surrounding tissue which could increase the risk of metal sensitization or even tumor formation [35]. This again is of great concern and must be closely observed in the long term.

## References

1. Ferguson M (1861) Excision of the knee joint: Recovery with a false joint and a useful limb. Med Times Gaz 1: 601
2. Verneuil A (1863) Resultats obtain for France par l'operation d'esmarch. Examen de couses d'insuccess et moyen d'y remedier. Gos Hebd Med Chir 10: 97
3. Putti V (1921) Arthroplasty, Am. J. Orthop Surg 19: 421
4. Brown JE, McGow WH, Shaw OT (1958) Use of cutis as an interposing membrane in arthroplasty of the knee. J Bone Joint Surgery 40A: 1003
5. Campbell WC (1921) Arthroplasty of the Knee: Report of cases. Am J. Orthop Surg. 19: 430
6. Baer WS (1918) Arthroplasty with the aid of animal membrane. Am J Orthop Surg 16: 171
7. Sampson JE (1949) Arthroplasty of the knee joint. J. Bone and Joint Surg 31B: 50
8. Kuhns JG, Porter TA (1951) Nylon arthroplasty of the knee joint in chronic arthritis. Surg Gynecol Obstet 91: 351
9. Gunston FH (1971) Polycentric knee arthroplasty prosthetic simulation of normal knee movement. J Bone Joint Surg 52B: 272
10. Insall JN, Kelly M (1986) The Total Condylar Prosthesis. Clin Orthop 205: 43
11. Ewald FC, Jacobs M, Miegel RE, Walker PS, Poss R, Sledge CB (1984) Kinematic total knee replacement. J Bone Joint Surg 66A: 1032
12. Willert HG, Ludwig J, Semlitsch M (1974) Reaction of bone to methlymethacrylate after hip arthroplasty. J Bone Joint Surg 56A: 1368
13. Linder L (1976) Tissue reaction to methylmethacrylate monomer. Acta Orthop Scand 47: 3
14. Linder L, Romanus M (1976) Acute local tissue effects of polymerizing acrylic bone cement. Clin Orthop 115: 303
15. Jefferiss CD, Lee AJC, Ling RSM (1975) Thermal aspects of self-curing polymethylmethacrylate. J Bone Joint Surg 57B: 511
16. Sloof TJ (1971) The influence of acrylic cement. Acta Orthop Scand 42: 465
17. Linder L (1982) The tissue response to bone cement In: Williams DF (ed) Biocompatibility of orthopaedic implants, vol 2. CRC Press, Boca Raaton, pp 1–23
18. Rhinelander FW, Nelson CL, Stewar RD, Stewart CL (1979) Experimental reaming of the proximal femur and acrylic cement implantation, vascular and histologic effects. Clin Orthop 14: 74

19. Rosenqvist R, Bylander B, Knutson K, Rydholm U, Rooser B, Egund N, Lidgren L (1986) Loosening of the porous coating of bicompartmental prothesis in patients with rheumatoid arthritis. J Bone Joint Surg 68A: 538–542
20. Hungerford DS, Krackow KA, Kenna RV (1984). Total knee arthroplasty, A comprehensive Approach, Williams and Wilkins, Baltimore, pp 1–335
21. Cameron HU, Pilliar RM, Macnab I (1973) The effect of movement on the loading of porous metal to bone. J Biomed Mater Res 7: 301
22. Ducheyne P, DeMeester P, Aernout E, Mulier JC (1977) Influence of a functional dynamic loading on bone ingrowth into surface pores of orthopaedic implants. J Biomed Mater Res 11: 811
23. Pilliar RM, Lee JM, Mancotopoulos C (1986) Observations on the effect of movement on bone ingrowth into porous surfaced implants. Clin Orthop 208: 108
24. Lee JM, Pilliar RM, Adulla D, Bobyn JD (1984) In vitro testing of porous coated orthopedic implant support in bone at 1 year: differences between fibrous tissue support and bone ingrowth. Transactions, Second World Congress on Biomaterials, Washington, D.C., April 27–May 1, 1984, p 1266
25. Howmedica (1984) The PCA primary total knee system. Howmedica, Rutherford
26. Kenna RV, Hedley AK, Hungerford DS, Habermann ET, Borden CS (1984): The PCA total hip system. Technical monograph. Harrington Arthritis Research Foundation
27. Ducheyne P, Hench CC, Koyan A, Martens M, Bursens A, Mulieer JC (1980) Effect of hydroxyapatite impregnation, on skeletal bonding of porous coated implants. J Biomed Mater Res 14: 225
28. Cook SD, Kay JF, Thomas KA, Anderson RC, Harding AF, Reynolds MC, Jarcho M (1986) Variables affecting the interface strength and histology of hydroxyapatite coated implant surfaces. Transactions Twelfth Annual Meeting of the Society for Biomaterials, Minneapolis, May 28–June 1, 1986, p 14
29. Thomas KA, Cook SD, Anderson RC, Haddad RJ, Kay JF, Jarcho M (1986) Biological response to hydoxyapatite coated porous titanium hips. Transactions Twelfth Annual Meeting of the Society for Biomaterials, Minneapolis May 28–June 1, 1986, p 15
30. Pilliar RM (1987) Porous surfaced metallic implants for orthopaedic applications. J Biomed Mater Res 21: 1
31. Brown IW, Ring PA (1985) Osteolytic changes in the upper femoral shaft following porous coasted hip replacement. J Bone Joint Surg 67B: 218
32. Engh CA, Bobyn JD (1985) Biologic fixation in total hip arthroplasty. Slack Inc., Thorofare
33. Ducheyne P (1983) In vitro corrosion study of porous metal fibre coatings for bone ingrowth. Biomaterials 4: 185
34. Margolion S, Pilliar RM, Weatherly GC (1981) Corrosion characteritics of porous surfaced cast Co-base implants—in-vivo and in-vitro studies. Transactions Seventh Annual Meeting of the Society for Biomaterials, Troy, NY May 28–31, 1981, p 82
35. Block J (1984) Systemic effects of biomaterials. Biomaterials 5: 11

# *Discussion*

*Bae* (Kyung Hee University Hospital): With regard to the design of the PCA knee, the amount of resection of the distal and posterior parts of the femoral bone must not be much greater than the replacement by the femoral component if adequate function of the posterior cruciate ligament in flexion and extension is to be achieved. In your cases, however, of flexion contracture or angular deformity, you cut more bone at the femoral part than that replaced by the femoral component.

*Hastings* (Wellesley Hospital): I seldom find it necessary to remove bone in a fixed flexion deformity. You are limited in the amount of bone you can remove from the femur because of the femoral insertion of the posterior cruciate ligament, but I think you are even more limited by the amount of bone you can remove from the tibia, because you get down below the tibial origin of the posterior cruciate and get into worse osteoporotic bone. So here, I think that the lesser of the two evils is to resect on the femoral side if this becomes necessary.

*Goodfellow* (Oxford University): There is a radiolucent zone underneath the tibial component in probably about 80% of these cases, since bone ingrowth occurs in about 20%. This is not evident on X-rays because of the metal lip all the way round, which is 1.5 mm deep. The radiolucent line will only become visible, therefore, if it is greater than 1.5 mm. Is that correct?

*Hastings*: Yes. However, even looking at the knees under a fluoroscope and trying to shoot at right angles to the tibial plate is extremely difficult. So when we are talking about radiolucent lines, we are clearly tending to underestimate the number of cases. I do not really know what is under the metal overhang.

*Goodfellow*: But you would believe it to be fibrous tissue? That is what all the rest of us would consider it to be.

*Hastings*: Yes I would expect it is. I have a great deal of experience with the Mackintosh prosthesis and when we took these out, we found a very good imprint of the face of the prosthesis. The prostheses function very well and I suspect that the tibial component might function very well in spite of what Dr. Miller says about having to have ingrowth.

*Goodfellow*: Yes, the evidence is that almost all implants are sitting on a layer of fibrous tissue and most of them seem to function very well in that mode.

*Hastings*: I am not so sure about the femoral component, especially on its anterior face; I think bony ingrowth may develop. We appear to be heading, as in total hips, toward a hybrid type of implant where the tibia is cemented and the femoral component can be inserted without cement, just as bone cement is not required for the acetabulum.

# Panel Discussion

*Ranawat* (Cornell University Medical College): Dr. Krackow indicated at the beginning of his talk that PCA, as its name would suggest, has a very anatomical design; it preserves the posterior cruciate ligament. You also said that the IB knee and Total Condylar had such unphysiological kinematics. Yet in the postoperative range of motion, you and the other panellists obtained a maximum of only 97°–108°. Why is the range of motion so small if the kinematics are so physiological?

*Krackow* (John Hopkins University): I think that the ultimate range of motion has relatively little to do with the prosthesis design if certain bad features are not present, i.e., if the tibial component does not run into a particular metal or bony block as the knee comes into flexion or inadvertent physical tightening of a cruciate or collateral ligament does not occur. Essentially, all the modern knee designs are theoretically capable of very great degrees of motion; even some of the older knee designs, e.g., Townley's knee, are capable of this. However, the ultimate range of motion in a knee is dependent on a great many factors, involving surgical technique, preoperative range of motion, postoperative hemorrhage, cement versus no cement in terms of postoperative hemorrhage, patient motivation, in addition to many others. I am thus not so surprised that one sees 105° or 107° of motion. Even with some of the Geomedic knees, aside from the considerations with the cruciate ligament, I am sure that many of those patients could have bent their knees a great deal farther. There is certainly not an inherent block to flexion in the PCA knee as compared with other knees.

*Goldie* (Karolinska Institute): It would be interesting to follow up this question with the problem of alignment. We generally relate this to the normal anatomy of the knee joint in a position when the knee is not loaded. There is another aspect to alignment and that is dynamic alignment, including the soft tissues; the latter includes not only the structures mentioned in the last presentation by Dr. Hastings but also the medial structures, the anterior structures, and, in particular, the patellar ligament. There is the question of how the patellar ligament is related to the joint line; what happens if so much bone is resected that the patellar pole becomes too distant from the prosthesis and joint line or too close to the joint line? Will this in any way interfere with the range of motion?

*Hastings* (Wellesley Hospital): In the early phases of PCA, we were doing relatively conservative patellar resections and inserting a thick patellar button, thereby advancing the whole extensor mechanism anteriorly and bringing about a major loss to flexion. This is one of the reasons I think why there is 8°–10° less than in the kinematic series. This problem has been dealt with recently to a certain extent by resecting more of the patella and by the new design of the patellar component with three buttons, which is certainly not as thick as the old PCA design of the patellar button.

*Krackow*: I can understand features of prosthetic design as they relate to ultimate range of flexion when those features involve, for example, portions of the tibial component abutting on some aspect of either the metal femoral component or residual bone in the posterior femur, or, as Dr. Hastings was alluding to, to the possibility really with any prosthesis that the extensor mechanism is felt to be tight as the knee comes to maximum flexion. That situation can result if the femoral component is a little large and/or the residual thickness of the patella in combination with the patellar replacement makes the extensor mechanism proud and distant.

I think all lf us have experienced knees at surgery which passively flexed perfectly freely to 110°, 120°, or even 125°. And yet the patient recovered after surgery and struggled for a week to achieve 80° or 90° and ultimately did not exceed 105° or 110°. Another patient essentially showing the same physical setting during the operation will go on to have 125° or 130° of flexion postoperatively—I do not have a answer for this.

*Goldie*: The question is whether the interference of the extensor mechanism might in any way explain the patellar problems that we found in certain of these patients that are operated upon.

*Hastings*: We used CPM on about one-third of our patients and not on the other two-thirds. It made no difference to the range of motion. A factor I think that is important is if the capsular closure is performed with the knee in flexion, there is less likelihood of capsular malalignment; impairment of flexion can be minimized in this way.

*Ranawat*: Pain in the postoperative period from whatever source is the main cause of reduction in range of motion. The joint line in the Total Condylar and IB knee is raised by 3–5 mm most of the time. In spite of that, the average range of motion with the IB knee after follow-up of 5 years or more was 115°. This indicates that there is some factor in the design which causes the patients to suffer less pain. With Total Condylar at present, about two-thirds of the patients are in the same range of motion of about 115°. This point is further seen in patients who have joint disease; the patients have very little pain and great range of motion.

*Goldie*: I would agree with you up to a point. However, when we operate on knees we have the patients on epidural block and continuously give them morphine intrathecally. The patients are thus absolutely pain-free, but we still cannot get the same flexion postoperatively as we achieved on the operating table. Perhaps 3 or 4 days after operation when the patients are no longer receiving this kind of pain relief, they may be subject to discomfort, rather than pain.

*Goodfellow* (Oxford University): Our statistical analysis shows a very close correlation between the preoperative and postoperative range of motion. That is the only correlation we have ever been able to find and it is very positive. If bilateral knee replacement is performed, there is a very close correlation between the range of motion obtained in the two knees: It is very seldom for one knee to bend a great deal more or less than the other. So I would say that the factors which limit range of flexion have little to do with design of the implant but have a great deal to do with the individual soft tissues of the individual preoperatively. In my presentation tomorrow, I will show a distribution curve of the flexion range preoperatively and postoperatively and it will be seen that they are almost identical. In a recent report from Sweden on a PCA unicompartmental device with an average postoperative range of flexion in excess of 120°, however, the preoperative range of motion was greater than 125°.

*Ogata* (Kyushu University Hospital): We tested the range of motion intraoperatively and we always found good flexion, but postoperatively if we did not use any cement, the patients complained of pain, could not do exercises, and ended up with poor range of motion. But when we used cement and encouraged early range of motion, the patients usually got good flexion. However, preoperative range of motion is a very important factor.

*Koshino* (Yokohama City University): The preoperative range of motion of patients is often very good in Japan, e.g., in rheumatoid arthritis it may be up to 110°, 120°, or even 130°. To obtain a good range of motion after surgery I never make a suture in the capsules, I just make a suture at the insertion of the muscles and then keep it open. This gives 120°–130° range of motion. Miller-Galante may have a slightly better range of motion than the Kinematics knee. Hemiarthroplasty using Marmor gives better flexion.

*Goldie*: So you do not suture the soft tissues around the joint, you just suture the skin?

*Koshino*: I make a suture in the investing layer and skin. I do parapatellar release. I go into the joint from the lateral side. I have done this in over a hundred cases and there have been no complications.

*Bontemps* (Fabricius-Klinik): We also use the lateral approach in all valgus deformities, i.e., most rheumatoid patients, and therefore of course in most cases a lateral release has to be performed; we leave it open at the end of the surgery. In other cases of lateral release, we have seen upon revision a few years after surgery callosity of the capsule on the lateral side. I would expect the same with this procedure with any prosthesis.

*Kurosaka* (Kobe University): I do not think that the difference between having 90°–95° flexion on one side and having 110° flexion is on the other side is very great in the daily life of the patient. What do the panel think about this?

*Krackow*: I would agree to a point. Normal walking requires about 5°–75°, stair-climbing a little more; height plays a role here too. However, getting out of a chair will be more difficult if a patient has had both knees replaced and can only bend 85°–90° on each knee. It would be very nice if the worst range of motion were at least 95° on one side. However, range of motion is not the ultimate goal here. Our experience with the GUEPAR type of prosthesis or other hinges has shown that if we wanted to achieve 120° flexion we would have to take out a lot of bone and put in a great deal of hinge. Obviously, we are not looking simply to maximize flexion.

*Matsui* (Nagoya City University): Loosening may occur so we have to gain the stability to remove that pain and for this 100° flexion is sufficient.

Miller (McGill University): We are seeking to create knees that are as normal as possible. Obviously, there are many factors that we try to optimize, such as pain, alignment, and stability. We must also try to get the best flexion possible. So it is wrong I think to say that we do not want the maximum range of motion possible.

We have heard a number of papers today in which it was stated that the Total Condylar type of knee achieves flexion of about 90°–95°. We have also heard that the PCA achieves 105°. So it cannot be said that the prosthesis design has no bearing on the range of motion because it clearly does on the basis of the data we have see today.

*Goldie*: With regard to bone ingrowth, bone grows into cement as it grows into all kinds of materials that are inserted into the human frame. Could Dr. Bontemps tell us a little more about his studies where a density of bone was found shortly after insertion of the prosthesis, but where resorption subsequently occurred more on the mediolateral side than centrally?

*Bontemps*: We had bone resorption underneath the metal tray and on the outer medial and lateral borders of the tray. This occurred during the first 1 or 2 years but then progressed no further. Under the central part between the pegs and around the medial pegs we found increased bone density. The bone density was most compact directly underneath the metal tray. In varus knees, it was mostly around the medial peg, from which there developed an increased trabecular structure going to the diaphyseal corticalis. We think this is because the bone is not stressed sufficiently at the outer portions of the tibial plateau and that stress protection occurs there. In the normal joint, the tibial condyles are mainly stressed; the bone is densest in the center and weakest on the tibial plateau. When we introduce the prosthesis, the bone is mainly stressed in the central part. Here, increased bone density is found, as I showed in my densitometric measurement slides, where it was evident from 3 months to 1 year that the bone density between the pegs was obviously increasing.

*Goldie*: What do you think of the physical properties, in particular the hardness, of this bone, knowing the Rank and Stear photogrammetric studies referred to in the last presentation show that there is clearly subsidence of the prosthesis to quite a large degree? This does not apply just to the PCA prosthesis; it applies to all prostheses.

*Bontemps*: These densitometric measurements have nothing to with bone ingrowth; they just indicate whether the bone might become strong enough with time so that no further displacement of the prosthesis will occur. With further standardization of this technique, it may become possible to state after, say, 2 or 3 years if little is happening in terms of bone density and osteolysis and that stabilization has occurred and the prosthesis been accepted. In this way we do not have to wait 10–15 years to see if the prosthesis is successful.

*Goldie*: Dr. Krackow you showed a slide on the X-ray of a PCA prosthesis, where the tibial plateau had subsided quite considerably or at least you said that there was an overgrowth of bone anterior to the superior part of the tibial tubercle. Is this in fact the case or is it because the prosthesis had sunk down, not having rested on the tibial cortical rim?

*Krackow*: That particular X-ray is an example of something we commonly see on the tibia, fairly commonly on the patella, and only occasionally on the femur. One sees an overgrowth of bone or at least the appearance of bone coming up from the level of the metal; this is at least 80%–90% overgrowth and not more than 10%–20% subsidence. On that particular view of the tibia, if we had imagined the tibial component to have started at the edge of where the bone was, the tibial component would have sloped down much more and it would have been much higher and farther away from the tibial tubercle. We have just completed a study of the patellar component, in which it is perfectly clear that essentially all the bone formed represents overgrowth bone and not subsidence. We do not see this appearance if the metal comes all the way to the edge, i.e., if we have a tibial component where the metal base plate is perfectly positioned and goes from the entire posterior to the entire anterior border. On the other hand, I am certain that in some cases that have been shown to me and perhaps a small number of our own cases, there has been some amount of subsidence anteriorly on the tibial component. We would certainly prefer the tibial component to cover the cut surface of the tibia as completely as possible.

*Goldie*: Do you find the same extent of bone ingrowth into the patella as you do into the tibia and femur?

*Krackow*: I am only referring to the phenomenon of bone overgrowth; I am not saying anything about bone ingrowth into the porous surface. Many of us have witnessed at least "spotty" bone ingrowth. I do not know if the absence of a lucent line implies bone ingrowth.

*Goldie*: In the new version of the patellar button, you have extended the pegs. Does this in any way jeopardize the circulation of the patella? The question has been raised as to whether some of the complications in the patella are due to avascular necrosis, and this in turn would have something to do with the osseous reaction to the implant.

*Krackow*: I share your concern regarding avascular necrosis, but I would not think that it would be solely due to the pegs being 2 mm longer. I think that avascular necrosis of the patella is a distinct possibility in situations where one has had to deal with very substantial lateral release and/or has too liberal a dissection along the margin of the tibia.

*Ranawat*: With regard to vascular necrosis of the patella following lateral release, to my knowledge only one or two cases have been reported. I have done hundreds and hundreds of lateral releases and I do not think it is a common entity at all. The best way to find out whether it is likely to occur is, when performing lateral release, to cut the lateral superior genicular artery; the tourniquet should be released to see whether the patella shows any signs of blood. If blood is flowing through the cancellous bone it proves that there is sufficient circulation in the bone. There are many reasons why the patella fractures, but I do not think that avascularity is an important contributing factor.

*Goldie*: Do you do your knees under a tourniquet?

*Ranawat*: Yes.

*Goldie*: And so you look at the circulation after you have released the tourniquet and when you have put the button into the patella[2].

*Ranawat*: I do not do it routinely, but if there is doubt it can be done. I do not think it is the cause.

*Goldie*: I think you are right there. The patella is in the center of a very rich vascular network, with vessels coming in not only from the lateral genicular artery but also from the rectus tendon and the medical retinaculi, with quite a number of small vessels penetrating the patella. Time will show if there is any truth to this fear of vascular necrosis.

*Yamamoto*: The concept of bone ingrowth was originally based on animal experiments. For example, if a piece of coated porous metal is implanted in the tibia under static conditions, the bone grows in perfectly. However, when a prosthesis is inserted into the human body the conditions are dynamic and to obtain early bone ingrowth initial immobilization is very important. The patella though is very difficult to immobilize and this may be one of the reasons why there are so many problems associated with it.

*Goldie*: It is amazing how the patient can walk around with the prosthesis not fixed with cement and yet still the bone grows in and fixes the prosthesis. This would seem to be the opposite of what one would expect: When a bone is broken it should be stabilized and kept still.

Could Dr. Engelbrecht comment on the use of hinge prostheses as a risk factor in increased infection in view of the popularity of this prosthesis in continental Europe?

*Engelbrecht* (Endo-Klinik): There is an increased risk of deep infection with the hinged knee. We treat these cases as we do in hip replacement by primary one-stage exchange procedures using antibiotic-loaded acrylic cement according to the antibiogram. In early infections, we do not do a primary exchange procedure because the infection is usually only present in the soft tissue and not at the bone-cement interface. Debridement and irrigation are sufficient in these cases in addition to a systemic antibiotic, given as perioperative treatment. We cannot prevent a deep infection in all cases. In some cases, the organisms are sensitive to the Gentamycin present in the bone cement.

*Goldie*: Dr. Kurosaka would you comment on the early treatment of infection? As Dr. Engelbrecht has said, there might just be a soft tissue involvement, which can be handled by antibiotics, debridement, and irrigation. However, if it has gone so far that bone may be interfered with and there is an infection of the sinuses down to the bone what would be your first action?

*Kurosaka*: If acute infection is suspected, we can debride the joint with retention of the prosthesis, because in the early phase most of the infection is limited to the soft tissues and does not invade to the bone-cement interface. If an infection exists at the bone-cement interface, it is probably very difficult to treat just by debriding the soft tissue and giving antibiotics. Judging whether an infection is present at the bone-cement interfaces can be very difficult. X-rays can be examined with fluoroscopy to see if there are any progressive radiolucent lines. Gallium scintigrams can also be used to judge whether there is any infection at the interface. In general, I would say that in the acute situation, i.e., within a couple of weeks of surgery, if infection is suspected the soft tissue can be debrided with retention of the prosthesis.

*Goldie*: But what would you do if you have an osseous infection, would you go for an arthrodesis immediately after removing the prosthesis or would you just wait for some time and reoperate with retention of the prosthesis? The question is how long do you actually wait to do an arthrodesis?

*Kurosaka*: If we have to remove the prosthesis, as in chronic infection, we give intravenous extensive antibiotics for 4–6 weeks and we have to wait until we are fairly convinced that the infection has subsided. After this, we would probably do two-stage reimplantation.

*Krackow*: Our decision whether or not to seek knee fusion rather than reimplantation would depend on the medical condition of the patient and the residual bone stock. If the patient could put up with several more operative procedures, we would probably prefer to treat by delayed revision; so there would be prosthesis removal, debridement, intraoperative check to ensure that all the cement had been used, and implantation of antibiotic-impregnated spacers as large and thin sheets to maintain the tissue planes. The wound would then be closed and the patient maintained on parenteral antibiotics for 3–6 weeks and reimplantation would be performed 3–6 weeks after the procedure. If the decision is made to carry out fusion, I see no reason not to do the fusion at the same time. I personally have performed 20 knee fusions in one stage and these have included patients with diabetes, patients receiving high-dose steroids, methotraxate, and all manner of antimetabolites; I have never failed to bring about perfect healing of the wound and have only failed once to produce healing of the fusion. In the latter case, there was healing following a simple reoperation and bone grafting. I think there is no need for two-stage fusion, but we do two-stage reimplantations most of the time.

*Goldie*: Do you find the healing time longer with these cases of arthrodesis than with ordinary cases of arthrodesis?

*Krackow*: I have very limited experience with ordinary arthrodesis. I think I have only ever performed two primary knee arthrodeses which did not have a prosthesis. I would be confident of these cases showing quicker healing. I personally allow 3 months of external fixation for a knee prosthesis arthrodesis followed by 2 or 3 months of cylinder casting.

*Matsui*: Fortunately, I have not had to deal with infections so much. In the case of infection to synovial areas, debridement and synovectomy under arthroscopy should be carried out. If there is a change in the bone itself, the artificial joint should be taken out and debridement conducted.

*Bontemps*: I would try to avoid arthrodesis in the case of infection. I would attempt one-stage replacement if the case were not too severe. If the case were more severe, I would explant it and introduce Gentamycin beads and intravenous therapy. After a few weeks, I would implant a second prosthesis. If this failed, I would repeat the procedure. After three or four failures, I would direct the patient to Dr. Engelbrecht.

*Hastings*: This question depends on the infecting organism, the status of the bone, and on the status of the patient. With a Gram-negative organism, the surgeon is not going to win and should proceed directly to arthrodesis as soon as the infection is under control. In the case of bone with draining sinuses and perforations of the cortex, again, an exchange will probably not succeed and a fusion should be performed. On the other hand, if the patient is old and frail and could not stand up to an arthrodesis, perhaps the exchange would be preferable.

*Engelbrecht*: The indication for arthrodesis in both infections and aseptic cases is not a severe defect or so-called problem organisms, but in our experience it is severe defects in the extensor apparatus. In these cases, we feel we have to perform an arthrodesis because there is no chance of obtaining good function or partially good function postoperatively. We may perform a primary exchange procedure.

# Part 4
# Cementless Total Knee Replacement II

# An Uncemented Alumina Ceramic Total Knee Prosthesis

H. Oonishi, A. Maeda, N. Murata, S. Kushitani, M. Aono, T. Nabeshima, K. Tsuyama, and Y. Takayama[1]

**Summary.** A prosthesis is presented in which the part in contact with the bone is made of alumina and the articulating part is made of a combination of alumina and UHMWPE; the stem is located at the center of the tibial plateau. The combination of alumina and ultra-high molecular weight polyethylene (UHMWPE) was compared with that of metal and UHMWPE. Test results with a knee joint simulator have revealed that the rate of wear of UHMWPE is more than ten times smaller in the combination with alumina than in that with metal.

Indication varies depending on the individual conditions of both the prosthesis and the living body. With respect to the prosthesis, design, initial fixation, and limitation in strength and brittleness of alumina, etc. are important. With the tibial side, when fixation without cement is performed "loosening" will be reduced if there is rest with external fixation and nonweight bearing is maintained for a certain period. In patients with severe bone atrophy or severe sclerotic bone on the surface contacting the prosthetic component over a large area, cement fixation is safer. Before insertion of a component, very finely crushed bone chips are spread over the surface of the bone at a thickness of 2–3 mm in order to fill the small grooves of the component and facilitate contact of the component with the bone over the whole area. The authors are now developing a new material by coating the surface with titanium alloy beads or alumina beads with hydroxy apatite (HAp) layer about 10 $\mu$m thick by means of a plasma spray. Compared with the untreated surface, HAp coating presents almost two to three times the adhesion rate and strength in the initial stage. When a polymethyl methacrylate (PMMA) bone cement is used, we put fine granules of HAp between the bone and bone cement, and we term this the interfacial bioactive bone cement technique.

**Keywords:** Alumina ceramics—Total knee prosthesis—Cementless—Hydroxyapatite coating—Porous materials

## Introduction

The alumina ceramic total knee prosthesis we developed, in which alumina ceramics are employed for the part that contacts the bone and a combination of alumina ceramics and UHMWPE is used for the sliding part, is a so-called total condylar type of prosthesis. Surgically, the anterior and posterior cruciate ligaments are removed.

The stem is positioned at the center of the tibial plateau and through the stem the load is transmitted to the cortical bone of the posterior part of the tibia. This design has proved to be excellent as a result of analyses by three-dimensional finite element method (FEM) of stress analysis and photoelastic method (Fig. 1) [1–10].

We performed a wear test by the pin-on-disc method on the combination of alumina ceramics and UHMWPE comparing it with a combination of metal with UHMWPE. The test results have shown that decrements of UHMWPE due to wear, including creep deformation, are much lower in the combination with alumina ceramics than in the combination with metal. A test with a hip simulator has demonstrated that the UHMWPE socket wears less in combination with alumina ceramics and that metal elements are precipitated in a lubricating solution in the combination with metal; in the combination with alumina ceramics aluminum is not precipitated [1–3].

## Simulator Test

In the present study, a wear test was performed with a knee simulator on our developed total knee prosthesis using the combination of alumina with UHMWPE in comparison with a total condylar type of knee prosthesis using the combination of metal Co-Cr-Mo alloy and UHMWPE with and without a metal tray. The three prostheses are similar in configuration. In the experiments, the maximum load was 1960 N (200 kgf), the forward and backward moving distance was 5 mm, the flexion-extension angle was 0°–15°, one cycle lasted 1.8 s, the number of repetitions was one million, and the sliding part was filled with saline solution. With equal loading to the bilateral condyles, as in the case

[1] Department of Orthopaedic Surgery, Artificial Joint Section and Biomaterial Research Laboratory, Osaka-Minami National Hospital, Osaka, Japan

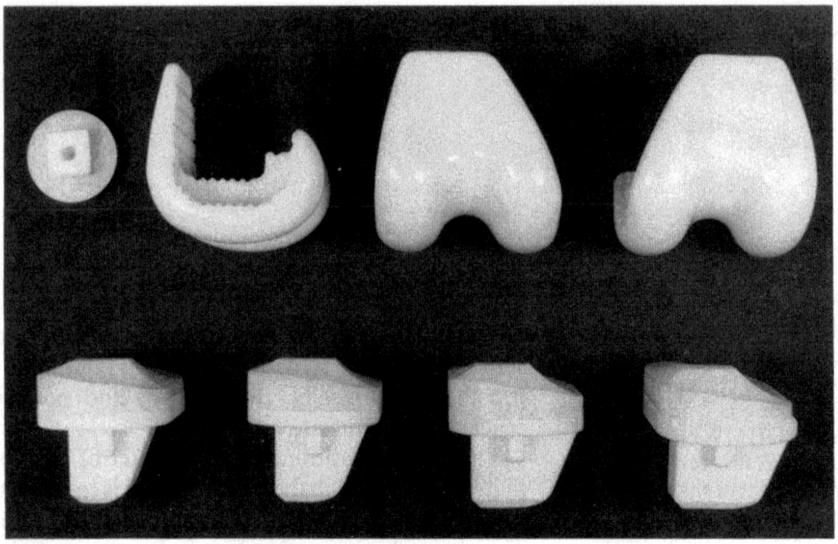

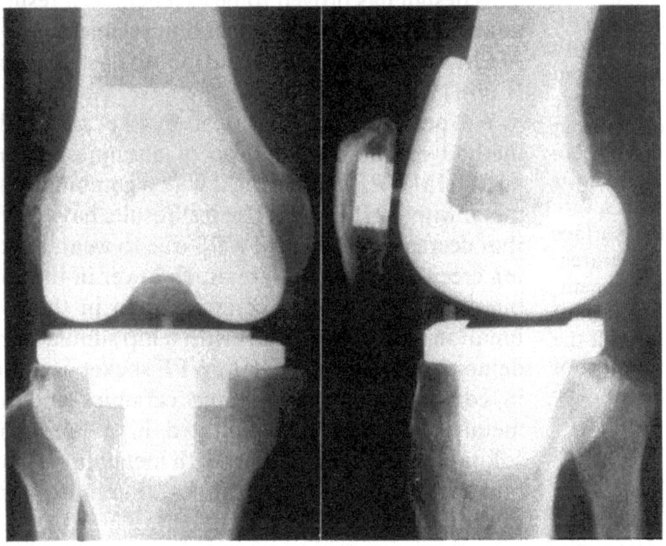

**Fig. 1.** **a** KOM cementless alumina ceramic total knee prosthesis, **b** X-ray after surgery

of combination with metal (total condylar), the maximum decrement of UHMWPE was 0.3 mm; in the combination with alumina, no decrements were seen in many parts. The decrement of UHMWPE in the combination with alumina was more than ten times smaller than that in the combination with metal (Fig. 2). In both cases, the decrease was more prominent in the anterior part. The friction-contact are of UHMWPE was not shiny in the combination with metal; macroscopically, numerous fine scars were observed. On the other hand, in the combination with alumina, the contact area was shiny and macroscopically only a small number of scars was seen. In the combination with metal, the decrement of UHMWPE showed slightly greater one-sided loading than equal loading to the bilateral condyles. In the combination with alumina, the differences observed between the two conditions of loading were almost imperceptible. In the combination with metal at the parts presenting deep scars polyethylene had been dug up and was projecting in numerous fine slivers set in arrays. Even at the parts showing relatively smooth scars, polyethylene was thinly scaled off in an irregular manner. In the combination with alumina, rough scars before use disappeared entirely and the whole surface became smooth. At the center of a worn area the surface did not show any minimal unevenness, was absolutely smooth, and presented no separation of polyethylene (Fig. 3) [11].

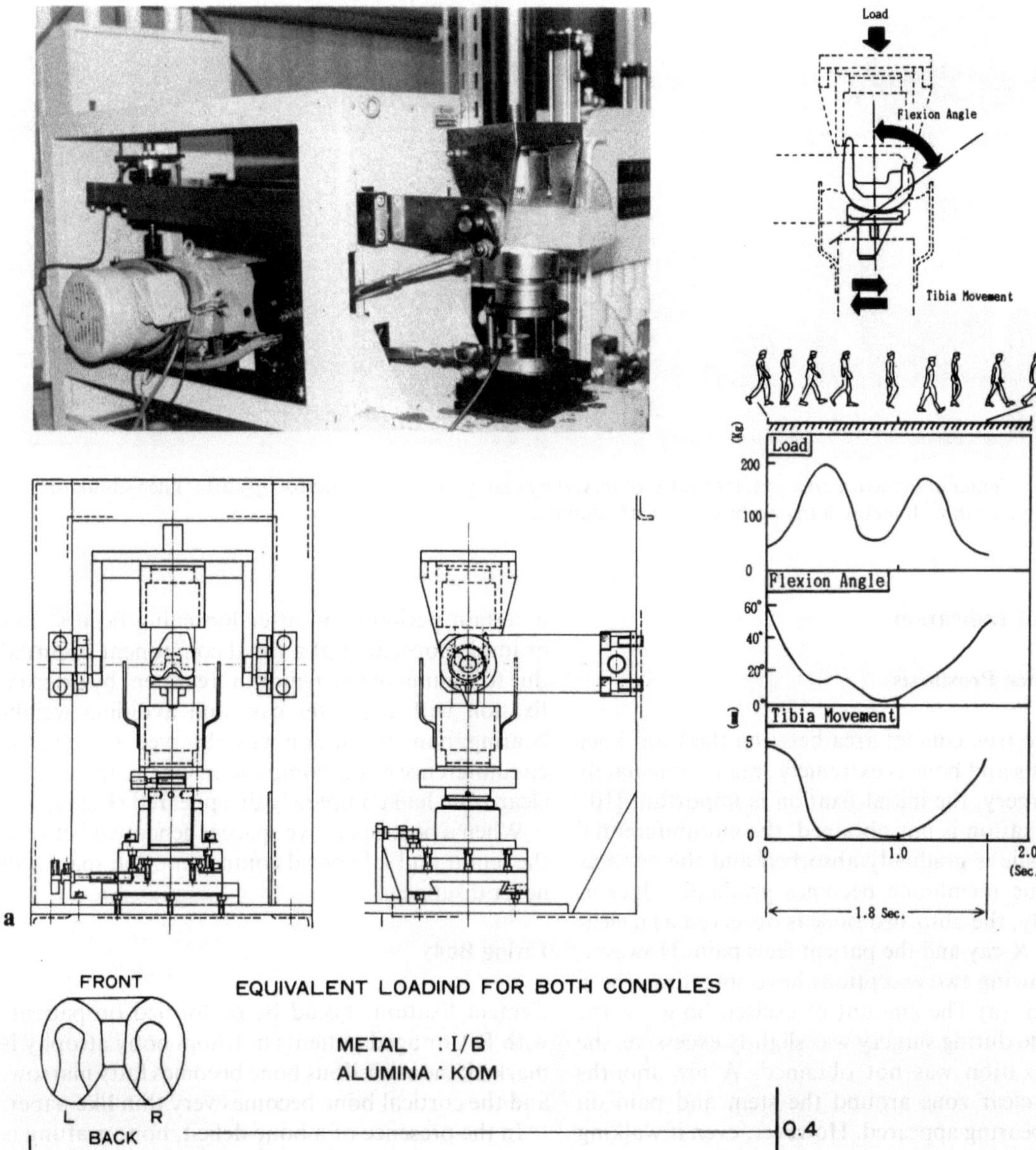


**Fig. 2a, b.** Simulator test of total knee prosthesis. The combination of alumina with UHMWPE (KOM total knee prosthesis) was compared with that of metal with UHMWPE (I/B total condylar). A physiological load cycle was reproduced. The maximum load was 1962N (200kgf) and the sliding part was always filled with saline solution. After one million repetitions, the amount of deformation due to wear, including creep deformation, was measured with a Contracer. **a** Knee simulator. **b** Simulator test results, showing maximum decrement of UHMWPE a 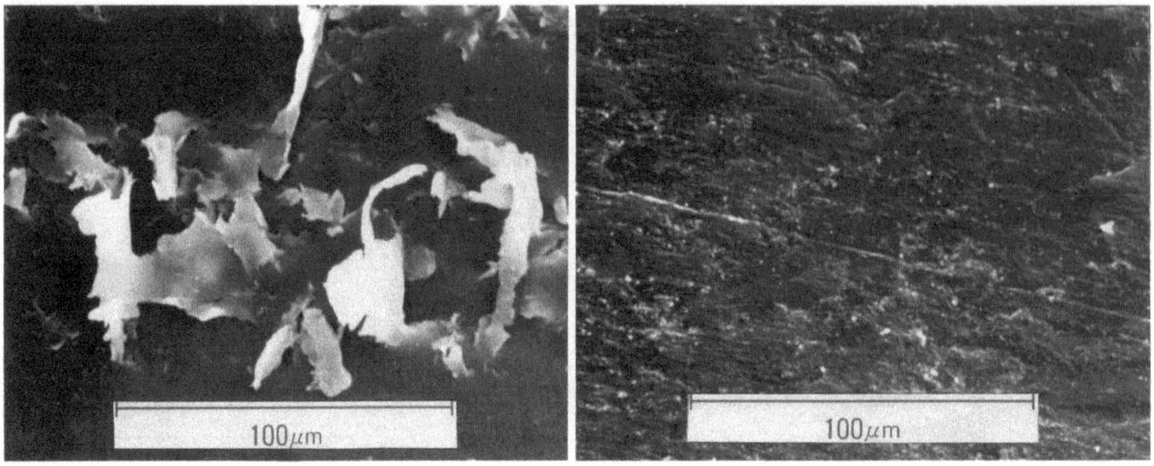 b


**Fig. 3a, b.** Center of the worn area of UHMWPE observed by scanning electron microscopy after knee simulator test. **a** In combination with metal. **b** In combination with alumina

## Limits of Indication

### Total Knee Prosthesis

Since the true contact area between the total knee prosthesis and bone is extremely small immediately after surgery, the initial fixation is important [10–13]. If fixation is not obtained, the circumferential bone tissue is gradually absorbed and the connective tissue membrane becomes gradually thicker. Clinically, the absorbed bone is observed as a clear zone on X-ray and the patient feels pain. However, the following two exceptions have sometimes been observed: (a) The amount of excised bone on the tibial side during surgery was slightly excessive, the initial fixation was not obtained. A few months later, a clear zone around the stem and pain on weight bearing appeared. However, even if walking with weight bearing was continued in this condition, bony formation occurred again and, finally, fixation to the bone was obtained. (b) The amount of excised bone was small and for this reason the range of motion was limited. However, since bony atrophy was severe, a tibial component sank by a few millimeters during walking on weight bearing; this increased the range of motion and induced the appearance of a painless and fine clear zone around the stem. After that, the component did not sink any more and the clear zone gradually disappeared. These phenomena are seen in patients developing bony atrophy such as those with rheumatoid arthritis (RA) (Fig. 4).

When cement fixation is not performed, "loosening," if it appears, can be rectified by rest and avoiding weight bearing, with external fixation for a certain period soon after loosening occurs. For example, loosening of a tibial component occurred due to trauma. After 1-month treatment by external fixation with a plaster cast and avoiding weight bearing, bone formation was observed again in the circumference of the component. One year later, the clear zone had completely disappeared (Fig. 5).

When a post-operative space is generated between the femur and a femoral component, the space will never disappear.

### Living Body

Cement fixation should be performed on patients with RA or aged patients in whom bony atrophy is marked; the cancellous bone becomes fatty marrow, and the cortical bone becomes very thin like paper.

In the presence of a bone deficit, bone grafting is carried out, and this does not always require the use of bone cement. When a bone defect is less than one-third on the outer side of a unilateral plateau, only a bone graft will suffice. When a bone defect exceeds the one-third limit, a bone graft only is extremely unstable and it is safer to use bone cement. If a bone defect is less than one-third on the outer side of a unilateral plateau, a bone chip can only be inserted using pressure. When a bone defect exceeds the one-third limit and a bone graft is performed, the following is one of the methods used: A cancellous bone with a cortical bone as a bone graft is used and the portion of cortical bone is placed on the most peripheral side so that it can support load. Thus, when the amount of bone deficit is large and bony atrophy slight, tibial osteotomy in the distal part can decrease the required amount of bone graft. However, when

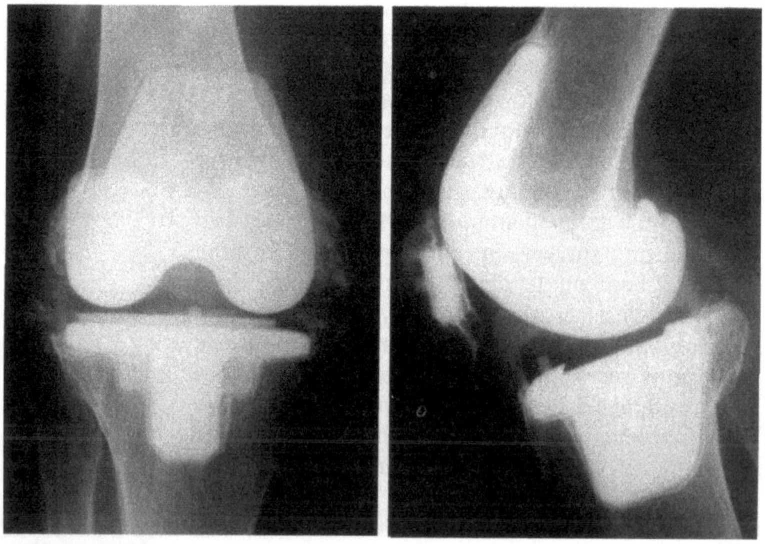

**Fig. 4.** Since bony atrophy was severe, the tibial component sank during walking on weight bearing, which induced the appearance of a fine clear zone around the stem.

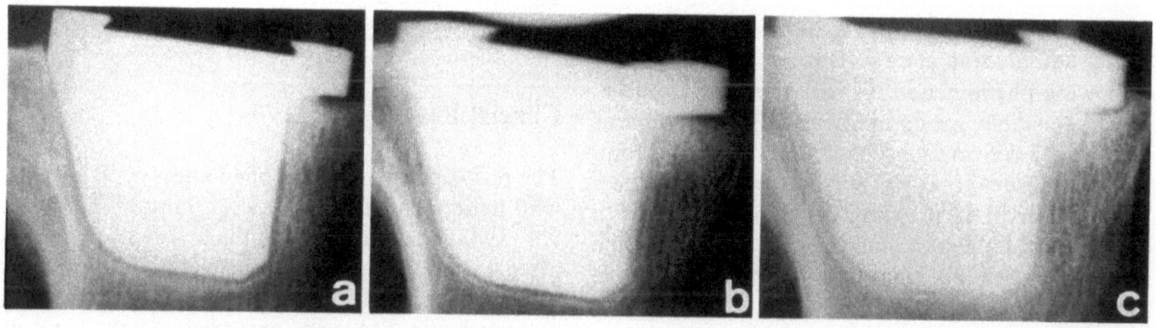


**Fig. 5a–c.** A painful clear zone due to loosening appeared around the stem after trauma; it disappeared, however, with rest and the use of a nonweight bearing plaster cast. **a** One month after trauma. **b** Six months after trauma. **c** Twelve months after trauma

bony atrophy is severe, it is important to reduce the amount of excised bone as much as possible, because the closer the osteotomy is to the joint end, the denser the bone is.

On the side of the femur, the anterior and posterior sides of the cortical bone of the femur should be in contact with a larger portion of the component. In particular, if the posterior side of the femoral condyle is in contact with the component only slightly, the component gradually moves forward, even though bone grafting has been carried out; as a result, a space is generated between the anterior side of the femur and the component. In addition, when the knee joint is flexed on weight-bearing it generates such force as to push the femoral component forward from behind and the component is thus made to move farther forward. If there is relatively marked bony atrophy at the distal end of the femur or many bone grafts are used, the component easily sinks.

## Conditions of Bone and Component in the Cementless Prosthesis

The stem is inserted into the tibia, whereas the femur is located inside the component [10–13]. Thus, the conditions are completely different in these two bones. The clinical reaction is also completely different. In the case of the stem, even though a clear zone appears after surgery, bone formation recurs, the clear zone gradually disappears, and around it a fine line of bone sclerosis appears. This is because sclerotic bone develops just below the thin connective tissue membrane. On the side of the femur, once a space between the femur and the component is generated on the anterior and posterior sides of the femur, bone formation will never recur and a line of bone sclerosis will seldom appear.

When a step made on the surface is small or the surface is made uneven only slightly, the initial fixation is extremely important. In the case of incomplete initial fixation, movement will enlarge a space, which will carry the risk of thick connective tissue being generated, followed by loosening.

In order to make the connective tissue membrane lying between the two structures as thin as possible and to prevent loosening, we fill the space generated between the component and the bone with crushed bone during surgery. Specifically, we place small pieces of bone on the metal tray that we developed on a trial basis, crush the bone by hammering, and spread it at a thickness of 2–3 mm over the surface of a bony recess just before installing the component, and then drive in the component. In future, we will use bioactive bone cement which is now under development for the cementless prosthesis.

## Contraindication

**Marked bony atrophy.** In the tibia, the component will gradually sink after surgery and the risk of the following phenomenon is high: The knee itself becomes unstable, the component loosens, and varus and valgus deformity occur. In the femur, the component loosens in a forward and backward direction or sinks in the proximal direction and there is a high risk of having the same results as those in the tibia (Fig. 6) [12]. Therefore, fixation with bone cement should be performed.

**Marked sclerotic bone.** If the space prepared by osteotomy or bone excision is a little too small for the component, fracture might occur on insertion since the bone is not deformed. Even though there is no problem on insertion, the contact area after insertion is extremely small and there are many spaces, which results in poor fixation. It cannot be expected that new bone formation will occur in the spaces, even though the spaces are filled with crushed bone, because the crushed bone will be frequently absorbed. Boring many holes through the sclerotic bone in an effort to prevent this risk has little effect. After high tibial osteotomy, bony sclerosis sometimes develops, and great care is thus required.

**A large amount of bone graft in the weight bearing part.** When a lot of bone graft is required, it is desirable to adjust it by the amount of excised bone. There is a high risk of the destruction of transplanted bone.

**Infection.** Even if osteomyelitis was cured a long time previously, there is a risk of recurrence.

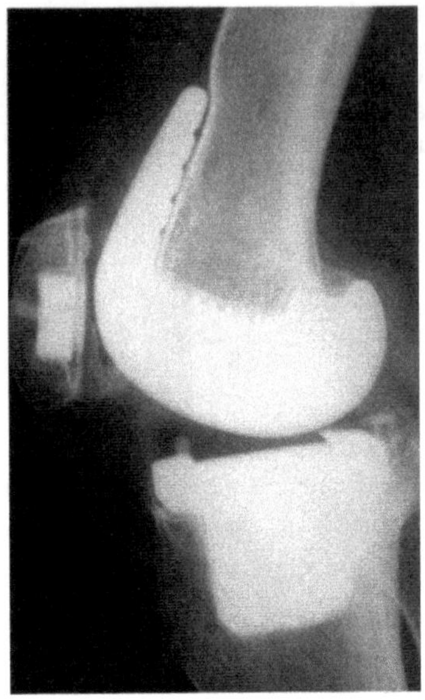

**Fig. 6.** A space appeared 3 years after surgery in the femur, but there was no complaint of pain

## Clincial Results

The post-operative results of 46 knees of 30 patients who underwent surgery between January 1982 and July 1983, i.e., 2 years 6 months to 4 years 6 months after surgery, are presented here [13]. Two patients developing late infection, one with RA and one with osteoarthritis (OA), are excluded. At the time of surgery, the patients were aged between 38 and 78 years (with a mean of 60 years); there were three knees of two males and 43 knees of 28 females.

In the RA group, consisting of 39 knees of 25 patients, there were three knees of two males and 36 knees of 23 females. At the time of surgery, the patients were aged between 38 and 78 years (with a mean of 57 years). Before surgery, the severity of RA was stage IIIb in 14 patients and stage IV in 11 patients (Fig. 7).

The OA group consisted of seven knees of five females. At the time of surgery, the patients were aged between 65 and 76 years (with a mean of 70 years). Before surgery, the severity of OA was stage IV in four patients and stage V in one.

The post-operative follow-up period lasted 2 years 6 months to 4 years (with a mean of 3 years 2 months). The results obtained are evaluated on the basis of the Knee Joint Function Evaluation Table (prepared by Okayama, Aichi, and Shinsu Universities; see Table 2 in Chap. 11).

With respect to the two patients developing late infection, one had a history of high tibial osteotomy about 6 years before and the other had a history of

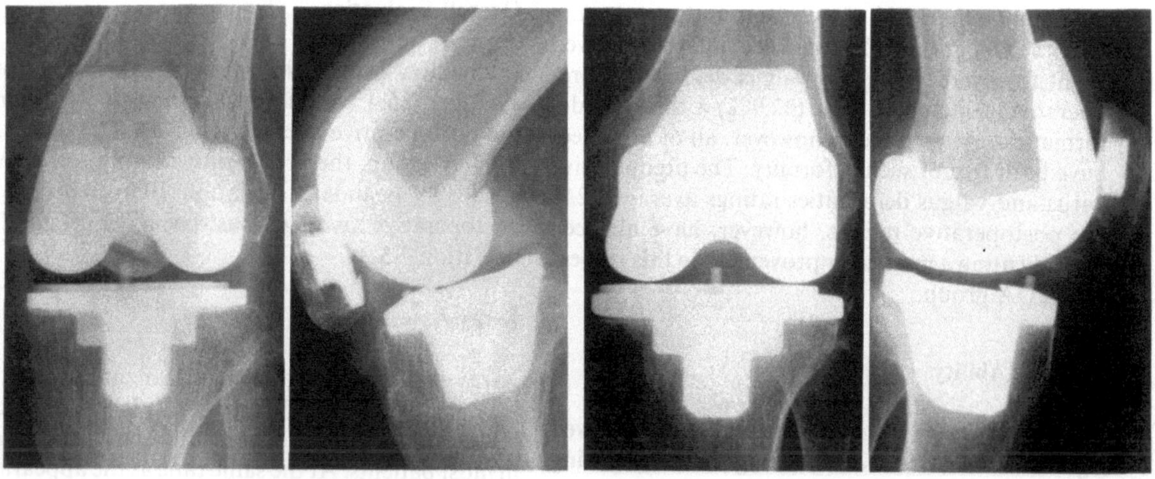

a b

**Fig. 7.** **a** X-ray taken 4 years 6 months after replacement in a patient with RA. The patient is now mostly confined to the house. **b** X-ray taken 4 years after replacement in a patient with RA. The patient now works in a factoy

osteomyelitis of the tibia on the same side about 20 years before.

**Pain**

In the RA group, significant or severe pain (rating 15 or below) was experienced by all patients preopertively, but after surgery 30 (77%) of the knees operated on showed no pain (rating 30), nine (23%) had slight pain (rating 25), and none had significant or severe pain (rating 15 or below), which means that all of the affected knees have improved to slight or better levels of pain. Whereas the preoperative levels of pain averaged 9.1, the postoperative average has been 28.0, indicating a remarkable general reduction in pain.

In the OA group, significant or severe pain was seperienced by all of the patients preoperatively, but after surgery five (71%) of the knees operated on had no pain, one (14%) slight pain, and one (14%) significant pain. Whereas the preoperative levels of pain averaged 13.6, the postoperative average has been 27.5, indicating a similar remarkable general reduction in pain in the OA group.

**Range of Motion**

Both preoperatively and postoperatively, 33 (85%) of the knees operated on in the RA group showed ranges of motion of 90° or more (rating 15 or above). Whereas the preoperative range of motion ratings averaged 17.2, the postoperative average has been 15.4, indicating a slight decrease.

In the OA group, all of the knees operated on showed ranges of motion of 90° or more both preoperatively and postoperatively. But whereas the preoperative range of motion ratings averaged 17.9, the postoperative average has been 16.4, indicating a slight decrease also in the OA group.

**Extension Lag**

In the RA group, all of the affected knees showed slight or more than slight (5 or below) extension lag preoperatively. After surgery, however, 36 (92%) of the knees have shown no extension lag (rating 10), and only three (8%) still show slight or worse extension lag. Also, whereas the preoperative extension lag failure ratings averaged 2.2, the postoperative average has been 9.6, indicating a marked improvement in extension lag.

In the OA group, all of the affected knees showed slight or worse degrees of extension lag failure preoperatively. After surgery, however, none of the knees have shown any extension lag. Whereas the preoperative extension lag ratings averaged 2.1, the postoperative average has been 10.0, indicating a marked improvement in extension lag in the OA group too.

**Varus and Valgus Deformities**

In the RA group, all of the knees affected showed slight to severe varus and valgus deformities (rating 5 or below) preoperatively, including two (5.1%) with severe deformation (16° or greater, rating 0). After surgery, however, all of the knees have been free of such deformity (rating 10). Though the preoperative varus and valgus deformities ratings averaged 4.7, the postoperative ratings have all been 10, indicating a marked improvement in this respect.

In the OA group, al! of the knees affected showed slight to severe varus and valgus deformities preoperatively, including three (42.9%) with severe deformation. After surgery, however, all of the knees have been free of such deformity. The preoperative varus and valgus deformities ratings averaged 2.9, the postoperative ratings, however, have all been 10, indicating a marked improvement in this respect in the OA group.

### Walking Ability

In the RA group, all of the knees affected showed significant or more severe walking difficulty (rating 10 or below) preoperatively. After surgery, however, three (7.7%) of the knees have been normal (rating 20) and 21 (53.9%) have had slight difficulty, while the number of knees with significant or severe difficulty has been reduced to 15 (38.5%). The preoperative walking ability ratings averaged 1.9; the postoperative average has been 13.5 indicating a marked improvement in walking ability.

In the OA group, all of the knees affected showed significant or severe walking difficulty preoperatively. After surgery, three (42.9%) of the knees have been normal and three (42.9%) have had slight difficulty; significant or severe difficulty has remained in only one case (14.3%). The preoperative walking ability ratings averaged 2.1; the postoperative average has been 16.4, indicating a marked improvement in walking ability in the OA group also.

### Activities of Daily Living

In the RA group, 21 (53.8%) of the knees had an activities of daily living (ADL) rating of 0, 18 (46.2%) knees were 5 or below, and no knees were 6 or above preoperatively. After surgery, however, 27 (69.2%) of the knees have been rated 6 or above , 12 (30.8%) knees rated 5 or below, and none rated 0. The preoperative ADL ratings averaged 1.3; the postoperative average, however, has been 6.0, indicating a marked improvement in ADL.

In the OA group, three (42.9%) of the knees had an ADL rating of 0, four (57.1%) knees were 5 or below, and none were 6 or above preoperatively. After surgery, five (71.4%) of the knees have been rated 6 or above, two (28.6%) knees rated 5 or below, and none rated 0. The preoperative ADL ratings averaged 1.3; the postoperative average has been 7.0, indicating a marked improvement in ADL in the OA group.

### Overall Evaluation

In the RA group, the preoperative rating totals averaged 36.4 (standard deviation 10.3), whereas the postoperative average has been 82.5 $\pm$ 7.1). In the OA group, the preoperative rating totals averaged 39.9 (standard deviation 10.0), whereas the postoperative average has been 87.3 (standard deviation 7.3).

### X-ray Assessment

X-ray examination revealed a clear zone around the stem in about 60% of the patients. It was not seen a few months after surgery but 1–2 years after surgery in most patients. At the same time as the appearance of the clear zone, a line representing bone sclerosis was seen just below the clear zone. The clear zone that appeared after trauma could be made to disappear by rest and avoidance of weight bearing.

When bony atrophy is marked, as in RA, and the tibial plate is too small, it frequently sinks 2–3 mm 6 months to 1 year after surgery. It sank more than 5 mm in some patients in whom the range of motion was reduced. In one patient with marked bone sclerosis after high tibial osteotomy, a wide contact area between the component and the bone was not obtained during surgery and for this reason the initial fixation was poor. As a result, micromovement appeared on weight bearing, the clear zone gradually increased, and the maximum width reached 5 mm. Slight pain appeared on weight bearing.

## Improvement and Future Prospects

It has been frequently reported that alumina is excellent in biocompatibility and binding to bone [14–19]. Our animal experiments have revealed the same result. However the follow-up X-ray examination on the clinically used alumina as an implant material has disclosed that alumina is not always so superior to metal or polymeric materials in binding to bone. Alumina is completely unreactive to the living body and extremely stable in vivo. On the other hand, titanium or titanium alloy stimulates the tissue only slightly and accelerates bone formation; it is, therefore, slightly better with respect to connecting to bone. In order to fix alumina to the bone firmly, as with other materials, a prosthesis with excellent mechanical fixation, such as the screw type or the porous type, is required. At present, the reason for the use of alumina is that wear resistance of ultra high molecular weight polyethylene (UHMWPE) is remarkably good in the sliding part,

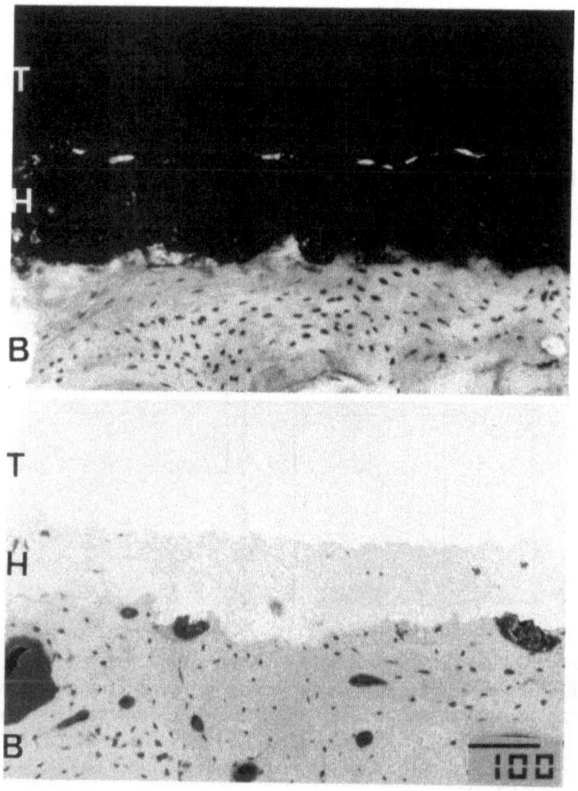


Fig. 8a, b. Titanium plates coated wih HAp were implanted into the tibial bone of beagles for 6 weeks. HAp bonded to the bone biochemically. **a** Light-microscopic image. Stained with Coal H and E. **b** Composite picture. *T* titanium, *H* HAp, *B* bone

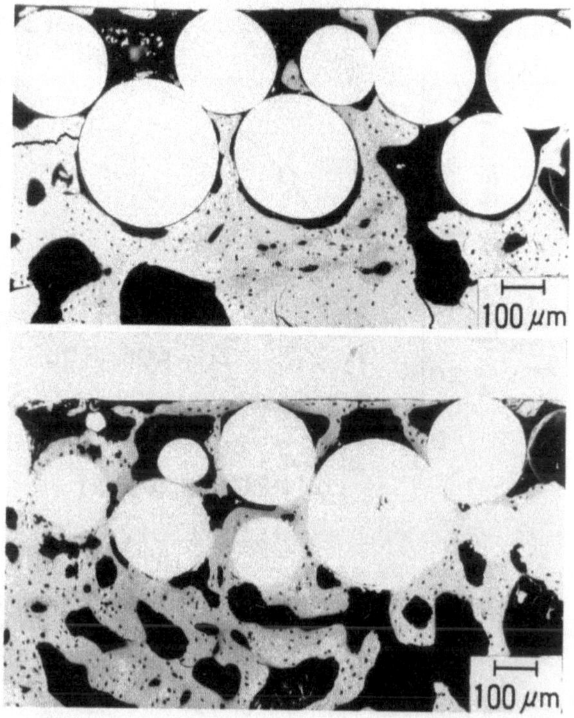


**Fig. 9. a** The implant material is a Ti-6A1-4V plate coated with Ti-6A1-4V beads; 4 weeks after implantation. **b** The implant material is another plate prepared by coating the surface of **a** with HAp; 3 weeks after implantation. The plates were implanted into the femoral condyle of rabbits. Though **b** is 1 week earlier than **a** the volume of the invaded bone into **b** is more than that in **a**. HAp coated on the beads is bonded to the bone biochemically

which is more important than that alumina be inert in vivo.

When cement fixation is performed, the component is strongly fixed immediately after surgery and in almost all patients pain can be immediately received. When cement fixation is not performed, a common problem is that about 20%–40% of patients complain of a slight pain and an oppressive feeling on weight bearing, especially at the stem of the total hip prosthesis, for a certain period after surgery. Mostly, the complaint gradually disappears with time. The cause of these phenomenon is that complete initial fixation is not obtained immediately after surgery, which is related to various factors, including design, condition of the bone, and operative procedure. However, when the long-term result in the interface is taken into account, it is not desirable to use PMMA cement which is currently employed. In order to resolve the problems that occur with cementless fixation, we are now developing a new material, which involves coating the surface of titanium alloy or alumina beads with a hydroxyapatite (HAp) layer, about 10 μm thick, with a plasma spray. As a means of cementless fixation, HAp coating obtains reliable fixation relatively early through chemical bonding (Fig. 8). Recently, porous metal has come to be used to allow early, strong fixation with bone, though for earlier and stronger fixation, apatite coating on the porous metal surface appears to be more useful (Fig. 9). However, when HAp is coated on a flat surface, problems with fatigue fractures of HAp and peeling-off of HAp from the basic metal are as yet unsolved. These problems do not appear when HAp is coated on the surface of beads. Our experiment has revealed that an HAp coating produces almost three times the adhesion rate and strength 2 and 4 weeks after implantation and twice the adhesion rate and strength 6 weeks after implantation. Three months after implantation, the difference almost disappears and is almost negligible

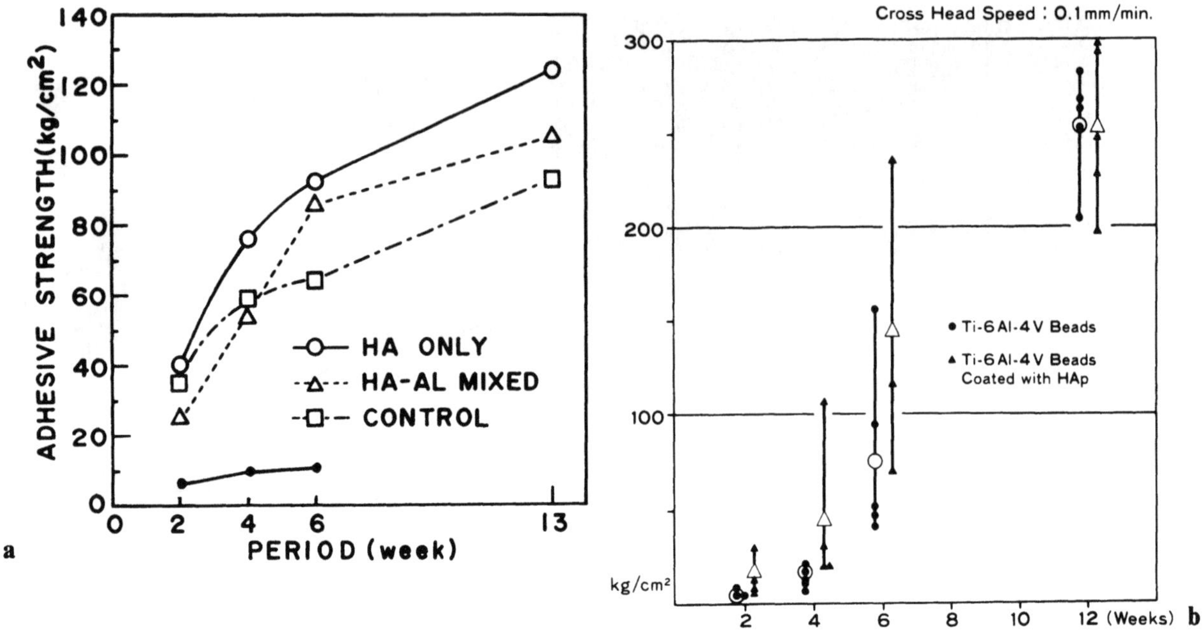


**Fig. 10.** **a** Experimental result of the same kind of material as in Fig. 9a. **b** Result with the same kind of material as in Fig. 6b. These materials were implanted into the tibial bone of a goat. After killing the animal, the bonding strength (shearing strength) of each sample was measured by a push-out test from the bone over a measured period of time. *HA ONLY* coated with 100% HAp, *HA-AL MIXED* coated with a mixture of 80% HAp and 20% alumina, *CONTROL* pure titanium applied with only shot blasting, *circles* represent samples coated with Ti-6A1-4V beads, triangles represent samples coated with HAp on the surface of Ti-6A1-4V beads

(Fig. 10).

At present, when bony atrophy is severe, long-term and stable fixation cannot be obtained unless fixation is performed with PMMA bone cement. Even though PMMA bone cement is used, the probability of loosening relatively early is high when bony atrophy is severe. We are now developing bioactive bone cement, which hardens within 10 min during surgery like PMMA bone cement and the strength of which after hardening is not inferior to that of PMMA cement. Specifically speaking, when αTCP powder is mixed with a citric acid solution during surgery, it is hardened within 10 min. The α-TCP in contact with the bone hydrates with the fluid in the body and is transformed into HAp, which is chemically bound to the bone. Thus, the connective tissue membrane does not exist in the interface with the bone. There are two ways of using the cement. First, although this is cementless fixation, all spaces can be completely filled with bioactive bone cement. Second, it can be used in the same manner as the present PMMA bone cement (Fig. 11).

The disadvantages of biological reactions on the interface between bone and conventional PMMA bone cement can be avoided by putting a thin layer of fine granules of HAp between the bone and PMMA bone cement during the cementing procedure. As a result, PMMA bone cement and fine granules of HAp become bonded mechanically, and HAp and bone become bonded biochemically. We have used this method in several cases of total hip replacement since 1984, and no clear zone has yet appeared on X-ray between PMMA bone cement and the bone. We term this the interfacial bioactive bone cement technique" (Fig. 12).

**Chemical bonding.** With either fixation with PMMA bone cement or cementless fixation, even though the connective tissue membrane is porous it always exists in the interface with the bone. More than 10 years after artificial joint replacement, as a reaction to wear particles of high-density polyethylene (HDP) or fine powder of PMMA, the bone tissue falls into necrosis through the connective tissue membrane existing in the interface with the bone. Necrosis starts at the joint and gradually moves in the distal direction. Despite the fact that the connective tissue membrane is porous, it induces the same phenomenon and loosening appears. However, when the bone is chemically bound to the bioactive materials and there is no connective tissue membrane in the

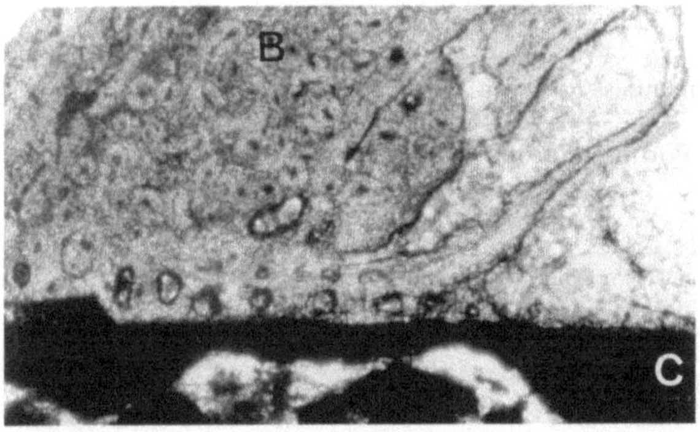


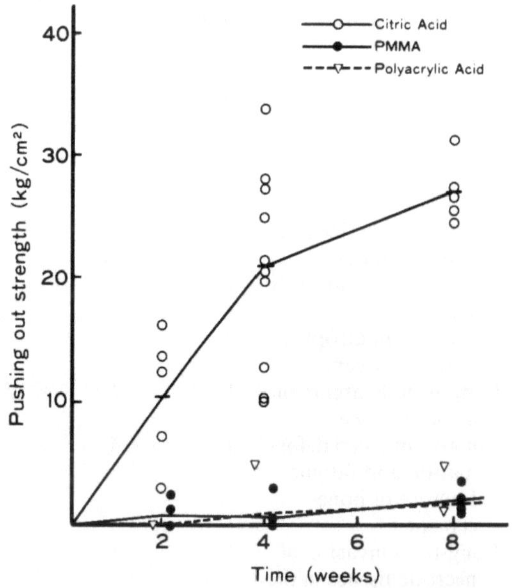


**Fig. 11.** Each test piece of several hardened bone cements was implanted into the femur of dogs. After killing the animals, the bonding strength (shear strength) of each test piece was measured by a push-out test over measured intervals of time after implantation. *Citric Acid* mixture of α-TCP powder and liquid citric acid, *PMMA* "Simplex" bone cement as a control, *Polyacrylic Acid* mixture of α-TCP powder and liquid polyacrylic acid liquid

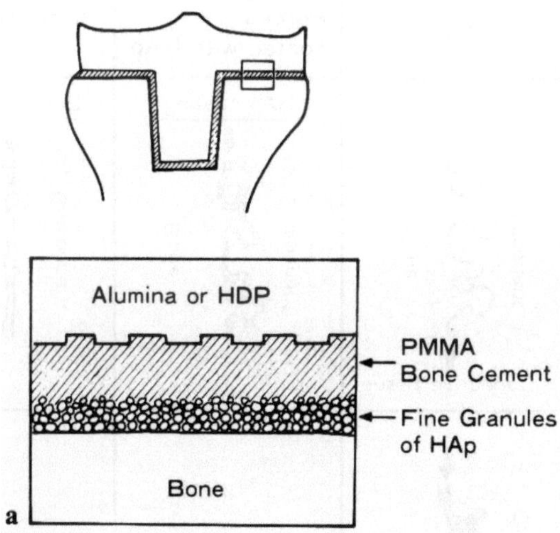


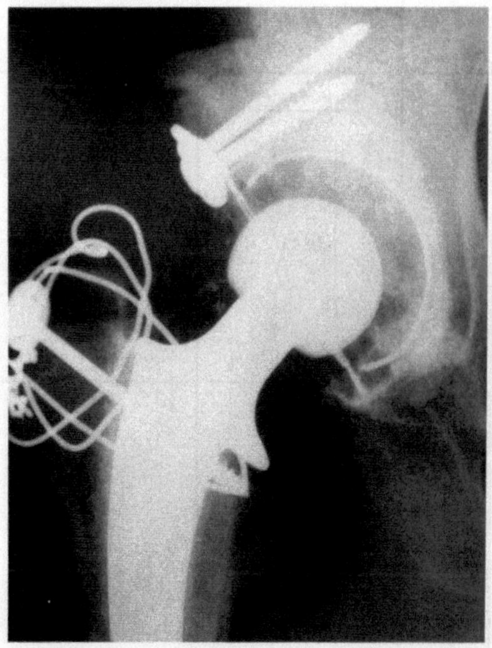


**Fig. 12a, b.** A thin layer of fine granules of HAp is put between the bone and PMMA bone cement during the cementing procedure. **a** Schematic diagram of the technique. **b** X-ray picture. This technique was used with the acetabulum and the femur

**Table 1.** Fixability of components

| | Cement fixation (PMMA) | Cementless | | | Bioactive bone cement |
|---|---|---|---|---|---|
| | | Nonporous | Porous | Porous coated with HAp | |
| Initial fixation (loosening at early stage) | 4 | 2 | 2 | 3 | 4 |
| Fixability after an early stage | 4 | 3 | 4 | 4 | 4 |
| Fixability on atrophic bone at surgery | 4 | 1 | 1 | 3 | 4 |
| Long-term fixability on atrophic bone | 1 | 1 | 3 | 3 | 3 |
| Long-term creep deformation and fatigue fracture of bone cement | 1 | 4 | 4 | 4 | ? |
| Long-term invasion of necrotic tissues in the interface | 1 | 1 | 1 | 4 | 4 |

*Figures 1–4* indicate decreasing order of merit

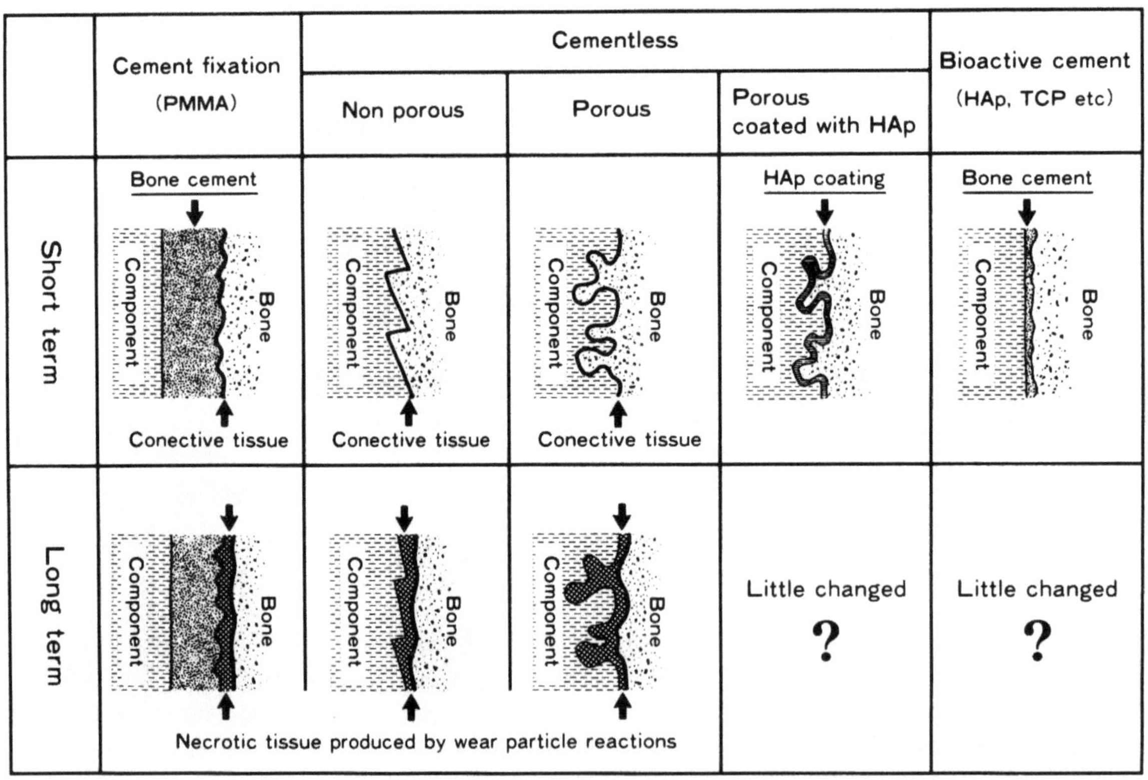


**Fig. 13.** Fixabilities and biological reactions of components using several fixation methods—a comparison of short- and long-term fixation

interface, this phenomenon does not occur and we believe that loosening in the interface can be avoided (Table 1; Fig. 13).

## Conclusion

Alumina ceramics are much superior to metal in the sliding part. However, alumina ceramics are not always better in contact with the bone. To resolve the problems with alumina ceramics, we are now developing titanium alloy beads and alumina beads coated with HAp and bioactive bone cement.

## References


1. Shikita T, Oonishi H (1980) Erfahrungen bei peripheren Osteosynthesen mit monokristallinen Alumina-Keramik-Schrauben. Z. Orthop 118: 975
2. Shikita T, Oonishi H (1981) Herstellung und klinishe Anwendung von Alumina-Keramik-Implantaten in der Orthopädie, Implantate und Transplantate in der Plastischen und Wiederherstellungschirurgie, Springer, Berlin-Heidelberg-New York, pp 244–248
3. Oonishi H, Shikita T (1981) Application de l'alumine ($Al_2O_3$) mono et polycristal à la chirurgie orthopédique. Rev Chir Orthop (Suppl II) 66
4. Oonishi H, Hasegawa T (1981) Cementless alumina ceramic total knee prosthesis. Orthopaedic Ceramic Implants 1: 157–160
5. Oonishi H, Kawaguchi A, Tatsumi M (1982) Biomechical analysis of the knee replaced with cementless alumina ceramic artificial knee joint—by means of 3D-FEM, Orthopaedic Ceramic Implants 2: 61–84
6. Oonishi H, Shikita T, Kitamura Y (1983) Application of supphire "single crystal alumina ceramics" to orthopaedic implants, Bull Japan Soc of Prec Eng 17, 2: 81–86
7. Oonishi H, Yunoki H, Komai T (1983) Mechanical analysis of the knee replaced with a cementless alumina ceramic total knee prosthesis—by photoelastic method, Japanese Orthopaedic Biomechamics 5: 103–107
8. Oonishi H, Maeda A, Murata N, Nabeshima T (1983) Designs and surgical technique of our cementless alumina ceramic total knee prosthesis, Jap J Rheum Joint Surg II: (1) 11–18
9. Oonishi H, Tatsumi M (1984) Some biomechanical considerations of finite element analysis of cementless alumina ceramic total knee prostheses, Biomaterials and Biomechanics 1983. Elsevier, Amsterdam, pp 49–54
10. Oonishi H, Okabe N, Nabeshima T, Kushitani S, Tsuyama K (1984) Some problems of cementless alumina ceramic total knee prosthesis and its solutions, Orthopaedic Ceramic Implants 4: 275–288
11. Oonishi H, Nabeshima T, Hanatate Y, Tsuji E (1984) Wear test of KOM-alumina total knee prosthesis by a knee simulator. Orthopaedic Ceramic Implants 4: 297–304
12. Oonishi H, Maeda A, Hamaguchi T, Nabeshima T (1984) Indications for cementless alumina ceramic total knee prosthesis and its limitation. Jap J Rheum Joint Surg III, 4: 311–322
13. Oonishi H (1985) Biomechanical analysis of cementless alumina ceramic total knee prosthesis with reference to clinical experience, Research MA J Vl, 2: 1–18
14. Okabe H, Tsuji E, Ike H, Oonishi H (1985) A study on the Fe-Cr-Al alloy as a biomaterial—mechanical properties, corrosion resistance and $Al_2O_3$ formation. J Jpn Soc Biomaterials, 3, 1: 55–63
15. Oonishi H, Okabe H, Ike T, Tsuji E (1985) Development of Fe-Cr-Al alloy with α-alumina layer diffused on the surface—Studies on biocompatibilities. J Jpn Soc Biomaterials, 3, 3: 125–133
16. Oonishi H, Tsuji E, Kohda H, Ishimaru H, Sugimoto T (1987) Studies on Ti-6A1-4V beads coated with HAp. Orthopaedic Ceramic Implants, 6
17. Oonishi H, Okabe H, Ike T, Tsuji E (1987) Development of Fe-Cr-Al alloy with alpha alumina layer diffused on the surface. New York Academy of Sciences
18. Oonishi H, Kohda H, Ishimaru H, Tsuji E (1987) Hydroxyapatite coating on Ti and $Al_2O_3$—Studies on the biological fixation. Advances in Biomaterials, Elsevier, Amsterdam
19. Oonishi H, Aoki H, Shin K (1987) Studies on development of α-TCP bioactive bone cement—material properties and biological reactions. Advances in Biomaterials. Elsevier, Amsterdam

## *Discussion*

*Bontemps* (Fabricius-Klinik Remsheid): If you have this sinking of 3–5 mm of your components, do you not have any laxity or varus-valgus instability?

*Oonishi* (Osaka Minami National Hospital): In sinking of more than 5 mm, range of motion decreases somewhat; instability does not, however, exist.

*Inoue* (Okayama University): We adopt a somewhat different type of ceramic prosthesis; we use surface replacement. The problem is the clear zone between the ceramics and bone. There is an increase in the rigid bone under the tibial component. But there is a layer of fibrous tissue between the ceramics and bone. There are cases which lead to loosening by a layer of fibrous tissue in ceramic cases. So far, however, we have witnessed no cases of serious bone absorption. Do you consider a clear zone to be undesirable or do you think this is permissible, including one layer of fibrous tissue?

*Oonishi*: Although we do observe the clear zone, we do not consider this to be sufficient grounds to carry out revision. After 10 or 20 years, we have to anticipate whether loosening will result. We must be prepared to accept some loosening after this amount of time.

*Inoue*: Using cementless prostheses, there is some discomfort with the total hip and knee. I think the fibrous tissue may be one of the reasons for this discomfort. There are also cases where the persons are free of pain. More studies are necessary into whether revision is necessary. I do not think that the clear zone is necessarily undesirable.

*Oonishi*: After the appearance of the clear zone, we have not conducted any revision of cementless cases. Generally speaking, including the hip, sensitivity to the cementless prosthesis may lead to complaints or discomfort. I do not think it is inevitable that patients with a cementless artificial joint are subject to greater discomfort. Our aim should be to produce cementless joints which reduce the pain.

*Bourne* (University of Western Ontario): We know that when porous surfaces are applied to metal prostheses, there is sometimes a deleterious effect in terms of the mechanical properties of the metal, e.g., notch sensitivity or metallurgical changes in the implant. We know that ceramics are somewhat brittle and there have been some problems because of fracturing. When you add a rough surface—plasma spray, etc.—does this also have a deleterious effect on the mechanical properties of the ceramic surface? Will we see more fractures with a porous ingrowth ceramic surface?

*Oonishi*: Since ceramics are rather brittle they have to be thicker in the design than metal. Apatite is similar to ceramics; when it is coated on a flat surface it will perhaps peel off. Ceramic or metal beads can be coated to encourage bone ingrowth into the porous surface. Coated beads are seen to induce three times the rate of ingrowth seen in uncoated beads. However, after about 3 months, the strength of the coated and uncoated aurfaces is very similar.

*Yamaga* (Nagoya University): After trauma, you had cases of loosening with no weight bearing and external fixation. What was the period of time here? Did the clear zone also disappear?

*Oonishi*: In one case, the patient came to me after a month and we applied a plaster cast. One month later, there was still pain; we removed the cast and allowed full weight bearing. Now, the pain has completely subsided and there is no clear zone whatsoever. There is some difficulty concerning the relationship between the clear zone and radiolucent line. In my opinion, the clear zone occurs because of micromovement.

*Yamaga*: In other words, after surgery, if there is no weight bearing and external fixation is maintained for about 1 month, would you expect the cases with clear zones to decrease?

*Oonishi*: Yes, 1 month after surgery with plaster fixation and no weight bearing, it would I think decrease even further. But perhaps the patients themselves would not be satisfied with such treatment.

*Hirohata* (Kobe University): What about the difference in terms of fracture between metal and ceramics?

*Oonishi*: I am not completely sure about this. When we use cobalt-chrome, the fracture tends to occur in the cobalt.

*Hastings* (Wellesley Hospital): When we do PCA total knees, we are very careful not to notch the front of the femur for fear of producing a distal femoral fracture. The alumina femoral component seems to be so thick that you have to notch the front of the femoral shaft in order to insert it. Do you have any incidence of femoral fracture for that reason?

Oonishi: We do not use thin ceramics and so we do not experience this.

# The Kodama-Yamamoto Knee Arthroplasty: A Long-Term Follow-Up Study of Non-Cemented Total Knee Replacement

S. YAMAMOTO, M. HACHINOTA, and Y. KONDOH[1]

**Summary.** The first operation for the Kodama-Yamamoto knee prosthesis was performed in 1970. The basic design concept of surface replacement and the noncemented approach have not changed from the original mark I to the present mark III. We reviewed the results of the Kodama-Yamamoto knee prosthesis mark II from 1975 to 1984. The study comprised 950 patients (1168 joints) in multicenter trials at 70 hospitals, including 300 patients (410 joints) at our own hospital.

Among the 950 patients (115 male, 795 female; 624 rheumatoid arthritis, 299 osteoarthritis, 26 others), the conditions of 805 patients (85%) were satisfactory and 75 (7.8%) were unsatisfactory. Of the rhematoid arthritis (RA) patients, 87% were satisfactory; 84% were satisfactory in the osteoarthritis (OA) group. For the other disease group, however, the rate was 73%. We must, therefore, carefully reconsider the indications of the procedure for diseases other than RA and OA.

The causes of unsatisfactory results were: infection in ten joints (0.85%), loosening or sinking in 20 joints (1.7%), and restriction of range of movement in 12 joints (1.0%). In addition, accurate surgical technique was recognized as an important factor.

**Keywords:** Kodama-Yamamoto knee prosthesis—Total knee replacement—Knee arthroplasty—Noncemented knee prosthesis

## Mark I Series

In 1970, the Kodama-Yamamoto Mark I was introduced. In 1972, preliminary results of a few cases were reported. The initial model was used from 1970 to 1974 (Fig. 1a). However, the results were not always satisfactory.

The concept at that time was as follows. The femoral side was replaced by an artificial physiological surface made of COP alloy and the tibial side was replaced by a comparatively flat tibial component made of high-density polyethylene. Bone cement was not used. This noncemented approach has been used consistently from the beginning and is still used in the present mark III. We reported the basic design concept at the Total Knee Replacement Conference held in London in 1974 [1]

The cause of variable initial results is attributed to the inability to gain effective range of motion and secure postoperative stability, although we were able to attain good postoperative pain relief. At that time, we performed surface replacement; however, we were unable to secure basic stability. This was considered to be the major cause of the unsatisfactory results.

## MarK II

Based on the limited experience obtained from the mark I series, we improved the prosthesis (mark II; Fig. 1b). The mark II was used for the next 10 years. We operated on 400 cases with the mark II and it is estimated that the mark II has been used in more than 4000 cases in Japan.

The mark II design was based on the results of research in biomechanics and biomaterials, including the surface design of the artificial joint, method of fixation, surgical technique, and selection of patients. We attempted to secure good knee stability from the experience with the mark I. The result was the stability of the mark II series; stability together with good alignment is the aim of total knee replacement. The initial results of the mark II were reported in 1979 [2] and 1981 [3].

## Mark III

It became clear after 10 years with the mark II that the long-term results of noncemented knee replacement were stable and even complications could be handled relatively easily. To improve the postoperative results even further, we partially altered the design of the prosthesis in 1985. At the same time, surgical instruments were also improved to achieve a more accurate surgical technique, as shown in

[1]The Centre for Rheumatic Disease, Matsuyama Red Cross Hospital, Bunkyocho, Matsuyama, Japan

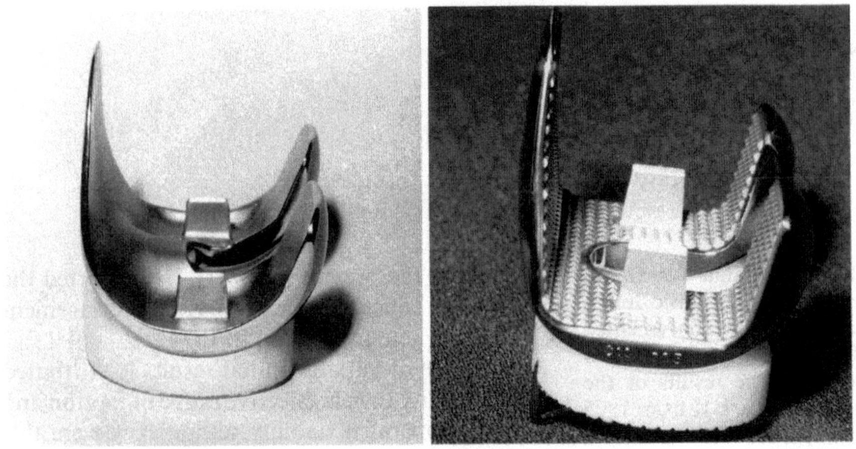

a b

**Fig. 1.** **a** Kodama-Yamamoto mark I, used from 1970 to 1974. **b** Mark II, used from 1975 to 1984

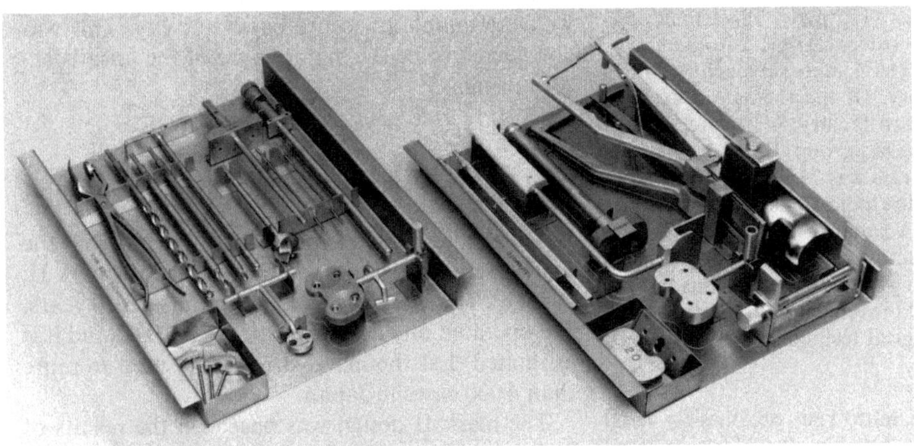

**Fig. 2.** Surgical instruments for the Kodama-Yamamoto mark III

Fig. 2. The new prosthesis is called the mark III (Fig. 3). The Mark III is produced by Thackray Co. Ltd. in England and consist of three components: the femoral component made of cobalt-chromium-molybdenum alloy, the tibial component made of high-density polyethylene (HDP) and with a larger surface contact area, and the patellar component also made of HDP.

The internal structure of the femoral component was improved to give a more parallel alignment of the anterior and posterior walls, thereby providing better fixation by press-fit. In the tibial component, the contact area with the tibial surface was enlarged and improvements were made to allow the use of a three-layer peg to provide stable fixation. Bone cement fixation proved to be totally unnecessary. Thus far, we have treated about 300 cases, and the results have been better than those with the mark II. The durability is better, and the flexion angle has been improved to an average of 105°.

## Ten-year Operative Results—1975–1984

### Subjects

We conducted multicenter trials at 70 hospitals all over Japan which used the Kodama-Yamamoto knee prostheses from 1975 to 1984. The total number of patients was 950 comprising 1168 joints. There were 795 females and 115 males. By disease, 624 patients had rheumatoid arthritis (RA), 299 osteoarthritis (OA), and there were 26 others. Regarding side of operation, right and left were almost equal in number (right 362, left 346) with bilateral surgery having been performed in 230 patients.

## Postoperative Results

We asked the surgeons of the 70 hospitals to divide the surgical results into three categories—satisfactory, unchanged, and unsatisfactory. In 300 cases from the Matsuyama Red Cross Hospital (MRCH), 94.3% were satisfactory and 3.3% unsatisfactory. The total of the other hospital groups (650 cases) shows 80.3% satisfactory results and 10.2% unsatisfactory. Among the 950 patients operated on between 1974 and 1984, satisfactory results were obtained in 805 (84.7%) and unsatisfactory in 75 (7.8%).

Figure 4 shows the operative results by disease. Our MRCH group had satisfactory results in 95.5% of RA patients. However, the results of the other hospitals for RA were 81.3%. As for OA, the MRCH group's satisfactory results were 90.5%, which is slightly below the figure for RA. Other hospitals had 81.7% satisfactory results, which is almost the same figure as for RA.

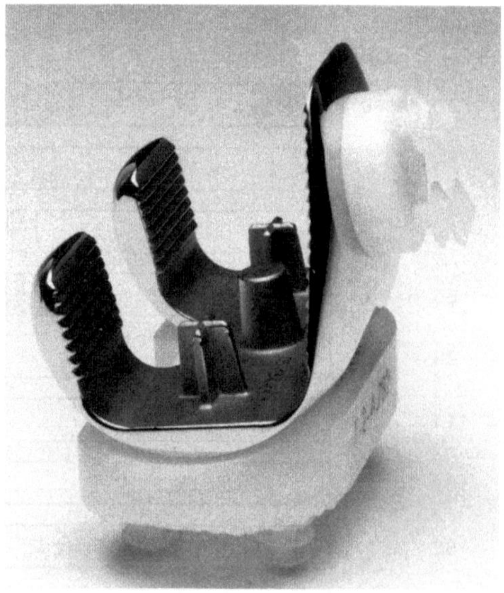

**Fig. 3.** The Kodama-Yamamoto mark III, which has been in use since 1985

Why is there this discrepancy? In the case of OA, which is different to RA, the influence from other joints is less and the postoperative evaluation became more stringent. In our hospital, the OA score is significantly higher than that of RA. However, in OA, the preoperative expectations are rather high, and if the actual results did not reach those expectations they were evaluated as unsatisfactory.

Indications other than RA and OA were osteonecrosis in three cases at our hospital and satisfactory results were obtained in all three. The satisfactory results in other hospitals, however, were 69.6% for indications other than RA and OA. This group of other hospitals included cases which had problems of indication or contraindication, such as paralysis of the lower extremities due to spinal damage, neuropathy due to diabetes, tumors such as pigmented villonodular synovitis, and infected arthritis. This may explain the difference.

As is shown in Fig. 5, during the follow-up period of 1–6 years the results are almost the same, with the average satisfactory rate of 90%. At 7, 8, 9, and 10 years, the percentage gradually decreases. Unsatisfactory results tended to concentrate in certain types of patients in certain hospitals. This led us to suspect problems of surgical technique and indications.

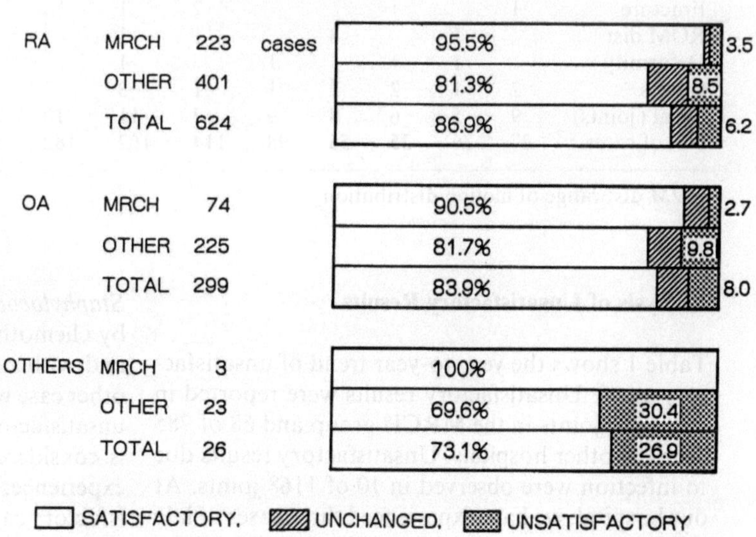


**Fig. 4.** The operative results by disease in Matsuyama Red Cross Hospital (*MRCH*) and other hospitals

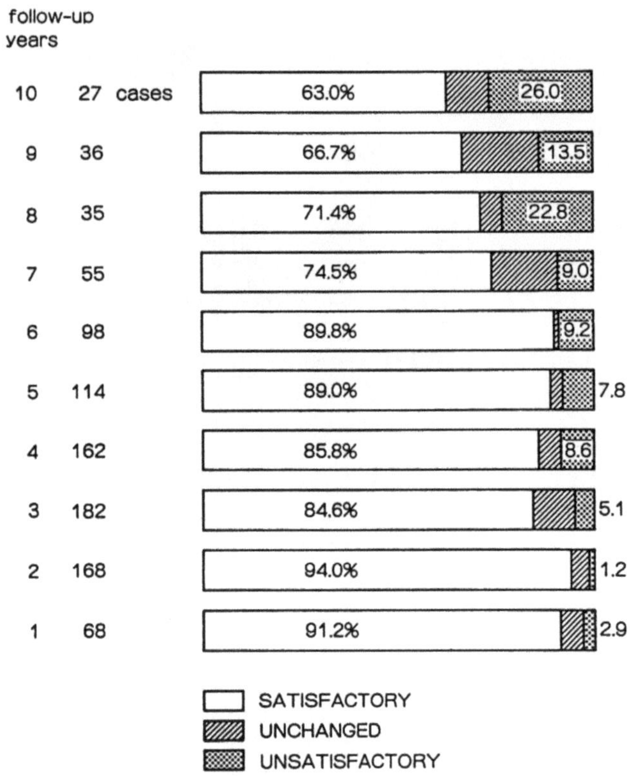


**Fig. 5.** The number of satisfactory cases at follow-up 1–10 years after the operation

**Table 1.** Unsatisfactory cases showing the year-to-year trend 1–10 years after surgery

| | Unsatisfactory cases (years) | | | | | | | | | |
|---|---|---|---|---|---|---|---|---|---|---|
| | 10 | 9 | 8 | 7 | 6 | 5 | 4 | 3 | 2 | 1 |
| Infection | 2 | 1 | | 1 | 2 | | 4 | | | |
| Loosening | 2 | 1 | 1 | 1 | 3 | 3 | | 1 | | |
| Instability | 2 | | 1 | | 2 | | 1 | 1 | | |
| Fracture | 1 | | 1 | | | 2 | 1 | | | |
| ROM dist | | 1 | | 3 | | 1 | 1 | 5 | | |
| Deformity | | 1 | 1 | 1 | 1 | | 1 | | 1 | |
| Others | 2 | 1 | 2 | 2 | 1 | 1 | 3 | 3 | 1 | 1 |
| Total (joints) | 9 | 5 | 6 | 8 | 9 | 7 | 11 | 10 | 2 | 1 |
| No. of cases | 27 | 36 | 35 | 55 | 98 | 114 | 162 | 182 | 167 | 68 |

*ROM* dist range of motion distribution

## Analysis of Unsatisfactory Results

Table 1 shows the year-to-year trend of unsatisfactory cases. Unsatisfactory results were reported in 10 of 410 joints in the MRCH group and 68 of 785 joints in other hospitals. Unsatisfactory results due to infection were observed in 10 of 1168 joints. At our hospital, we have experienced three cases of late infection, two of these had infection caused by *Staphylococcus aureus* and were successfully treated by chemotherapy without removing the prosthesis and with no decrease in range of movement. The other case was *Candida* infection, and the result was unsatisfactory. Infection in 10 of 1168 joints (0.85%) is considered to be a small percentage. From our experience, it can be said that even with the unsatisfactory cases due to infection, early chemotherapy could provide good prognosis in most cases.

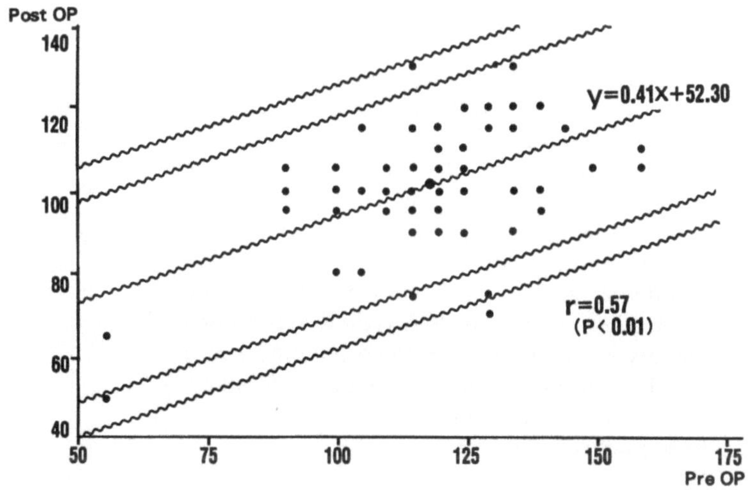


**Fig. 6.** The postoperative range of flexion correlated to the preoperative range of flexion

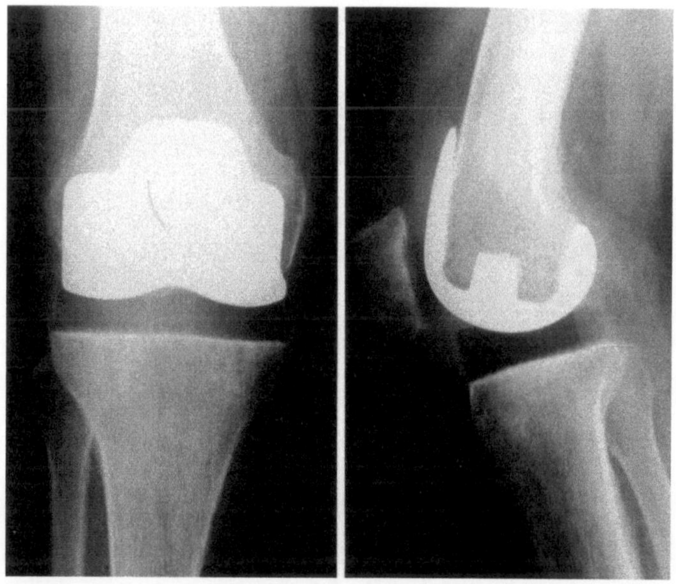

**Fig. 7.** X-Ray after surgery with the Kodama-Yamamoto mark III

Aseptic loosening or sinking are the most serious problems with artificial joints. Twenty cases of loosening included eight cases from our hospital. We experienced seven loosenings of the femoral component and one case of sinking of the tibial component. The causes of loosening are multiple. A systematic and comprehensive approach, including the careful selection of biomaterials, processing method, component design, surgical technique, selection of patients, and other related matters, is required to solve these problems. Most of our loosening cases were RA patients and they had rather severe osteoporosis, probably due to their preoperative bedridden condition. It is possible to treat the loosening of the component by revision surgery with bone grafting if revision is performed at an early stage. This is one of the important merits of the noncemented knee prosthesis.

There were many causes of postoperative supracondylar fracture. Our approach to this fracture is to preform intramedullary fixation with the Rush Pin from distal end of the femur. These results were favorable.

The postoperative degree of flexion is correlated to the preoperative degree. (Fig. 6). This was confirmed statistically in our series. That is, if preoperative flexion is good, we can expect good flexion postoperatively; conversely, if preoperative flexion is not good, good flexion cannot be expected postoperatively. Some RA cases, however, showed a drastic reduction of flexion angle and we do not have an effective countermeasure for this condition.

Several residual deformity cases, such as varus or valgus deformity and flexion contracture, were reported as unsatisfactory results.

It is considered that the major cause of problems is inadequate surgical technique. Surgical technique is one of the most important factors in improving the results of surgery. Figure 7 shows a typical postoperative X-ray of the Kodama-Yamamoto mark III. As seen in the X-ray, the first condition of surgery is the accuracy of the osteotomy and next are the issues of accurate alignment and stability. These are the most important factors in artificial knee-joint surgery.

## References

1. Kodama T, Yamamoto S (1975) Total knee prosthesis without Hinge, Total knee replacement. Institute of Mechanical Engineering, London
2. Yamamoto S (1979) Total knee replacement with the Kodama-Yamamoto knee prosthesis. Clin Orthop 145: 60–67
3. Yamamoto S, et al. (1981) The Kodama-Yamamoto knee prosthesis, its design and clinical results, Ryumachi 21: 21–28

# Discussion

*Iseki* (Keio University): With the mark III, you removed both cruciates. Did you observe any difference between the group of patients in whom the cruciates were removed and those in whom the cruciates were preserved?

*Yamamoto* (Matsuyama Red Cross Hospital): At the very early stages of the mark II, we used to preserve the cruciates, but in 99% of the cases we removed both cruciates. In the mark II and III we removed them.

*Iseki*: But what differences did you observe between the preserved and nonpreserved cases?

*Yamamoto*: In rheumatoid arthritis and asteoarthritis with some deformities, I think that the cruciate ligaments are a hindrance rather than a structure that should be preserved. The cruciates, collateral ligaments on the medial side, and the lateral popliteal tendon should be released before bone resection. Knee movement should then be increased.

*Bae* (Kyung Hee University Hospital): Your design is unconstrained and you sacrifice the posterior cruciates ligament; does you design have features to compensate for the resultant lack of stability?

*Yamamoto*: The most important factor, I believe, in total knee replacement is obtaining stability. Design of the prosthesis and operational technique are both important in achieving stability.

*Bae*: In cases with upper tibial bone defects, we often graft the bone and use cement. Rehabilitation is then as with usual patients. You, however, did not use cement. Could you give details of your postoperative management, such as when you begin weight bearing?

*Yamamoto*: Bone grafting is a new technique for us. There are some problems associated with it. The bone graft should lie perpendicular to the shaft of the tibia; it should lie on the cortex of the tibia, not in the cancellous bone. If the block is not so large as to overcome the weight-bearing line of the medial femoral condyle, I do not think that there is any problem. If the block is very small, we begin weight bearing immediately after the operation, i.e., after 3 days.

*Bae*: But in large defects with 50% or more than the one tibial platform or the height is 1 cm or more than if you graft without bone cement, when do you start weight bearing? Bone union is after about 4–6 months.

*Yamamoto*: If the grafted bone overcome the weight-bearing line, the patient is allowed to start weight bearing after 6 weeks.

*Yamamuro* (Kyoto University): You used HDP-type pegs. With HDP, when load is applied creep deformation may occur. In PCA or recent Total Condylar models, a metal tray is attached and in this way creep deformity prevented. When no deformity occurs, there is an interface between the hard material and bone, and interface problems may occur. Do you think that the contact between HDP and bone is better than between metal and bone?

*Yamamoto*: This is a very important point. We have experience of only a few cases of a tibial component with a metal tray. In our current cases using HDP only in the tibial component, we have not experienced many problems. In some cases with metal trays, there has been some loosening and inclination. I find a combination of high-density polyethylene and bone to be better than the metal-bone combination. This question really is one that has to be solved by engineers. Engineers try to anchor the prosthesis as firmly as possible; however, bone and the soft tissues change a great deal from day to day. Do the engineers take this changeable nature of the body into consideration in their designs?

*Walker* (Orthopedics Biomechanics Laboratory Brigham and Women's Hospital): I think that engineers and surgeons are trying to achieve the same aim in prosthesis design, and I do not really think that there is such a great difference in their approach. The problem as I see it is how do we achieve a stress distribution on the bone surface that is as normal as possible, avoiding areas of stress concentration and tension and avoiding micromotion? Engineering research indicates that metal is better than polyethylene, i.e., given the same design of prosthesis, the metal interface provides better bone tolerance. This has to be tested in clinical series.

With the MacIntosh prostheses, the interface develops in a similar manner to that with yours—a fibrous membrane and then a thick subchondral sclerotic layer. These prostheses seem to be very stable with time: I have seen follow-up reports of up to 10 years. You note a deterioration with time and I wonder if that is due to constant sinkage because of the flexibility of the plastic? Is there any connection between deterioration clinically and sinkage or resorption of bone?

*Yamamoto*: After 10 years, we see a sclerotic line in direct contact with the tibial component. In satisfactory cases, there is almost no sinking and no inclination. Unsatisfactory cases after 6 years are mainly due to surgical technique and loosening of the femoral component.

*Tsukamoto* (Kitasato University): The mark II was stable and fixation was good. Loosening was observed in only 14 cases, which is less than 1%, and it occurred mainly with the femoral component. So, tibial component problems did not occur in my interpretation of your presentation. With the mark III, you attached four short pegs. Why did you do this?

*Yamamoto*: In tibial component design, we did not really face any big problems. The lateral part of the mark II is quite small and so osteoporosis is often found; the posterior part of the tibial component may sink. So, we needed to increase the lateral part in the mark III. In bone grafting, we use four pegs and this allows us to apply pressure from above.

*Tsukamoto*: I am in favor of removing the ligaments. In axial loading, the loading is related to the tension of the body. With replacement of parts of the body by a prosthesis, the deformity volume is different and so normal function cannot be expected.

*Ranawat* (Cornell University Medical College): With the prostheses that you removed 7–10 years after implantation, which I assume were aligned properly, did you notice any signs of increased wear or any other kind of mechanical damage on the plastic articulating surface? I ask this because Dr. Walker in his Key Note Lecture implied that failure of the plastic will be a big problem for the future. I am of the opinion that if the joint is aligned properly and the load is not eccentric on the plastic, wear in the knee will be less than in the hip, contrary to what Dr. Walker said in his talk. Of the 112 knees we examined, we could not detect any wear with the radiograph. There is some difference here in the engineering prediction based on retrieved knee joints and clinical observation of knees functioning satisfactorily.

*Yamamoto*: In reoperation cases, I found the surface of the high-density polyethylene to be very smooth. This is not just a surface problem though; there is also the question of the bone-prosthesis interface.

*Drobny* (Klinik Wilhelm Schulthess: If I understand you correctly, you use a medial approach in your operative technique and the prosthesis has quite a flat femoropatellar surface. Do you not have more problems with subluxation and femoropateller difficulties?

*Yamamoto*: The radius is 38, but we have had no dislocation between the tibia and femur.

*Hoshino* (Tokyo Medical and Dental University): Dr. Oonishi and others have discussed direct bonding with the bone, but some type of fibrous material is present to achieve fixation. You have achieved good results without obtaining bone ingrowth, do you think then that it is not necessary to obtain bone fixation in noncemented prostheses?

*Yamamoto*: I do not think that fixation without bone ingrowth is completely satisfactory. At our center, we now use press-fit and microanchoring techniques. With microanchoring, you use a porous-coated surface. What kind of surgery should be used here? Immediately after the operation, there is a very good fixation between the prosthesis and bone. Our current system is not perfect, but it seems to us to be the best we have at present.

*Bontemps* (Fabricius-Klinik Remscheid): I think there was some misunderstanding with the question from Dr. Drobny. He was asking you if there was subluxation of the patella because the patellar groove is very flat on the your femoral component.

*Yamamoto*: The patella may move laterally and so I cannot make a central groove on the anterior flange of the femoral condyle. If there is no groove and the anterior flange of the femoral condyle is flat, I think this situation is acceptable.

# Part 5
# New Designs of Total Knee Prostheses

# Yoshino-Shoji Total Knee System: Its Features and Postoperative Results

S. Yoshino[1] and H. Shoji[2]

**Summary.** The Yoshino-Shoji (YS) total knee system instrumentation for controlled soft tissue balance both in 90° flexion and full extension is used together with the prosthesis, which was designed to take into consideration kinematic aspects of full flexion. We performed 161 YS total knee replacements (103 patients) in the Department of Joint Disease, Nippon Medical School. Tokyo. Seven patients had died of causes unrelated to the operation before the time of follow-up. The subjects of this study included 151 joints (96 patients) with follow-up of at least 1 year. The preoperative diagnosis was osteoarthritis in 27 joints (16 patients) and rheumatoid arthritis in 124 joints (80 patients).

According to the Hospital for Special Surgery evaluation scale, the average score before operation was 53.6 ± 12.2, while after operation it was 89.9 ± 7.3 ($P < 0.01$). The average range of motion before operation was 99.4° ± 28.9°, while after operation it was 121.5° ± 15.9° ($P < 0.01$). In addition, of 80 rheumatoid patients (124 joints) eight patients (12 joints) became able to squat fully in Japanese style.

Based on the above results, YS total knee replacement was able to achieve a good stability and a better average range of motion than systems reported in the past.

**Keywords:** Yoshino-Shoji total knee system—Full flexion (full squat)—Bilateral soft tissue balance

The purpose of total knee replacement is to achieve relief of pain, improved ambulatory ability, and good range of motion among other benefits. With regard to pain relief and improved ambulatory ability, good results have been obtained with almost all types of total knee prosthesis. However, range of motion is not so satisfactory.

## Features

At least 90° of flexion is required for the ordinary activities of daily living such as going up and down stairs and so on; the swing phase of walking requires a mean of 67°, climbing stairs 83°, descending stairs 90°, and rising from a chair 93° [3]. We, therefore, developed the Yoshino-Shoji (YS) total knee system, which enables flexion of at least 90° after surgery [4, 5]. The YS total knee system also provides better stability than conventional knee prostheses.

To achieve smooth posterior roll-backing together with deep flexion, the posterior articular surface of the tibial component is completely flattened (Fig. 1). Using a knee distractor set, the tension balance of the soft tissue is reestablished so as to fit the inserted total knee prosthesis. The following surgical technique was developed so that equal tension of the bilateral soft tissues can be obtained over a range from the phase of full extension to the phase of maximum flexion.

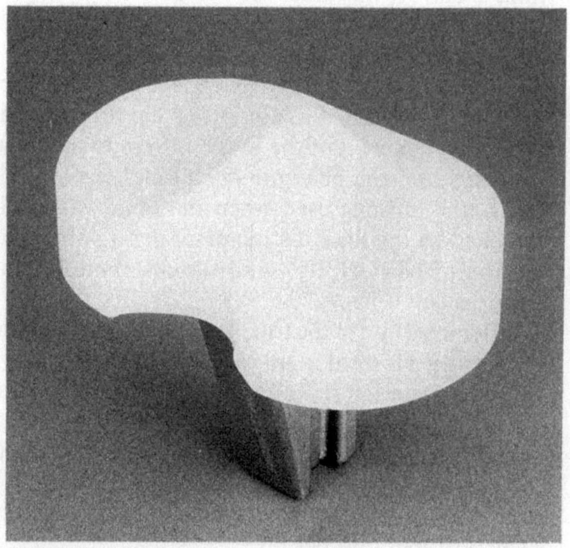

**Fig. 1.** YS knee tibial component. The articular surface is flattened posteriorly to allow rotation freedom in deep flexion

[1] Department of Joint Disease, Nippon Medical School, Tokyo, Japan
[2] Department of Orthopaedic Surgery, Louisiana State Medical Center, New Orleans, LA, USA

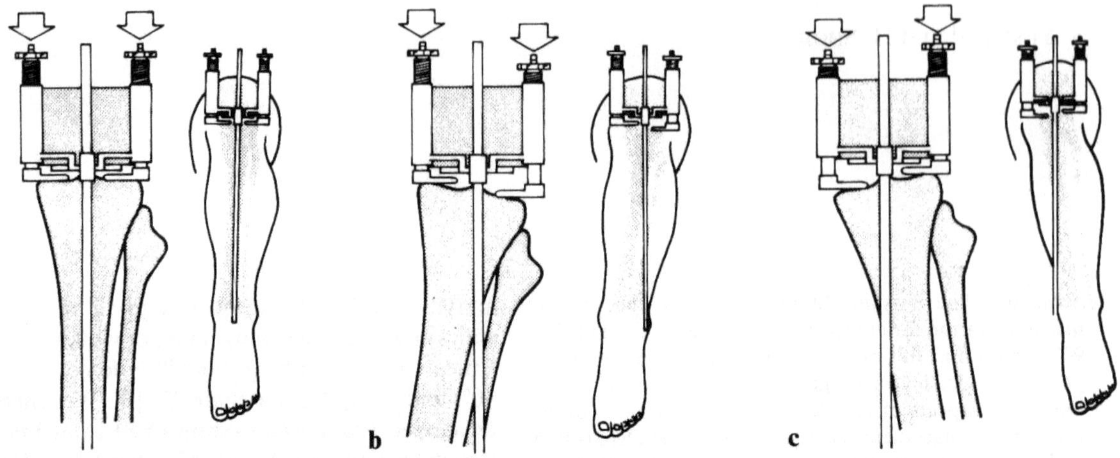


**Fig. 2.** **a** Soft tissue balancing is achieved with creation of normal alignment **b** Medial soft tissue is shorter than lateral with persistent varus deformity. **c** Lateral soft tissue is shorter than medial with persistent valgus deformity. When **b** or **c** is noted, soft tissue release has to be continued until **a** is achieved.

### Surgical Technique

After cutting the anterior and posterior condyles of the femur, a knee distractor is inversely inserted against the cut surfaces of the posterior femoral condyles while keeping the knee joint at 90° flexion. Under equal bilateral soft tissue tension of 45 N (10 lb), soft tissue release is performed until accurate alignment is obtained (Fig. 2). Next, a bushing with the thickness of the tibial component is attached to the knee distractor, and the articular surface of the tibia is cut. At this time, the operator should strive to preserve as much as possible of the subchondral bone of the tibia.

The knee joint is fully extended, and the knee distractor is inserted again. After confirming that accurate alignment of the lower extremity has been obtained and the bilateral soft tissue tensions are equal, the bushing used when the tibia was cut is attached to the knee distractor under a soft tissue tension of 68 N (15 lb), and the distal end of the femur is cut.

After insertion of the total knee prosthesis, lateral release is performed in all cases in order to achieve smooth posterior sliding of the medial collateral ligament together with flexion [6] and reproduction of a joint cavity the same as that of the normal joint.

To avoid intra-articular adhesion as far as possible after surgery, flexion exercise is started in the early postoperative period.

## Materials and Methods

One hundred and three patients (161 joints) had undergone YS total knee replacement at the Department of Joint Disease, Nippon Medical School as of June 1986. Of these patients, seven had died before the time of the first follow-up study due to diseases not directly related to the operation. The subjects of the present study were the remaining 96 patients (151 joints). They consisted of 80 patients (124 joints) with rheumatoid arthritis and 16 patients (27 joints) with osteoarthritis. The mean age of the patients was 59.4 years (23–78 years), and the male to female ratio was 15:81. The mean follow-up period was 2.0 years (1.0–3.0 years). The postoperative results were mainly evaluated according to the evaluation system developed at the Hospital for Special Surgery [1].

## Results

### Total Cases

The mean preoperative total score (normal, 100 points) was 53.6 ± 12.2 points, while the mean postoperative total score was 89.9 ± 7.3 points (Table 1). Thus, the mean total score improved with a statistically significant difference ($P < 0.01$). When the postoperative scores of the subjects were rated by a four grade system, 128 joints were rated as "excellent" and 22 joints were rated as "good" (Table 2).

The range of motion was found to be as follows: preoperative mean extension, 17.1° ± 17.8°; postoperative mean extension, 0.9° ± 2.8°, preoperative mean flexion, 116.6° ± 20.8°; postoperative mean flexion, 121.4° ± 15.2°. Thus, the improvements in both extension and flexion were statistically significant ($P < 0.01$, $P < 0.05$). Regarding postoperative

**Table 1.** Results of YS total knee replacement

| | Before surgery | After surgery |
|---|---|---|
| Average evaluation scores (HSS) | 53.6±12.2 | 89.9±7.3* |
| Average range of motion | | |
| Extension | 17.1°±17.8° | 0.9°±2.8* |
| Flexion | 116°±20.8° | 121.4°±15.2** |
| Average arc of motion | 99.4°±28.9° | 120.5°±15.9°* |

*$P < 0.01$
**$P < 0.05$

**Table 2.** Postoperative evaluation scores

| Rating (score) | No. of joints |
|---|---|
| Excellent (≥85) | 128 |
| Good (70–84) | 22 |
| Fair (60–69) | 1 |
| Poor (<60) | 0 |

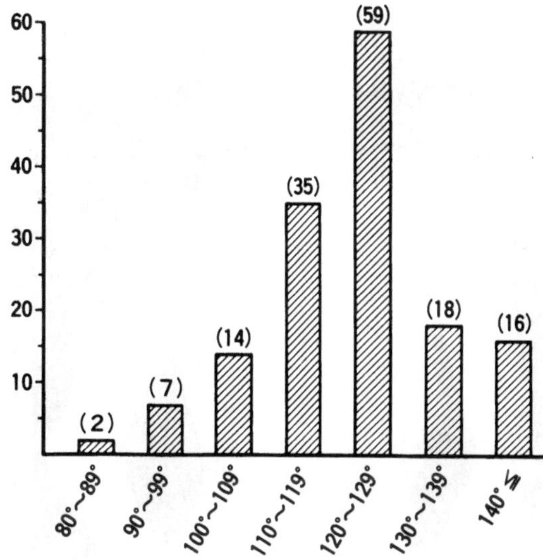


**Fig. 3.** Range of postoperative flexion

flexion, 93 joints (61.6%) had more than 120°; the minimum flexion was 80° (Fig. 3).

It had been anticipated that the postoperative flexion value would be affected by the preoperative flexion value, but there was no significant correlation between these two values.

With respect to the stability score (normal, 10 points). The mean preoperative value was 6.0 ± 3.1 while the mean postoperative value was 9.8 ± 0.6. Thus, the stability was significantly improved after operation ($P < 0.01$). However, while a posterior drawer sign was seen in all joints, an anterior drawer sign was seen only in two joints.

The mean functional score (normal, 22 points) was 7.2 ± 5.5 before operation and 16.2 ± 4.9 after operation. Thus, the improvement in the functional score was statistically significant ($P < 0.05$).

**Patients Able to Squat Fully**

Eight patients (12 joints) were able to squat fully on the floor, which is a common sitting posture in Japan after YS total knee replacement. They were all rheumatoid arthritis patients. The male to female ratio was 4:4, and their mean age was 53.9 years (45–69 years). The mean time required to become able to squat fully after surgery was 10.6 weeks (3–32 weeks). The average duration of follow-up was 2 years (1–3 years). In all the patients, good stability against valgus stress and varus stress was noted. However, although an anterior drawer sign was seen, no posterior drawer sign was detected in any of the joints. All the patients were able to move, without any aid, from a squatting to a standing position and from a standing to a squatting position.

**Case Report**

The patient was a 50-year-old male with rheumatoid arthritis. Before operation, the patient was limited to walking indoors due to severe pain in both knees. Simultaneous bilateral total knee replacement was performed. As a result, the patient became able to squat fully in Japanese style in the 4th week after the operation (Fig. 4).

**Discussion**

If a good range of motion is desired for a total knee prosthesis, the joint surface must have a great degree of freedom biomechanically. However, on the other hand stability becomes worse as the freedom increases. Thus, range of motion and stability are incompatible factors. We believed that this problem could be solved if we utilized the tension of the bilateral soft tissues (bilateral collateral ligaments) as the source of stability. On the basis of this idea, we successfully developed a new surgical technique using a knee distractor. The characteristic of this

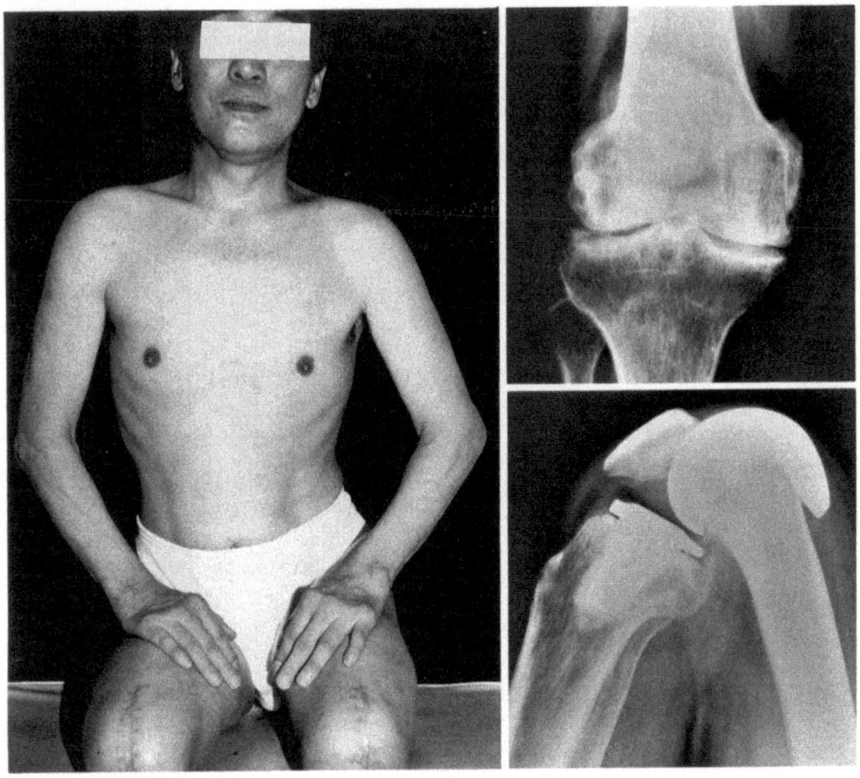

a b c

**Fig. 4.** **a** The patient in full squatting position **b** Radiograph of antero-posterior view of the knee before surgery showing remarkable pathological changes. **c** Radiograph of the knee in full flexion after surgery

surgical technique is that at 90° flexion, equal tension of the bilateral soft tissues and accurate alignment of the leg can be achieved simultaneously. Where equal tension of the bilateral soft tissues and accurate alignment of the lower extremity are achieved at full extension, balance in the soft tissue tension is sometimes lost as the degree of flexion increases. However with our method in which equal tension of the bilateral soft tissues and accurate alignment of the leg are achieved at 90° flexion, the tension in the bilateral soft tissues is balanced during the motion from full extension to full flexion, and the stability of the prosthesis is also good. In addition, our surgical technique enables greater freedom of movement of the joint surface of the total knee prosthesis, thereby providing a larger range of motion. Our idea has proved to be correct since: (a) the postoperative results indicated a mean range of motion of $120.5° \pm 15.9°$, which is much better than the value obtained with other types of total knee prosthesis, (b) eight patients are now able to squat fully in the Japanese style. It has been reported that the ability to kneel on the floor Japanese-style squatting cannot be fully performed without good stability and good muscle strength [2]. From this viewpoint, it is also apparent that our surgical technique achieves good stability.

There is always a concern that loosening of knee prostheses may occur in the future. To date, however, findings from roentgenograms have revealed no lucent zone in any joint. We believe that there seems to be little likelihood of accelerated loosening of the YS total knee prosthesis inserted by our technique even though the time of follow-up is short.

## References


1. Insall J, Scott N, Ranawat C (1979) The total condylar prosthesis. A report of two hundred and twenty cases. J Bone Joint Surg 61-A: 173
2. Iwakura H, Yoshida K, Ito M, et al. (1982) The role of knee joint muscles in Japanese sitting activity. Orthop Traum Surg 25: 13 (in Japanese).
3. Laubenthal KN, Smidt GI, Kettelkamp DB (1972) A quantitative analysis of knee motion during activities of daily living, Phys Ther 52: 32
4. Shoji H, Yoshino S, Komogamine M (1987) Improved range of motion with the Y/S total knee Arthroplasty system, Clin Orthop 218: 150
5. Yoshino S, Shoji H (1985) The newly designed total knee system-preliminary report, J, Joint Surg 4: 155 (in Japanese).
6. Yoshino S, Shoji H (1986) On bilateral soft tissue tensions and movement of medial collateral ligament after total knee replacement, Orthop Traum Surg 29: 1811 (in Japanese).

# *Discussion*

*Ranawat* (Cornell University Medical College): It is amazing that a with a prosthesis like this, such a range of motion can be obtained. It is a challenge to all those present who sacrifice or preserve the posterior cruciate ligament and who design knees on more anatomical principles and who have not been able to achieve more than 105°–110°. Yet here is a design that is very similar to the Total Condylar except for opening of the posterior plastic to a little flatter surface and this range of motion is the result.

*Niwa* (Aichi Medical University): Newly developed prostheses have differences in terms of configuration, but they are all based upon the same design principle. By fully utilizing your surgical techniques I wonder if we could improve the range of motion?

*Yoshino* (Nippon Medical School): As you say, recently developed artificial joints do not have so many differences, yet in terms of the tibial component flatness is of great importance.

*Bourne*: Yesterday, we learned that perhaps it is not only prosthesis design which leads to good range of motion, but also our handling of the soft tissues. Could you describe your approach to the knee and how you handle the extensor mechanism?

*Yoshino*: As I said, the balance of the soft tissue and alignment are conducted at 90° of flexion. Most surgeons, however, do these measurements at extension. This is a big difference I feel.

*Bourne*: Do you do a medial peripatellar incision, a lateral peripatellar incision, and a retinacular release routinely? Are there any differences in your soft tissue approach to total knee replacement?

*Yoshino*: We use a medial approach and have no experience of a lateral approach. At the flexion degree of 90°, we measure the balance in alignment compared with the position in extension. The tension from the medial to the posterior and in addition the semimembranes can be measured at 90° flexion. The tension cannot be easily measured at extension.

# The Oxford Knee: The Role of a Meniscal Bearing Arthroplasty

J. W. Goodfellow and J. O'Connor[1]

**Summary.** Modern trends in prosthesis design have moved from constrained hinges towards semi-constrained implants, preserving the natural ligaments for stability. The ideal implant would be completely unconstrained, depending for stability in all directions upon preservation of the ligaments. This implies the necessity of preserving the cruciates as well as the collaterals and of restoring them to their natural tensions. The cruciate mechanism requires the femur to roll backwards and forwards upon the tibia during flexion and extension; only a flat tibial plateau can accommodate this movement and only a meniscal bearing can confer congruity between the prosthetic articular surfaces. Meniscal bearings allow the tension in the ligaments to be accurately restored. The Oxford Meniscal Knee, a completely unconstrained implant, has been in use since 1976 and its indications and limitations have been defined. It is unsuitable when disease has progressed to distort the ligamentous apparatus. The failure rate in knees in which the anterior cruciate ligament was damaged was much higher than in knees in which the ligament was intact.

Since 1982 the device has been used increasingly for unicompartmental replacement. Osteoarthritis commonly first affects one compartment (usually the medial) and remains limited to that one compartment for many years before involving the other. Before this happens unicompartmental arthroplasty is an attractive alternative to tibial osteotomy or total condylar replacement.

In early arthritis progressive destruction of the joint can be halted and the physiological function of the ligaments restored by timely surface replacement with a completely unconstrained prosthesis. In osteoarthritis usually only one compartment needs resurfacing.

**Keywords:** Oxford meniscal knee arthroplasty—Cruciate ligament—Design—Clinical trial—Unicompartmental knee arthroplasty

The modern trend in prosthesis design is away from constrained, hinged devices towards semiconstrained implants which preserve the natural collateral ligaments for stability in the medio-lateral plane. A logical continuation of this trend is to restore the natural function of the joint in the antero-posterior plane as well. This requires the preservation both of the cruciate ligaments and the collaterals, for it is the cruciate mechanism which mainly controls the antero-posterior stability of the knee joint [1]. In the first part of this paper we examine the anatomy and mechanics of the natural human knee in the sagittal plane with particular reference to the cruciate ligament mechanism. From this analysis we deduce the need for meniscal bearings in any prosthesis which seeks to preserve the cruciates and restore them to their natural functions. Lastly, we describe some results of the clinical use of the Oxford Meniscal Knee over a period of 10 years.

## Kinematics of Knee in Sagittal Plane

During flexion and extension, the femur does not rotate about a fixed transverse axis, like a hinge, but about an axis which moves backwards with respect to the tibia during flexion and forwards during extension. Movements of this axis are accompanied by a combination of rolling and sliding movements between the articular surfaces of the bones so that the area of contact between them moves from the front of the tibial plateau in full extension to the back of the plateau in full flexion. These movements are ordained by the cruciates. These ligaments, with the tibia and the femur, form a crossed four-bar linkage. As the joint flexes and extends, the shape of this linkage changes. Figure 1 shows stills from a computer animation with the linkage in four different positions. Figure 2a shows, in kinematic form, the changing pattern of the cruciates during flexion of the femur with the tibia held still; in Fig. 2b, the femur is held still and the tibia moves through the range of flexion.

In Fig. 3 the computer has drawn diagrammatically the movements of the bones upon one another which the changing shapes of the cruciate linkage ordain.

[1] Nuffield Orthopaedic Centre, Oxford University, Oxford, UK

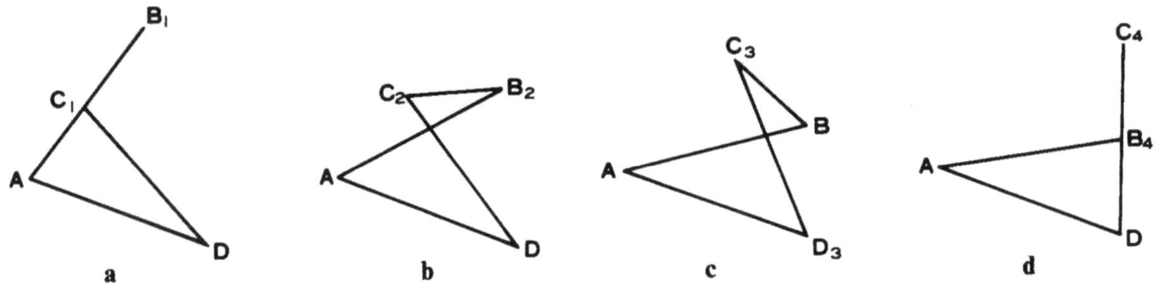


**Fig. 1a–d.** Planar four-bar linkage simulating relative position of the tibia (*AD*), which is taken to be stationary. *B* and *C* on the femur represent the origins of the cruciate ligaments, *A* and *D* their insertions. **a–d** Configurations of the linkage though a flexion range of 140°

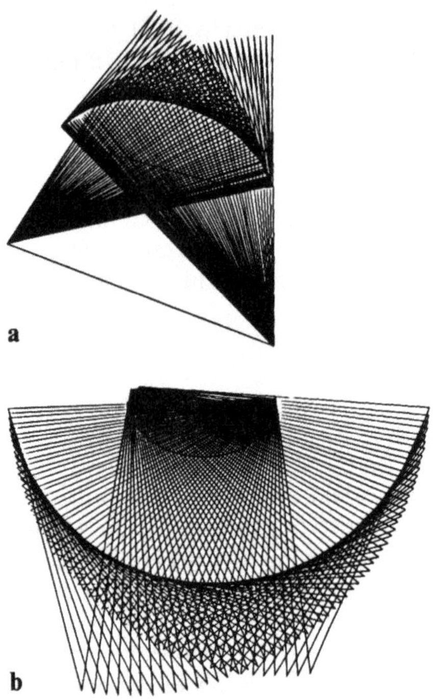


**Fig. 2a, b.** Computer simulation of the positions of the cruciate ligaments. **a** The tibia is stationary while the femur flexes. **b** The positions of the cruciates are shown during tibial flexion on a fixed femur

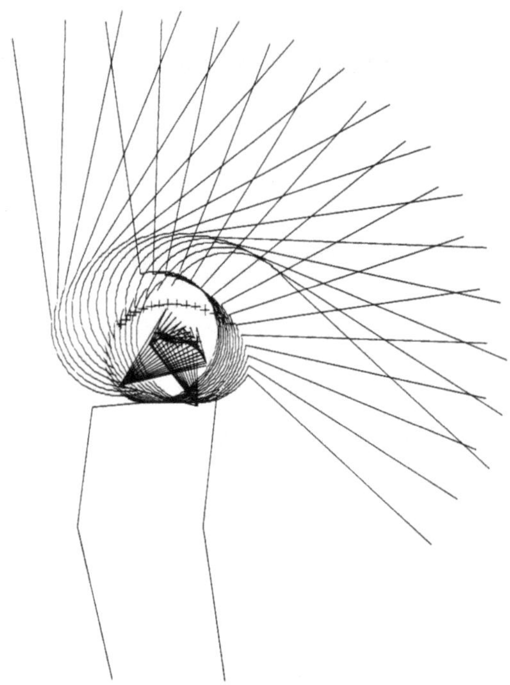

**Fig. 3.** Computer simulation of relative movements of tibia and femur ordained by the model cruciate linkage

It is an important feature of the crossed four-bar linkage that the instantaneous centre of joint movement, the point about which the bones are rotating at any time, is always situated at the point of cross-over of the anterior and posterior cruciate ligaments. The fact that this point moves backwards and forwards during flexion and extension has profound effects both upon the kinematics and upon the mechanics of the joint. In Fig. 4 the computer diagram has lines added to represent the extensor and flexor muscles. The lever arms employed by these muscles are also shown (BQ and BT for the quadriceps tendon and patellar tendon; BG and BH for the gastrocnemius and hamstrings). All these lever arms radiate from the instant centre of rotation of the joint, the cross-over point of the two cruciates. As the joint flexes and extends the lengths of the lever arms of all the muscle groups alter. Figure 5 demonstrates some effects of these changes upon the forces which the muscles exert at varying angles of flexion.

## Shapes of Articular Surfaces

The articular surfaces of the human knee, when seen

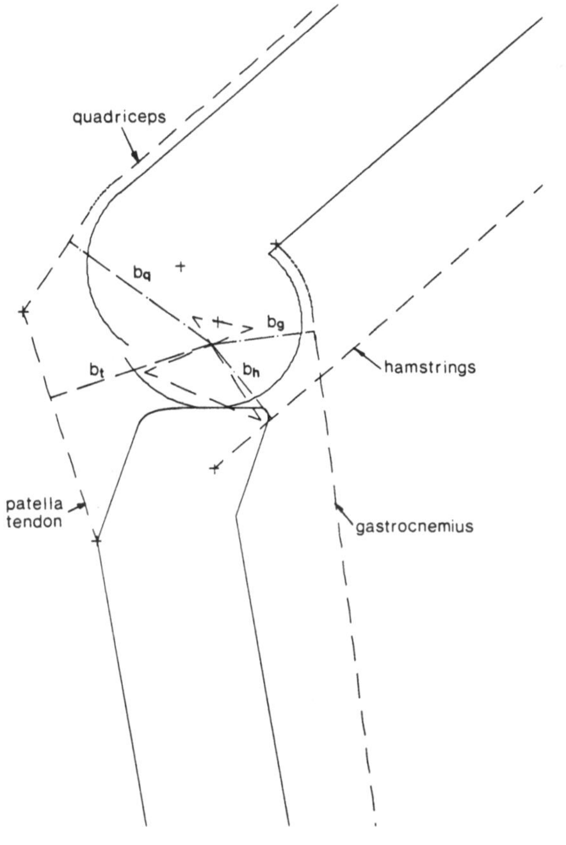


Fig. 4. Lever arms of extensor and flexor muscles drawn to the instantaneous center of the four-bar linkage

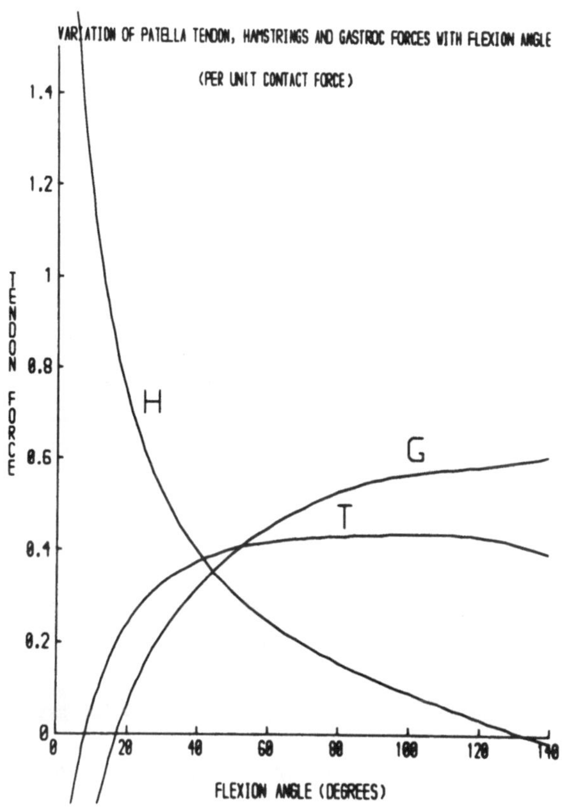


Fig. 5. Variation of patellar tendon (T), hamstrings ($H$), and gastrocnemius ($G$) forces with flexion angle (per unit contact force)

from the side, are completely incongruous. The tibial plateaux are flattened to allow the backwards and forwards rolling movement of the femur which the cruciate mechanism commands.

The convex curves of the femoral condyles are usually described as having a helical form with a radius of curvature which is larger anteriorly than posteriorly. We believe that this description is inaccurate and is based upon a confusion between the patello-femoral and tibio-femoral joints. Figure 6 is an antero-posterior section made through the trochlear sulcus. Such a section clearly defines the patellar facets of the femur, which are quite distinct, from the tibial facets. Once the tibio-femoral facets are clearly distinguished from the patellofemoral facets, the former are found to be approximately spherical, varying from perfect sphericity by less than 10%.

Such an incongruous articulation between spherical and flat articular surfaces must provide very small areas of contact, insufficiently large to allow the heavy loads expected at the knee to be transmitted at pressures which the articular surfaces could withstand. The menisci are the natural solution to the problem. By matching the dissimilar surfaces, they spread the applied load over a large area but, because they are mobile, they do not limit the movements of the femur on the tibia but passively follow the femoral condyles.

Although we have only discussed the movements which the femur makes on the tibia during flexion and extension, the very same mechanism allows for their movement during tibial rotation. During that movement the femoral condyles move backwards and forwards upon the tibial plateaux reciprocally, one forwards and one backwards. The flattened shape of the tibial plateaux allows such reciprocal movements and the mobile meniscal bearings continue to perform their load-bearing function (Fig. 7).

It will be noted that we do not attribute the pattern of observed movement to the shapes of the articular surfaces but to the design of the ligaments. The articular surfaces merely allow these movements. Their shapes maintain the cruciate ligaments at a constant length in all positions of the knee.

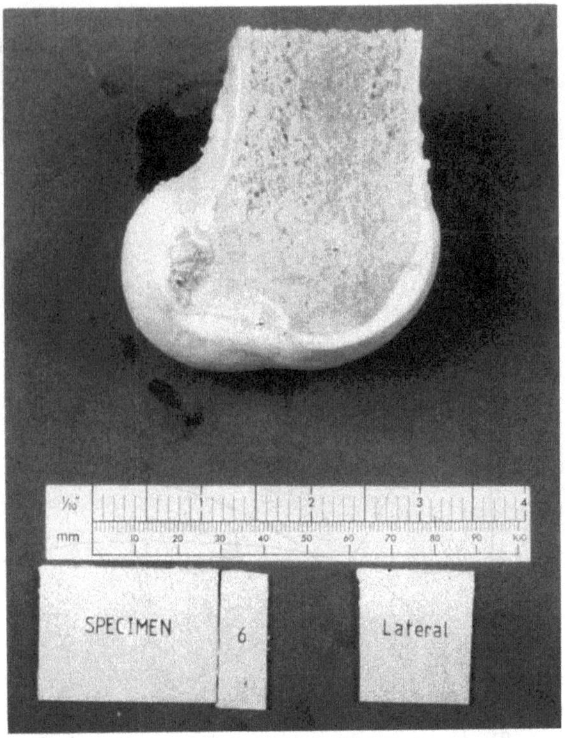


**Fig. 6.** Central sagittal plane section of the femoral condyles

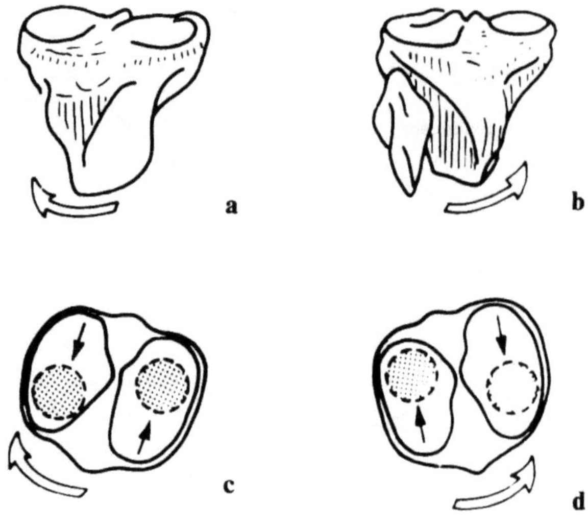


**Fig. 7a–d.** Movement of meniscal bearing during **a**, **c** outward rotation and **b**, **d** inward rotation

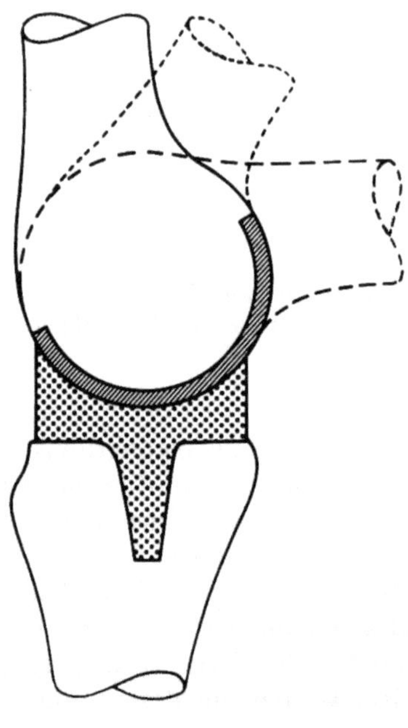

**Fig. 8.** Type of joint replacement design with a concave tibial plateau matching exactly the convex surface of the femoral component at different angles of flexion

## Prosthesis Design

How can the designer of artificial articular surfaces deal with these facts? One solution is simply to discard the cruciate ligaments or ignore them and to produce an altogether simpler type of knee joint. In Fig. 8 the tibial plateau is made concave to match the femoral surfaces. A large area of contact is then available for the transmission of load, but the joint is fully constrained in the antero-posterior plane and has no kinematic advantages over a hinged joint with an axle. Most of the currently popular forms of total condylar replacement employ some degree of concavity of the tibial plateau to control antero-posterior instability. Figure 9 shows a compromise solution, in which the joint components interpenetrate enough to produce stability but are not perfectly congruous. However, under the heavy loads of weight bearing, the femoral condyle must settle at the bottom of any such concavity and it is doubtful whether the function of this design is any more physiological than that shown in Fig. 8.

The alternative is shown in Fig. 10. Flat tibial surfaces are employed and the femur is therefore able to roll and slide upon them in a natural manner. However, the area of contact must be small and the load per unit area very high. Such a design might be expected to fail in the long term from the effects of creep and wear.

The solution to the designer's dilemma is the introduction of a third element into the prosthesis, an analogue of the naturally occurring meniscus. Figure 11 shows how a free bearing introduced between the articular surfaces can maintain them fully congruous throughout the range of movements and yet allow the joint to remain free to move as the ligaments dictate.

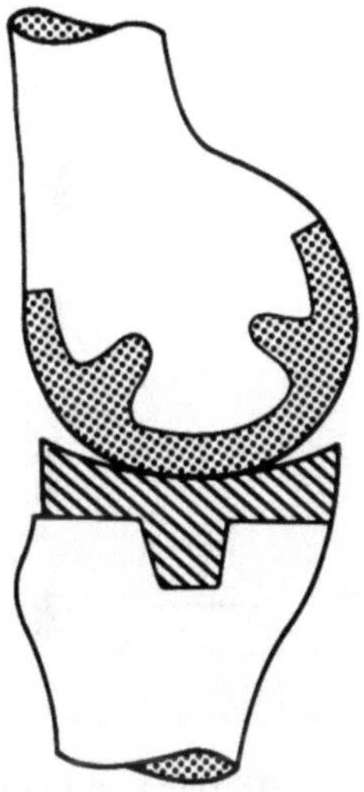

**Fig. 9.** Type of joint replacement design with a concave tibial plateau engaging with a convex surface on the femur haveing a smaller radius

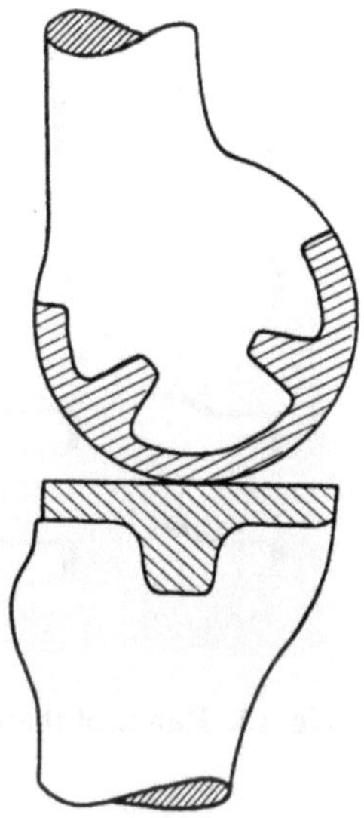

**Fig. 10.** Type of joint replacement haveing a flat tibial plateau in contact with a convex femoral component

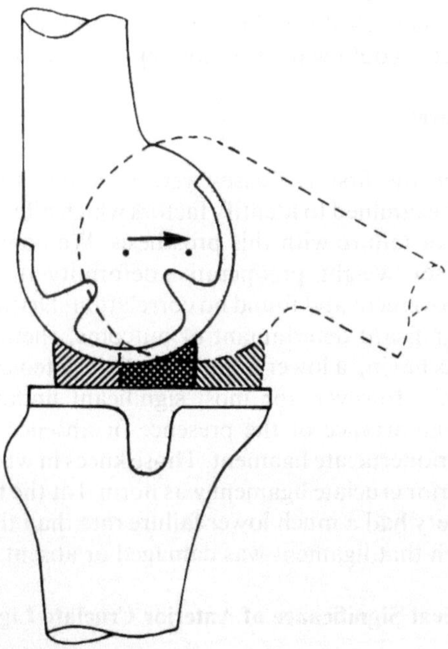

**Fig. 11.** Freedom of anteroposterior movement between a flat tibial plateau and a convex femoral component by the use of a sliding component (*shaded area*)

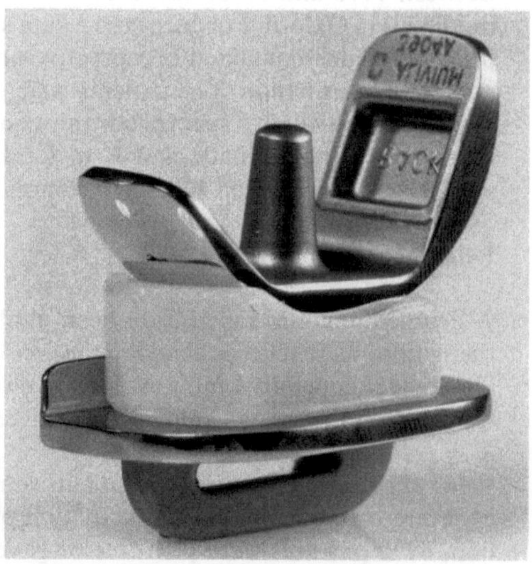

**Fig. 12.** Components of the Oxford Meniscal Knee

## Oxford Meniscal Knee

Figure 12 shows the components of the Oxford Knee assembled. The femoral component is spherical and the tibial component is flat. The meniscal bearing is spherically concave above and flat below to match the metal surfaces. The bearing is held in place by the tension in the ligaments which span the joint and its movements are otherwise unconstrained.

The bearings are available in eight thicknesses varying in 1 mm steps (Fig. 13). The thickness of bearing is chosen by trial and error *after* the metal components have been fixed to the bones. All the ligaments are thereby restored to their natural tension.

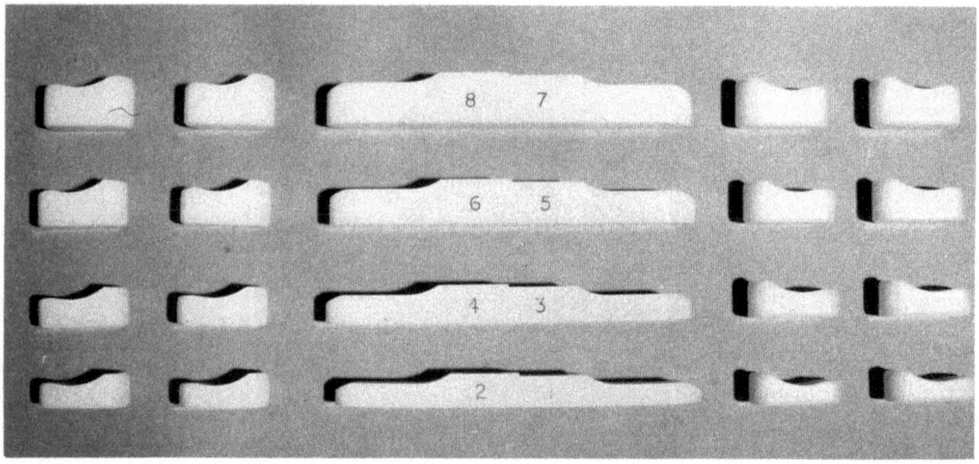


**Fig. 13.** Range of thicknesses in which the Oxford Meniscal Bearing is available

## Clinical Trial

Between 1976 and 1985, 321 knees were operated (by JWG) in Oxford. For each case a data sheet was prepared which contained preoperative and intraoperative information. The patients were reviewed at annual intervals at a special monthly clinic where measurements were made and X-rays taken. The data base is stored in an ICL 2988 computer.

## Relief of Symptoms

A detailed analysis has already been published of the symptomatic relief achieved in the first 125 cases [2]. Some preoperative and postoperative values, as recorded on the assessment chart, are given below.

**Relief of pain.** Preoperation, all patients complained of severe or moderate pain in activity. Postoperation, 89% of knees were pain-free or gave rise, at most, to mild pain in activity.

**Range of movement.** Preoperation, the mean flexion range was 104°. At follow-up, the mean range was 99°.

**Flexion deformity.** Preoperation, the mean flexion deformity was 14° in rheumatoid patients and 10° in osteoarthritics. At follow-up, a mean deformity of 7° persisted in both groups.

**Varus/Valgus deformity.** Preoperation, deformities ranged from 30° of varus to 30° of valgus. At follow-up correction to within 5° of neutral was achieved in 86% of rheumatoid knees and 80% of osteoarthritics.

**Recovery of function.** Walking distance improved in 75% of patients; 73% of the operated knees were habitually used for climbing stairs and 82% of the patients could walk at follow-up without sticks.

## Failures

When the first 125 cases were reviewed, the data were examined to identify factors which affected the rate of failure with this prosthesis. We considered age, sex, weight, preoperative deformity and range of movement and found no correlation. Disease was a significant determinant of outcome, rheumatoid joints having a lower failure rate than osteoarthritic joints. However, the most significant finding was the importance of the presence or absence of the anterior cruciate ligament. Those knees in which the anterior cruciate ligament was normal at the time of surgery had a much lower failure rate than those in which that ligament was damaged or absent.

## Clinical Significance of Anterior Cruciate Ligament

We have now reviewed the data of all the meniscal knee replacements performed by JWG in Oxford between 1976 and 1985. The state of the anterior cruciate ligament at the time of surgery had been recorded in almost every case and two groups could be identified (Table 1). The table shows the demography of the two groups. The mean follow-up time was very similar in both and the distributions of men to women, osteoarthritis to rheumatoid arthritis and unicompartmental to bicompartmental do not differ significantly. Survival tables have been constructed according to the method described by Tew and Waugh [3] and Armitage [4]. "Success"

**Table 1.** Details of patients and implants

| | Mean elapsed time (months) | Nos. of patients | | Disease | | Prosthesis | | | |
|---|---|---|---|---|---|---|---|---|---|
| | | Male | Female | OA | RA | Prototype | Oxford bicondylar | Oxford uni-compartmental | |
| | | | | | | | | Medial | Lateral |
| Anterior cruciate ligament absent (125 knees) | 56 | 21 | 104 | 78 | 46 | 16 | 83 | 18 | 8 |
| Anterior cruciate ligament intact (160 knees) | 54 | 41 | 119 | 101 | 57 | 13 | 97 | 36 | 14 |

*OA* osteoarthritis, *RA* rheumatoid arthritis

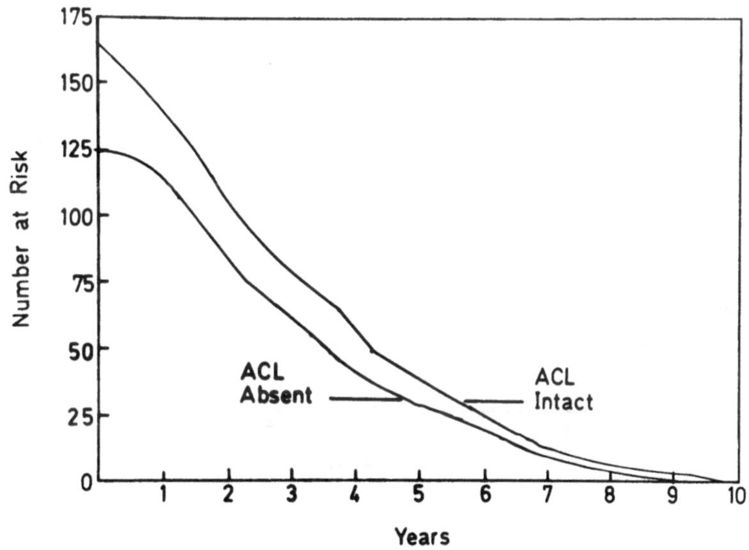


**Fig. 14.** Numbers of patients at risk. Operations before November 1985, reviewed at March 1987, based on conversion operations. *ACL* anterior cruciate ligament

means that the original prosthesis was still functioning at the time of follow-up and "failure" that the prosthesis had been removed and replaced by some other device or an arthrodesis performed. "Reoperation" refers to any surgical procedure which had to be undertaken following the primary implantation, even if the original prosthesis was not replaced. The reoperation figures include those cases in which a dislocated bearing was re-inserted or a loose component was recemented. Figure 14 shows the number of knees at risk over the 10-year period. Beyond 7 years the numbers are still too small for comparisons to be valid.

In Figs. 15 and 16 the cumulative success rate in the two samples, those with and those without an anterior cruciate ligament, are compared. Both the failure rate and the re-operation rate differ highly significantly.

Using the same data we have compared the effect of disease upon the two groups. In Table 2 the figures are given for knees with rheumatoid arthritis. In those knees which lacked an anterior cruciate ligament the failure rate was four times as high as in those in which the ligament was intact. However, the failure rate at 7 years was so low in both groups that the differences are not significant. Table 2 also shows the figures for osteoarthritic knees. It is in this group that the difference in outcome between those with and those without an anterior cruciate ligament is most marked.

## Discussion

Both rheumatoid arthritis and osteoarthritis are progressive diseases in which the knee joint suffers

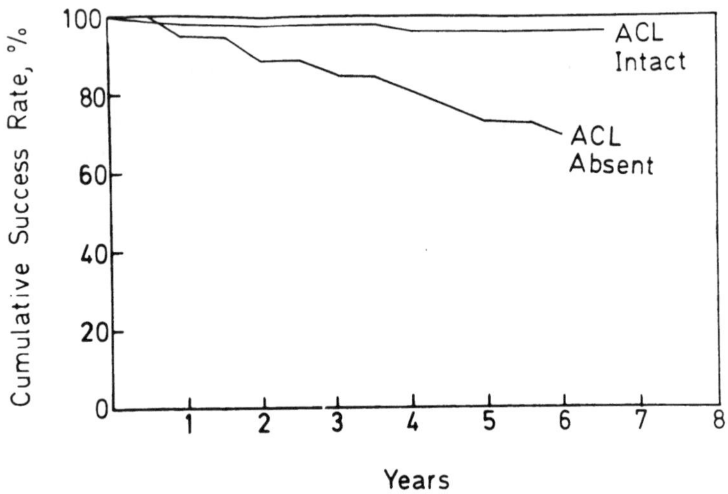


**Fig. 15.** Survival curves. Conversion operations at March 1987

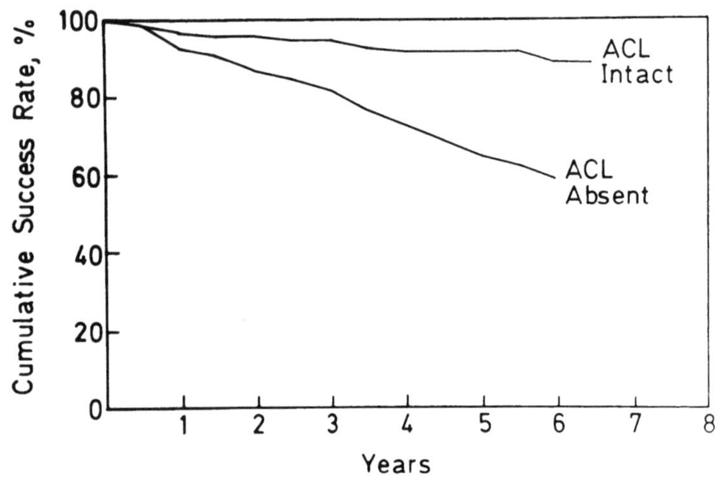


**Fig. 16.** Survival curves. Reoperations at March 1987

increasing destruction with time. Initially, in both diseases, the articular surfaces are affected. Failure of the articular cartilage and then of the underlying bone renders the ligaments slack and results in instability of the joint which frequently lapses into varus or valgus. Beyond this stage the ligaments become involved and it seems that usually the anterior cruciate is the first to rupture. Eventually the collateral ligament on the convexity of the deformity stretches and the collateral on the concavity may become secondarily shortened.

The theoretical analysis proposed at the beginning of this paper would suggest that a totally unconstrained prosthesis would only be appropriate at that stage in the disease process when the articular surfaces have been destroyed but the ligamentous apparatus has not yet been damaged. It has been our experience, both in rheumatoid arthritis and in osteoarthritis, that the anterior cruciate is the first of the ligaments to fail. It was found to be damaged or absent in rather less than half the knees that came to arthroplasty. By contrast the posterior cruciate ligament was almost never damaged. Our theoretical analysis suggests that the anterior and posterior cruciate ligaments act together as a four-bar linkage and that the absence of either must have serious effects upon the mechanics and kinematics of the knee. The results of our clinical review seem to support this theory. In those knees in which both cruciates were intact, reconstruction with the totally unconstrained components of the Oxford Meniscal Knee was very successful, providing success rates at 7 years of 98% and 95% in the rheumatoid and osteoarthritic groups respectively. However, in those joints which lacked an anterior cruciate ligament, the failure rates were much higher and, in osteoarthritis, compare poorly with the outcome reported for semiconstrained designs of total con-

**Table 2.** Effect of the presence or absence of the anterior cruciate ligament on the success of joint replacement surgery

| Disease | Ligament | Success | | Failed | | Success | | Reoperated | |
|---|---|---|---|---|---|---|---|---|---|
| | | % | No. | % | No. | % | No. | % | No. |
| Rheumatoid arthritis | Intact | 98 | 56 | 2 | 1 | 89 | 51 | 11 | 6 |
| | Absent | 91 | 42 | 9 | 4 | 83 | 38 | 17 | 8 |
| Osteo-arthritis | Intact | 95 | 98 | 5 | 5 | 93 | 96 | 7 | 7 |
| | Absent | 78 | 61 | 22 | 17 | 70 | 54 | 30 | 24 |

In rheumatoid knees the presence of the ligament is not significant ($P < 0.1$ in both cases). In osteoarthritic knees the absence of the ligament is significant ($P < 0.002$) in the patients where first implant failed and highly significant ($P < 0.0001$) in those having reoperation

dylar replacement.

We conclude that in the early stages of rheumatoid arthritis and osteoarthritis a completely unconstrained meniscal bearing implant achieves a high success rate and may be preferred in such cases to total condylar replacements, which are less physiological and more invasive. However, if ligamentous damage has supervened, a semiconstrained total condylar implant is preferred.

**Unicompartmental Replacement**

Since 1982, we have performed unicompartmental replacement in osteoarthritis of the knee with increasing frequency. The medial and lateral tibiofemoral joints are mechanically separate though they occupy the same synovial cavity. The best evidence for this statement is the observation that one of these joints can undergo severe degeneration while the other remains healthy (Fig. 17). Under these circumstances it is logical to perform a total replacement of the damaged compartment while preserving the others intact. The wholly unconstrained meniscal bearing prosthesis has obvious advantages in this context. The components of the Oxford Meniscal Knee, having no preferred axis of movement of their own, can accommodate the movements of the retained compartment. The appropriate choice of bearing size is made *after* the fixed components have been implanted, minimising the technical problems of the procedure. The ball and socket form of the menisco-femoral articulation accomodates minor errors of alignment without loss of articular surface congruity in the mediolateral plane (Fig. 18).

It has been our observation that in the majority of osteoarthritic knees the process of destruction commences in one compartment only, usually the medial, and remains more or less localised to that compartment as long as the anterior cruciate ligament remains intact. The osteoarthritic knees which are most suitable for a meniscal bearing prosthesis (because the anterior cruciate ligament is intact) therefore usually require only one compartment to be replaced.

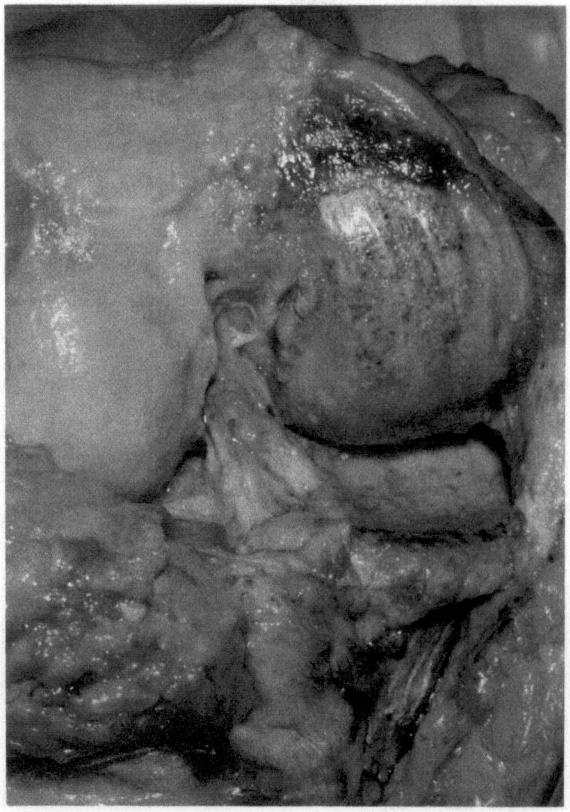

**Fig. 17.** Severe erosion of medial compartment of knee joint found at operation

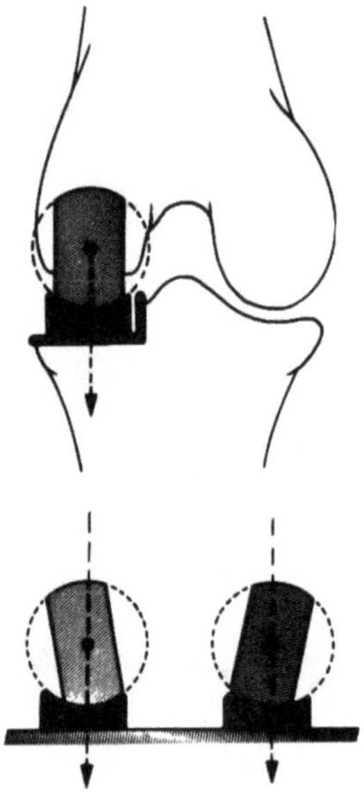

**Fig. 18.** Use of a matching meniscus accomodates minor errors of implant alignment without losing congruity

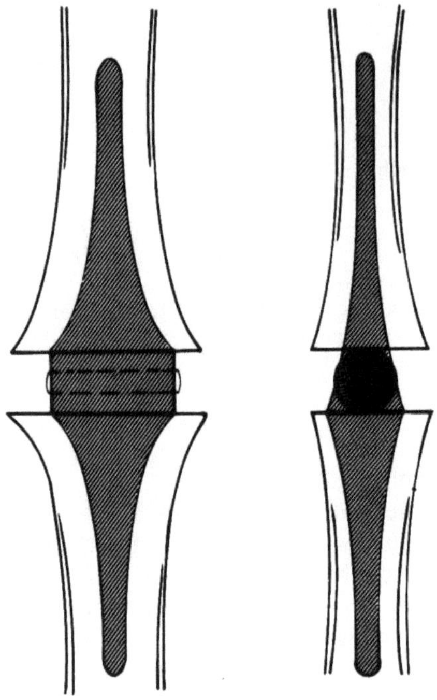

**Fig. 19.** Fully constrained hinged arthroplasty

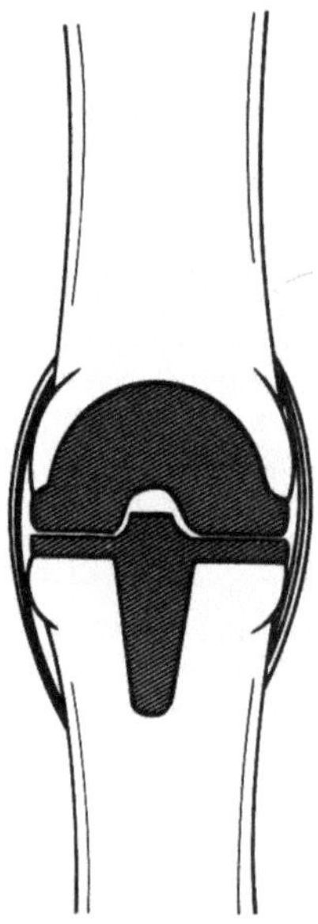

**Fig. 20.** Semiconstrained total knee replacement

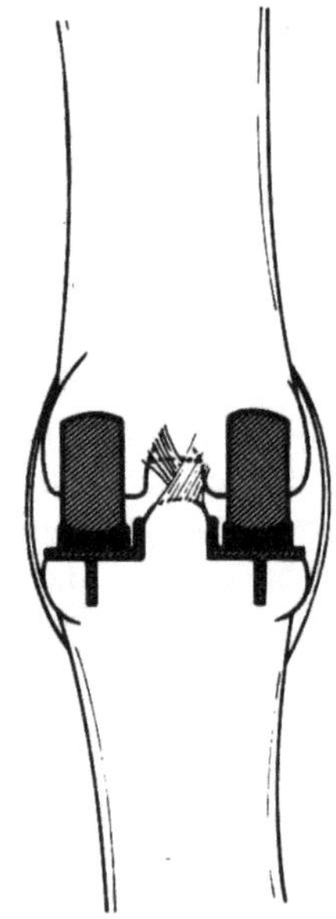

**Fig. 21.** Bicompartmental Oxford Meniscal Knee

## Conclusion

Treatment of the several stages of joint destruction which arise from rheumatoid arthritis or osteoarthritis requires a range of prostheses with differing degrees of constraint.

If neither the collateral nor the cruciate ligaments are present, nothing less than a fully constrained hinged arthroplasty will suffice to provide stability in the medio-lateral and antero-posterior planes (Fig. 19).

If the collateral ligaments are intact but the cruciate ligaments are damaged, a semiconstrained total condylar type implant is required (Fig. 20).

If the collateral and the cruciate ligaments are intact, i.e., *both* cruciate ligaments, not just one, then the Oxford Knee with its meniscal bearing offers a more physiological and less invasive alternative. In such cases it relieves the symptoms and conserves joint function with a high likelihood of success (Fig. 21).

Lastly, in early osteoarthritis, unicompartmental arthroplasty provides a reliable alternative to tibial osteotomy and is the least invasive of all such procedures (Fig. 22).

In our experience, about half of the patients who require arthroplasty for the relief of their symptoms have an intact cruciate ligament mechanism and are therefore suitable for treatment with the unconstrained meniscal bearing prosthesis.

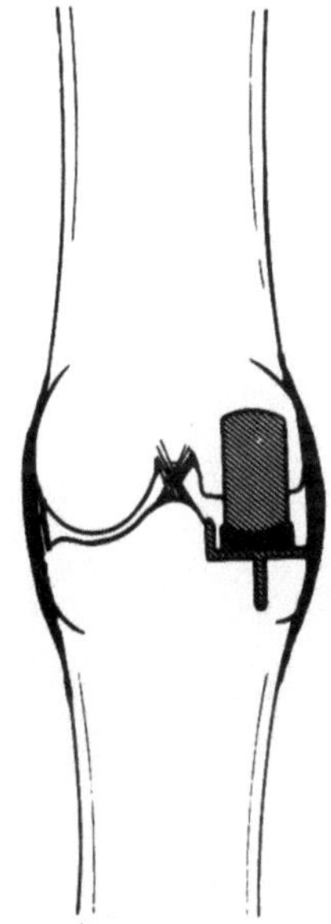

**Fig. 22.** Unicompartmental Oxford Meniscal Knee

## References


1. Goodfellow J, O'Connor J (1978) The mechanics of the knee and prosthesis design J Bone and Joint Surg. 60-B: 358–369
2. Goodfellow J, O'Connor J (1986) Clinical results of the Oxford Knee. Clin Orthop 205: 21–42
3. Tew M, Waugh W (1982) Estimating the survival time of knee replacements. J Bone and Joint Surg 64-B: 579
4. Armitage P (1971) Statistical methods in medical practice. Blackwell, Oxford

## *Discussion*

*Paul* (University of Strathclyde): You say that you adjust the tension in the cruciates by selection of the appropriate thickness of meniscus. Is any release of the collaterals required to accomplish this?

*Goodfellow* (Oxford University): No; we do not do the operation in patients in whom varus or valgus deformity has become fixed. Prior to surgery, we examine the knee in varus and valgus stress under the image intensifier. If the varus or valgus deformity can be corrected and the collateral ligaments do not need to be released, we perform this operation. We find that this is the state of affairs in most cases of rheumatoid arthritis and about half the cases of osteoarthritis. If ligamentous release has to be performed, the condition has passed beyond the possibilities of this kind of physiological reconstruction.

*Ranawat* (Cornell University Medical College): If we apply the meniscal bearing implant to unicompartmental disease on the medial side with normal anterior cruciate ligaments, the indications for the procedure become very narrow; if on top of that we add, as you stated, that there should be no fixed deformity we are talking about a very select group of patients. There are at least three reports in the literature on unicompartmental replacement and all indicated good results at 5-year follow-up in 90% or more of cases. Your failure rate is around 11% at 2-year follow-up. How can you justify the indication for this procedure in light of the high failure rate in such a short period of time?

*Goodfellow*: This device is only suitable for patients in whom the ligamentous apparatus is more or less intact. It will, therefore, compete probably very little with devices that we now use for total joint replacement. However, its main area of applicability is in those patients in whom at present a tibial osteotomy is performed. I find that the results I have presented here are in fact very considerably better than those which most of us have achieved with tibial osteotomy. I believe that this implant is useful between the two extremes of tibial osteotomy and total condylar replacement.

With regard to the number of patients for whom this would be suitable, the current volume of the Journal of Bone and Joint Surgery gives a report from Lund in Sweden. In that country, about half the total jont replacements performed for osteoarthritis are cases of unicompartmental arthroplasty. That has been my experience too: A very large number of patients who have received total joint replacements are actually suitable for unicompartmental arthroplasty.

As to why this device should be used in light of the results with devices that do not have a meniscal bearing, if the same criteria are applied to the choice of patients that are now applied to bicompartmental cases a very high success rate is obtained—1 of 49 cases is a failure rate of 2%. The theoretical basis for it of course depends upon its prospects in longevity. It seems to me very unlikely that articular surface components in a unicompartmental knee which only make contact over a very small area can possibly last for the 10 or 20 years that we must expect of them.

*Ranawat*: Does that mean that surgeons in the USA are doing unicompartmental procedures for a very extended indication? The designs that these surgeons are using do not move, do not have a meniscal bearing, and yet they are seen to be more durable. How do you explain that?

*Goodfellow*: I think there may be some problems of interpretation here. We heard yesterday of a very extensive series in Germany where the failure rate in sledge implants increased with the passage of years. The follow-up time was a little longer than my 7 years, but in fact the decline in their success rate was considerable and it fell well below that of hinged arthroplasties. That may be because they were perfomed in a mixture of patients, some of whom lacked the anterior cruciate ligament while others had the ligament. Our, admittedly, shorter follow-up strongly suggests that if you employ a totally unconstrained device in patients in whom the anterior cruciate ligament is intact, results are obtained after 7 years that are as good as or even better than those with hinged arthroplasty.

*Bourne* (University of Western Ontario): The bicompartmental nature of the Oxford knee may be a disadvantage. I would be interested in your comments in this regard. Can you foresee your design being altered to accept some of the advantages of the Total Condylar type concept, perhaps with a mobile bearing?

*Goodfellow*: I think that the notion of implanting a bearing into the knee joint is capable of almost endless variation. There are already to my knowledge eight designs on the market that include meniscal bearings in one form or another. I do not know whether all of them will prove applicable. I suspect that those designs that involve implantation of a meniscal bearing and yet do not preserve the anterior cruciate ligament may meet with failure, as ours did. It does not make sense to me to insert a meniscal bearing unless there is also something to control the anteroposterior movements.

With regard to the bicompartmental nature of the device, as you see when used in appropriate cases the bicompartmental device works very well and in the long term. But the number of patients for whom it is suitable is limited to those where the ligamentous apparatus is intact.

*Bontemps* (Fabricius-Klinik M): You stress limitation of the normal kinematics of the joint. Why do you not have decreasing radii on the dorsal part of the femoral components? Do you not have any conflict with your cruciate ligaments?

*Goodfellow*: The diameter of the tibial facets of the femur is more or less constant; it varies by less than 10% from a sphere. The articular surface of the femur is a composite: It consists of the tibial-femoral articulations and the patellar-femoral articulations, and the two are then blended into one another. The articular radii of the true tibial facets of the femur are found to vary very little from a sphere; they are on a smaller radius than the patellar facets, which then run into the tibial facets. If sections are taken through the femur, not through the condyles but through the center of the bone, the two curves are seen quite separately. If the tibial facets of the femur are measured, they are found to be so little different from a sphere that a spherical implant is a perfectly satisfactory replacement. The best test of this is in the cadaveric joint; here, we have cut off the natural surfaces in many instances, replaced them with a spherical surface, and observed the kinematics of the joint to be preserved. The notion that the ligaments are tightened up and relaxed by a camlike effect of the posterior part of the femur is not, in fact, in keeping with observations.

# GSB—14 Years of Experience with Total Knee Arthroplasty

N. GSCHWEND, T. DROBNY, and D.I.-RADOVANOVIC[1]

**Summary.** The GSB knee was introduced for clinical use in 1973. In 1978, a few changes in the prosthesis design were made; since 1978, the design has remained unchanged. The prosthesis is of a semiconstrained, low-friction type. While for the patellar component cementless fixation is appropriate, the stems of the femoral and tibial component are cemented into the intramedullar cavities of the femur and tibia. There is almost no deformity, bone loss, or other difficulty which would not permit the use of GSB implants. The simple semiconstrained prosthesis system gives the prosthesis inherent stability and allows it to function in a similar way to the kinematics of a normal knee joint. The instrumentation technique is quite easy and does not demand a great deal of specialization on the part of the surgeon. The overall long-term results are very satisfactory in terms of improvement in walking distance, pain relief, and range of motion postoperatively. The survival time and cumulative success rate of the GSB prosthesis are also surprisingly high compared with other systems. There is a good possibility for arthrodesis in cases where the prosthesis fails.

**Keywords:** Total knee arthroplasty—Patellar subluxation—Rigid hinge prosthesis—Semiconstrained knee—Clinical results—Titanium net—Patellar replacement

In 1972 the first type of GSB prosthesis (Gschwend, Scheier, Bähler), mark I, was implanted at the Clinic Wilhelm Schulthess in Zurich. This prosthesis can be placed as a floppy or physiological semiconstrained hinge in between the so-called condylar or nonconstrained prostheses and the fully constrained hinges. We tried to combine the advantages of both systems and hoped to avoid their disadvantages.

The loosening rate within 5–9 years was less than 2%. We modified this type to the present GSB prosthesis mark II for the following reasons residual pain at the level of the patella and metallosis due to a metal to metal contact where both components were linked to a hinge-like system. The new model is even more adapted to physiological movement, at least in the sagittal plane. Moreover, the femoral component now has a proximal flange to articulate with the posterior surface of the patella, which is also replaced by a high-density polyethylene prosthesis fixed without cement. One of the great advantages of this prosthesis is the simplicity of the operative technique which eliminates more sophisticated instruments. Furthermore, there is reduced risk of loosening even when residual deformities due to technical errors remain, especially in situations in which a condylar prosthesis inevitably leads to failure. The mobility has a mean range exceeding 100°. All types of deformities, regardless of the degree, can be corrected.

We analyzed the results of the last 3 years from the point of view of pain, range of motion, and walking capacity. These results were obtained by 13 surgeons of our clinic, including residents without specialized training.

The problem of patellar subluxation in some cases has not been definitely solved in spite of the fact that a great improvement has been achieved since we have been using a lateral approach to the knee joint without disturbing the vastus medialis, in particular its oblique component. These residual problems led to some modifications of the patellar and tibial component in 1987.

The simplicity of the operative technique, a range of motion exceeding 100° with full stability, and the minimum risk of loosening are great advantages, particularly for surgeons who do not have much experience with knee replacement.

Finally, we present the reoperation GSB prosthesis for salvage cases, where other types of prosthesis have led to failure and where the surgeon instead of using a hinge joint prefers to utilize a semiconstrained joint with almost physiological kinematic properties.

The results of 696 primary GSB knee replacements were analyzed by the method of survivorship. A prosthesis was considered to have failed if it was removed or persistently caused severe pain. The cumulative 5-year success rate was 91%—90% in osteoarthritis patients (OA) and 94% in rheumatoid arthritis (RA) patients. The cumulative survival rate at 7 years was 85% (OA group 84%, RA

[1] Klinik Wilhelm Schulthess, Zurich, Switzerland

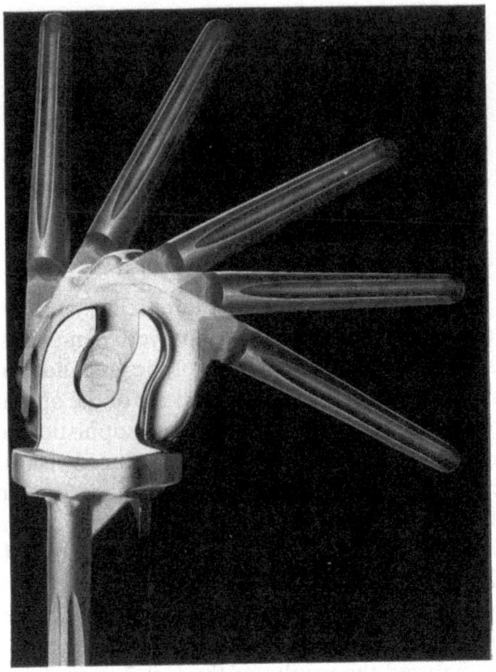

**Fig. 1.** The first prototype of the GSB total knee arthroplasty with the migrating axis. Used between 1973 and 1978

**Table 1.** Pain reported by patients receiving the first model GSB total knee arthroplasty (follow-up 5 years)

| Pain | Preoperative | | Postoperative | |
|---|---|---|---|---|
| | No. | Percent | No. | Percent |
| Severe | 80 | 68 } 98 | 6 | 4.5 |
| Moderate | 36 | 30 } | 22 | 18.5 |
| Slight/occasional | 2 | 2 | 33 | 28 } 76 |
| None | — | — | 57 | 48 } |

**Table 2.** Range of motion with first GSB total knee arthroplasty (>5 years; $n = 109$)

| Range of motion | Preoperative | Postoperative |
|---|---|---|
| Maximum flexion | 130° | 130° |
| Minimum flexion | 20° | 70° |
| Average | 90° | 104° |
| Maximum extension deficit | 70° | 45° |
| Minimum extension deficit | 0° | 0° |
| Average | 18° | 4° |

There were eight cases of arthrodesis and one of amputation
The average postoperative gain was 28°

94%), at 10 years 70% (OA group 70%, RA 76%), and the cumulative 12-year success rate was 48% (OA group 44% and RA 57%). The difference between the OA and RA groups of patients is highly significant after 5 years.

## First GSB Model

Fifteen years ago, when we developed the first GSB prosthesis, we were influenced by the negative results obtained with rigid hinge systems like the Shiers prosthesis (Fig. 1). A brief experience with a gliding prosthesis like the St. Georg type led us to the conclusion that the rigid hinge type of prosthesis was unable to produce simultanously good mobility and satisfactory stability as this kind of arthroplasty had a relatively restricted indications in the presence preexisting deformity and lesions of the ligaments. The purpose of the GSB prosthesis was to combine the advantages of both systems without suffering from their drawbacks. With a mobile axis and large condylar surfaces working under the low-friction principle, the kinematics of the prosthesis were almost physiological. In the event of failure, the minimal amount of bone resection permitted a withdrawal without difficulty. The movement between femoral and tibial components permitted reduction of the forces exerted on the intramedullary anchorage. The relatively simple operative technique, combined with the broad spectrum of indications (almost every deformity could be corrected), gave to any surgeon, especially those who are less well trained, the possibility of implanting a total knee arthroplasty. The study we performed 8 years ago shows that the first GSB knee prosthesis accomplished the functions we expected (Tables 1–5).

One striking aspect is the mobility of more than 100° in flexion, which is essential for patients suffering from bilateral OA or RA. One of the negative points was the relatively large percentage of patients suffering from patellar pain, having difficulty in getting up from a chair or climbing stairs. The percentage of re-operations due to patellar problems (over 12%) was also important. The rate of loosening more than 6 years post-operatively was only 1.7%, but the infection rate was 6.7%. Most of the infections appeared 4–6 years after the arthroplasty, half of them being hematogenous in origin. Were these infections provoked by metallosis due

**Table 3.** Use of mobility aids by rheumatoid arthritis and osteoarthritis patients treated with first GSB total knee arthroplasty (5-year follow-up)

| Reason for surgery | Aid | Preoperative | | Postoperative | |
|---|---|---|---|---|---|
| | | No. | Percent | No. | Percent |
| RA ($n = 48$) | No crutches | 3 | 7 | 24 | 50 |
| | One stick/crutch | 24 | 50 | 21 | 44 |
| | Two sticks/crutches | 20 | 41 | 2 | 4 |
| | Bound to wheelchair | 1 | 2 | 1 | 2 |
| OA ($n = 52$) | No crutches | 7 | 13 | 19 | 37 |
| | One stick/crutch | 27 | 52 | 21 | 40 |
| | Two sticks/crutches | 18 | 35 | 12 | 23 |
| | Bound to wheelchair | — | — | — | — |

**Table 4.** Walking capacity of patients with OA and RA treated with first GSB total knee arthroplasty (5-year follow-up)

| Disease | Walking capacity | Preoperative | | Postoperative | |
|---|---|---|---|---|---|
| | | No. | Percent | No. | Percent |
| RA ($n = 48$) | >1 km | 1 | 2 | 20 | 42 |
| | 1 km | 14 | 29.1 | 21 | 44 |
| | <100 m | 32 | 66.6 | 6 | 12 |
| | Unable to walk | 1 | 2 | 1 | 2 |
| OA ($n = 52$) | >1 km | 8 | 15.4 | 38 | 73 |
| | 1 km | 25 | 48 | 11 | 21 |
| | <100 m | 19 | 36.5 | 3 | 6 |
| | Unable to walk | — | — | — | — |

**Table 5.** Early and late complications in first GSB total knee arthroplasty (5-year follow-up)

| | Total ($n = 118$) | Rheumatoid arthritis ($n = 57$) | Osteoarthritis ($n = 61$) |
|---|---|---|---|
| Early complications | | | |
| Hematoma | 5 | 2 | 3 |
| Delayed wound healing | 4 | 2 | 3 |
| Transient palsy sciatic nerve | 1 | 1 | — |
| Fat pulmonary embolism | 2 | — | 2 |
| Total | 12 (10%) | 5 (4.2%) | 7 (5.8%) |
| Late complications | | | |
| Infections | 8 | 2 (3.5%) | 6 (9.8%) |
| Loosening | 2 | 1 | — |
| Breaking of implant | 3 | — | 3 |
| Implant incompatibility | 1 | 1 | 1 |
| Femoral fracture | 2 | 1 | 1 |
| Total | 18 (13.5%) | 5 (4.2%) | 11 (9.3%) |

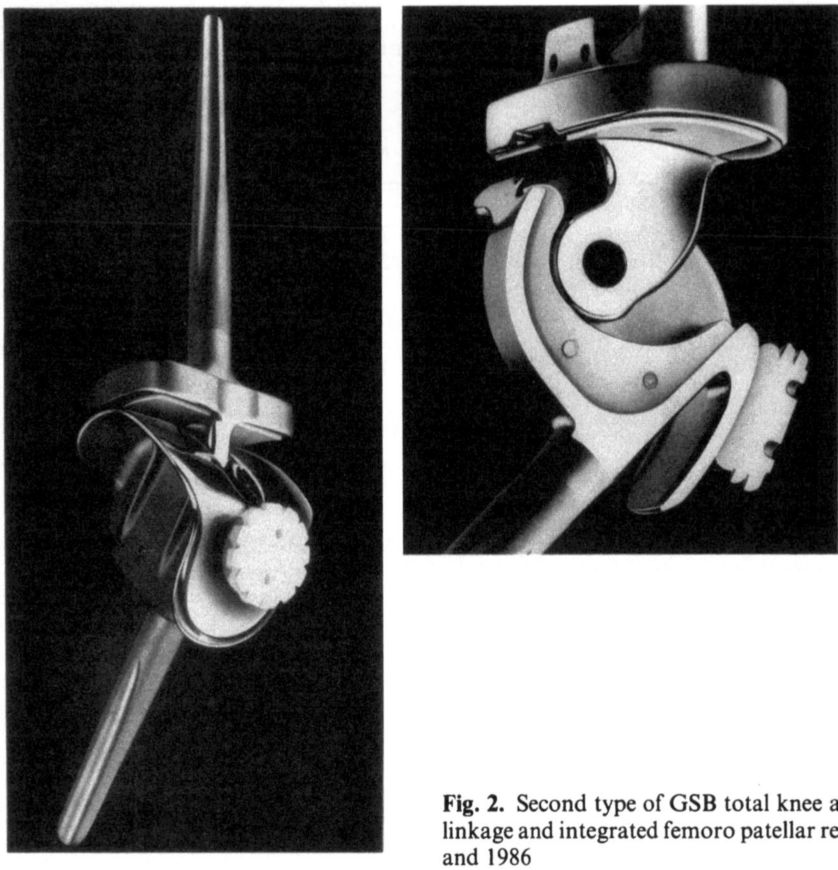

**Fig. 2.** Second type of GSB total knee arthroplasty with a loose-hinge linkage and integrated femoro patellar replacement. Used between 1980 and 1986

to the hinge, or through a diminished resistance of the bone due to disturbed blood circulation as a consequence of the intramedullary fixed implant? Two female patients, aged over 80 years, in a poor general condition died—one 3 h after operation from fat embolism, the other from thrombo-embolic disease 3 weeks after operation. Two fractures of the femur were observed after a fall, both of them were cured through osteo-synthesis. The original prosthesis fractured three times; as a consequence, an intermediate type was built with reinforcement of the hinge part. In eight cases, an arthrodesis had to be performed after failure of the arthroplasty. In all cases, radiological follow-up showed consolidation.

The above facts led us to review the concept of the first prosthesis and modify it to obtain the present model.

## Second GSB Model

The following are characteristic *features of* the new GSB prosthesis (Fig. 2): (a) Disappearance of the mechanical hinge, avoiding metal to metal contact. The hinge is only virtual and the surfaces in contact are of polyethylene and metal. (b) The kinematics of the prosthesis (Fig. 3) are almost the same as in the normal knee in the sagittal plane. This is particularly striking in flexion when the femur slides back to the posterior part of the tibial plateau, just as with the normal knee. (c) The femoropatellar joint has been completely modified with the insertion of a femoral shield and a patellar prosthesis. Anchorage of the patellar prosthesis with cement was abandoned, with care being taken not to implant it too deeply into the bone so as to reduce the possibility of lesions or fractures to the patella. The femoral shield, which originally had a plane surface now has a smooth concavity (Fig. 4).

## Operative Technique

The operative technique was improved and simplified with the development of new instruments (Fig. 5). Compared with other operative techniques, (e.g., condylar prosthesis) it is still relatively simple and within the capabilities of less-trained sugeons.

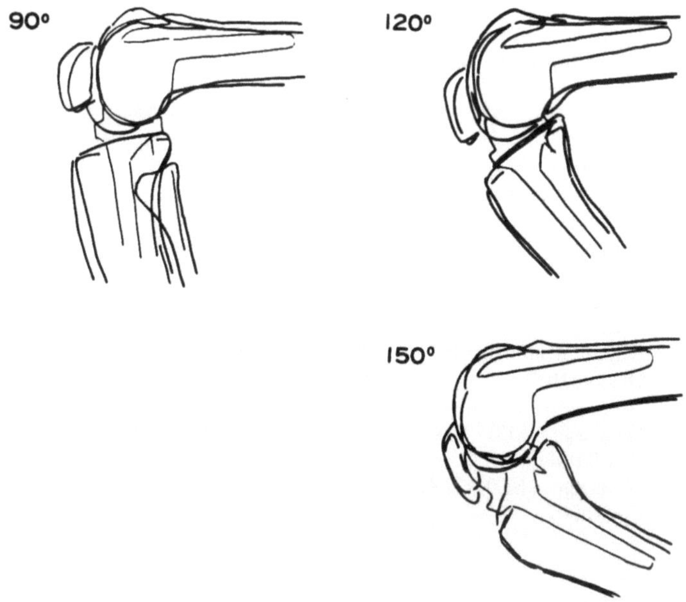


**Fig. 3.** Kinematics of the new GSB total knee prothesis are almost physiological

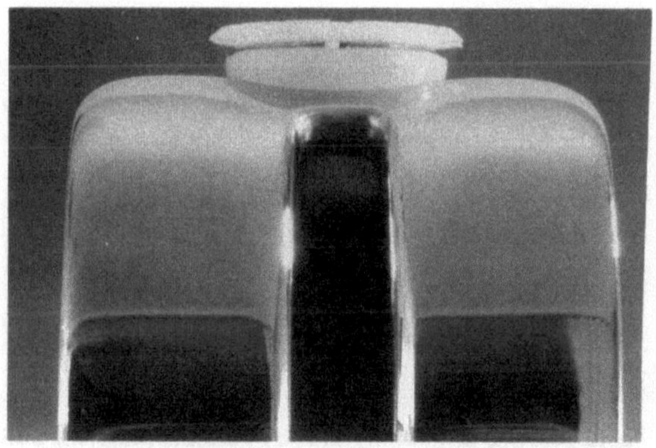

**Fig. 4.** Replacement of the femoropatellar joint in the GSB total knee arthroplasty (1979–1986); the patella is made of polyethylene and has been designed for cementless anchorage. The femoral shield is slightly concave

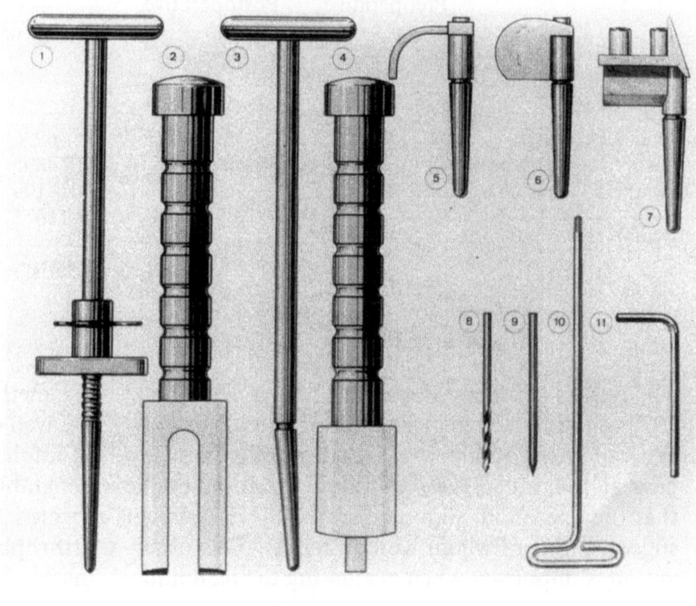


**Fig. 5.** Only these instruments are used for precise implantation of GSB total knee arthroplasty

**Table 6.** Statistics of patients receiving the second GSB model total knee arthroplasty (1980–1983)

| | Number | Percent | Age (years) |
|---|---|---|---|
| Total patients | 139 | 17.99 | |
| Male | 25 | 17.99 | |
| Female | 114 | 82.25 | |
| Total knee joints | 153 | | |
| Right | 83 | 54.25 | |
| Left | 70 | 45.75 | |
| Rheumatoid arthritis | 34 | 24.46 | 24–80[a] |
| Osteoarthritis | 105 | 75.54 | 53–85[b] |

[a] Average (SD) 59.41 (12.51); significantly different $P < 0.001$
[b] Average (SD) 72.43 (5.92); significantly different $P < 0.001$

**Table 7.** Numbers of knees in patients receiving the second model GSB total knee arthroplasty over the period 1980–1983 which had previous operations (total number of knees in series = 153)

| | Number | Percent |
|---|---|---|
| Synovectomy | 11 | 7.19 |
| Osteotomy | 17 | 11.11 |
| Meniscectomy | 7 | 4.57 |
| Ligamentous reconstruction | 1 | 0.65 |

**Table 8.** Pain reported by patients receiving second model GSB total knee arthroplasty (1980–1983)

| Pain | Preoperative | | Postoperative | |
|---|---|---|---|---|
| | No. | Percent | No. | Percent |
| Severe | 125 | 82.78 | 2 | 1.31 |
| Moderate | 23 | 15.23 | 20 | 13.07 |
| Slight/occasional | 3 | 1.99 | 43 | 28.10 |
| None | 0 | | 88 | 57.52 |
| Total | 151 | | 153 | |

**Table 9.** Walking capacity of patients receiving second model GSB total knee arthroplasty (1980–1983, number in series = 145)

| Walking capacity | Preoperative | | Postoperative | |
|---|---|---|---|---|
| | No. | Percent | No. | Percent |
| > 100 m | 69 | 43.31 | 4 | 2.68 |
| > 500 m | 52 | 34.9 | 13 | 8.72 |
| > 1 km | 20 | 13.42 | 21 | 13.08 } * |
| < 1 km | 8 | 5.37 | 111 | 74.5 } |

* Satisfactory results were obtained in 87.58% of cases

**Table 10.** Use of mobility aids by patients receiving second model GSB totak knee arthroplasty

| | Preoperative | | Postoperative | |
|---|---|---|---|---|
| | No. | Percent | No. | Percent |
| No crutches | 22 | 14.38 | 69 | 45.09 } 83.65 |
| One stick/crutch | 69 | 45.1 | 59 | 38.58 } |
| Two sticks/crutches | 58 | 37.91 | 25 | 16.33 |
| Bound to wheelchair | 4 | 2.61 | 0 | |

**Table 11.** Range of flexion in knees of patients receiving second model GSB total knee arthroplasty (total number of knees = 148)

| Range of flexion | Preoperative | | Postoperative | |
|---|---|---|---|---|
| | No. | Percent | No. | Percent |
| 0°–69° | 10 | 6.76 | 2 | 1.35 |
| 70°–89° | 16 | 10.81 | 2 | 1.35 |
| 90°–109° | 50 | 33.78 | 60 | 40.54 } * |
| > 110° | 72 | 48.65 | 84 | 56.76 } |

* Satisfactory results were obtained in 97.3% of cases

The results of all cases operated between 1980 and 1983 are summarized in Tables 6–15 and Figs. 6–9. We will later consider what kind of differences appear at 1, 2, and 3 years of follow-up. It is notable that the operations were performed by 13 different sugeons, nine of whom were residents. This observation is important when evaluating the technique.

If a method is so demonding that only sugeons who are well trained in the special technique are capable of implanting the prosthesis without mistake, it is debatable whether the technique should be performed by less well-trained surgeons, who do an arthroplasty fewer than ten times a year. It is a matter of fact that the insertion of many prosthesis

**Table 12.** Range of motion in the knees of patients receiving the second model GSB total knee arthroplasty

| Range of motion | Preoperative | Postoperative |
|---|---|---|
| Active[a] | | |
| Flexion | 30°–140° ($\bar{x}$ = 102.16° ± 20.87°) | 30°–130° ($\bar{x}$ = 107.73° ± 14.41°) |
| Extension (lack of) | 0°–40° ($\bar{x}$ = 11.28° ± 9.15°) | 0°–60° ($\bar{x}$ = 3.22° ± 8.21°) |
| Passive[b] | | |
| Flexion | 70°–130° ($\bar{x}$ = 107.36° ± 18.37°) | 30°–135° ($\bar{x}$ = 111.68° ± 16.12°) |
| Extension (lack of) | 0°–30° ($\bar{x}$ = 8.11° ± 6.32°) | 0°–30° ($\bar{x}$ = 0.77° ± 2.91°) |

[a] Preoperative total is 148; postoperative total is 152
[b] Preoperative total is 53; postoperative total is 86
The gain in flexion was 5.5° ($P < 0.01$) and that in extension 8.1° ($P < 0.001$). The total gain was 13.6°

**Table 13.** Follow-up of patients receiving second model GSB total knee arthroplasty at 1, 2, and 3 years

| | Follow-up | | |
|---|---|---|---|
| | 1 year (%) | 2 years (%) | 3 years (%) |
| Pain | | | |
| Improved | 91.67 | 100 | 96.83 |
| Satisfactory | 91.67 | 88.89 | 79.36 |
| Failure | 0 | 0 | 1.58 |
| Range of motion | | | |
| Improved | 32.35 | 28.3 | 29.51 |
| Satisfactory | 94.12 | 98.11 | 98.36 |
| Failure | 0 | 1.89 | 0 |
| Walking capacity | | | |
| Improved | 91.17 | 81.13 | 93.1 |
| Satisfactory | 85.29 | 88.68 | 87.93 |
| Failure | 2.94 | 0 | 0 |

The *numbers* indicate the percentage of the total number of knees (153) in each category of each assessment criterion
Loosening occurred in one case (0.65%). Perforation occurred in two cases (1.31%)
*Staphylococcus aureus* infection occurred in two cases (1.21%). The onset was 2 and 22 months postoperation. Treatment was by arthrodesis and aspiration and drainage

**Table 14.** Analysis of the effect of surgical approach on patellar subluxation in the knees of patients receiving second model GSB total knee arthroplasty (1980–1983, total number of knees = 153)

| Approach | Dislocation | Extreme subluxation | Medium subluxation |
|---|---|---|---|
| Medial ($n$ = 90) | 8 | 11 | 20 |
| Lateral ($n$ = 63) | 1 | 1 | 0 |
| Statistical significance | 0 | $P < 0.005$ | $P < 0.005$ |

Overall statistical significance $P < 0.001$

**Table 15.** Revision and mobilization procedures undertaken on the knees of patients receiving second model GSB total knee arthroplasty (1980–1983, 153 knees)

| | Number | Percent |
|---|---|---|
| Patellectomy | 1 | 0.65 |
| Removal of patellar component | 1 | 0.65 |
| Realignment of patella | 6 | 3.92 |
| Arthrodesis | 1 | 0.65 |
| Hematoma | 1 | 0.65 |
| Total | 10 | 7.83 |
| Mobilization under general anesthesia | 13 | 8.5 |

is very demanding technically and does not allow the smallest mistake. The statistics of authors showing the results of patients they have operated on personally should be considered critically. What is more important is the global result with patients who were treated with a well-defined technique.

Considering a series of 153 knees, treated with the new GSB prosthesis, presenting a follow-up of 1–3 years, we can observe that 75% of the patients suffered from OA, whereas 25% suffered from RA. The mean age of patients with OA (72.43 ± 5.92 years) was 13 years greater than the mean age of

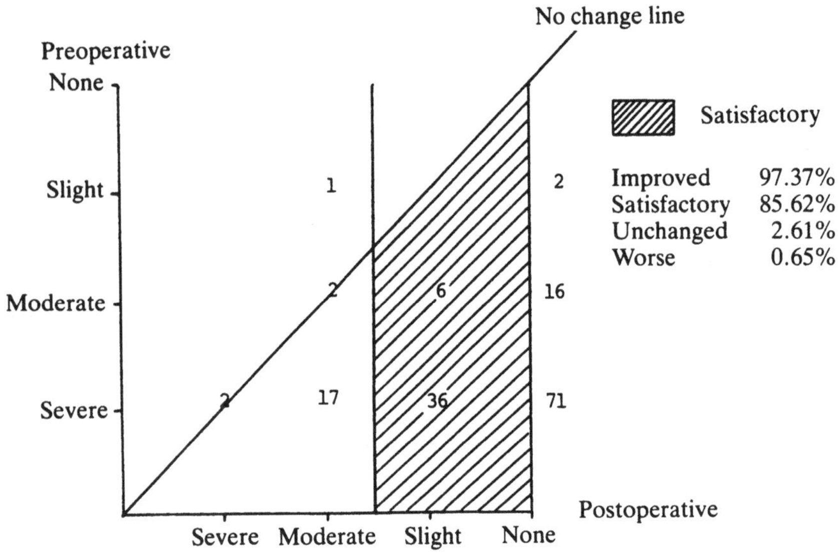


**Fig. 6.** Pain in second model GSB total knee arthroplasty (1980–1983; number of knee 3 = 153). The numbers indicate the knees in each category

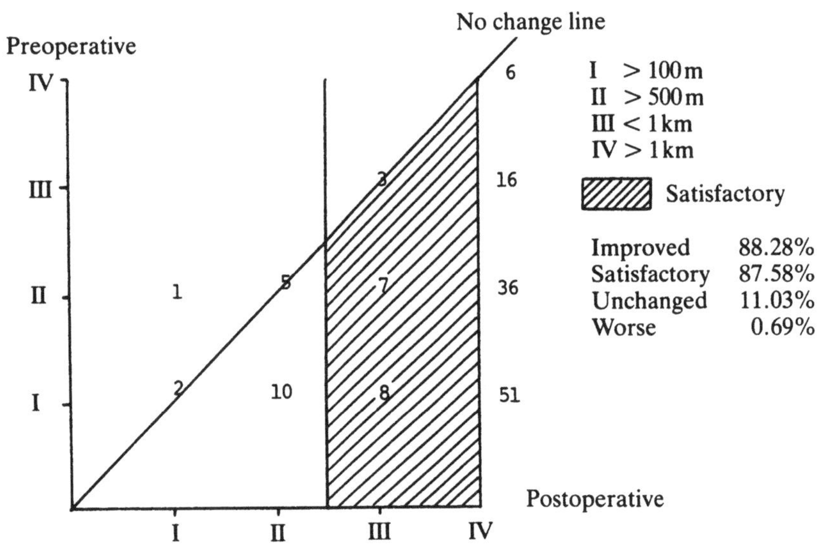


**Fig. 7.** Walking capacity of patients receiving second model GSB total knee arthroplasty (1980–1983; 145 patients). The *numbers on the graph* indicate the patients in each category

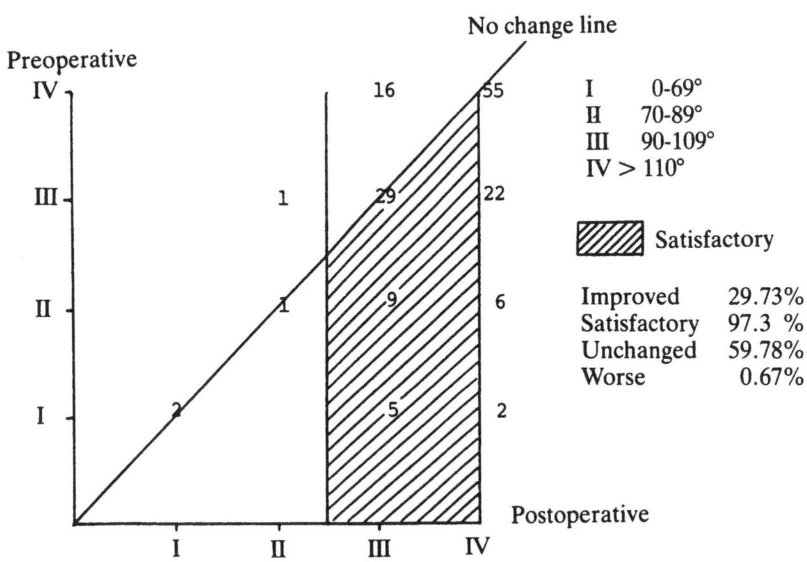


**Fig. 8.** Range of flexion of knees of patients treated with second model GSB total knee arthroplasty (1980–1983; 148 knees)

patients with RA (59.41 ± 12.61 years) (P 0.001). There were 82% female patients in this series and the results are as follows.

## Pain

### Results

Of the patients, 97.37% reported less pain after the operation, and 85.62% were generally satisfied: They no longer felt pain or the pain did not interfere with their daily activities. In 2.61% of patients, the pain was unchanged and it was worse in 0.65%.

### Walking Capacity

The walking capacity was ameliorated in 88.21% of all cases; 87.58% of the patients were satisfied with the functional gain and were capable of walking 1 km or for more than 30 min without feeling pain. Preoperatively, 85.02% of the patients had to use one or two sticks for walking, and four patients were bound to a wheel-chair. Postoperatively, 45.09% of the patients could walk without sticks whereas 38.56% were using one stick.

### Range of Motion

One of the greatest advantages of the method is the great mobility of the second model GSB prosthesis, with a mean range of flexion of 107.73° ± 14.51° actively and 111.68° ± 16.12° passively. There is a small lack of extension of 3.97°. This good range of motion is particulary helpful in rising from a chair and sitting down without difficulty. Patients suffering from bilateral OA or RA are handicapped if the mobility of the knee is less then 100°.

The global gain of mobility (13.67%; $P < 0.001$) after GSB arthroplasty does not interfere with the stability, as is often observed with patients after condylar arthroplasty. If the axial deformity is present preoperatively it can easily be corrected. Genu varum, which was encountered in 50% of cases preoperatively, was only observed in 1.59% of the cases postoperatively. Until recently, it was not possible to compare the results obtained with different techniques of arthroplasty. This is due to the different criteria used for each method. In view of this we tried with Aubriot and Freeman, to get homogeneous results.

These results are still very variable, even within our own series, if they are compared at 1, 2, and 3 years of follow-up. The percentage of patients suffering from RA is quite different in the three follow-ups and can, therefore, influence the overall results. The advanced age of the patients suffering from OA should be taken into account in addition to whether an arthroplasty of the other knee or of the hip has already been performed. If we consider the disappearance of pain, significant differences in the three series (at 1, 2, and 3 years) are evident. At 2 years follow-up, 100% of the patients declared they had shown improvement as a result of operation. This percentage falls to 91.67% at 1 year follow-up. How can we interpret the fact that at 3 years follow-up only 79.36% are classified as "little or no pain," whereas at 1 year follow-up 91.67% of the patients are in this category and at 2 years 88.89%? We could explain this phenomenon as an adaptive process of the soft tissue around the prosthesis which would bring a diminition of painful sensation after 1 or 2 years. On the other hand, at 3 years follow-up 41.94% of patients suffer from RA and the mean age is 52.18 years, whereas at 1 year follow-up only 26.32% of patients had RA, the mean age being 51.79 years. These observations should lead us to be careful with our conclusions.

The difference in the results is less significant with respect to knee mobility but it increases from the functional point of view.

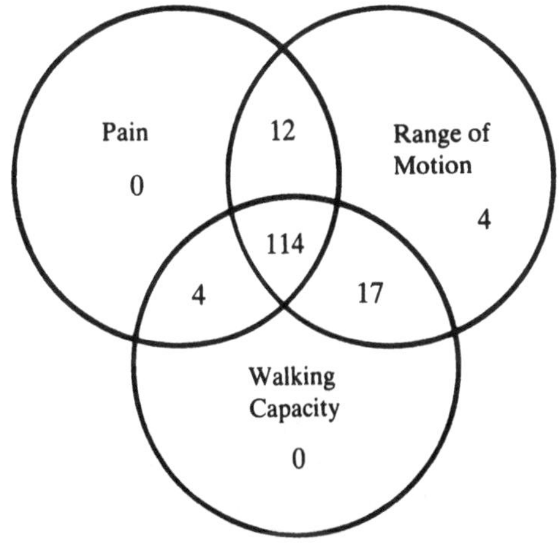


**Fig. 9.** Venn diagram indicating number of patients whose results of treatment are satisfactory assessed in different ways. *Data* refer to second model GSB total knee arthroplasty in 151 knees

### Complications

The value of each method has to be appreciated in terms of the complications it can produce. An operative technique should be called into question if the resulting complications show a specific character, the origin of which cannot be found or which cannot be solved by modification of the prosthesis.

The major complications that have to be considered are those that endanger the life of the patient or compromise the future of the prosthesis. This means infection and/or loosening. We did not observe any deaths as a direct consequence of the intervention in the series of 153 patients. Prevention of thromboembolism through early mobilization and anticoagulant therapy seems to play a vital role.

Loosening of the prosthesis, which was rare in the GSB I model, was encountered in only one case with the new GSB II arthroplasty.

Infection is still much too frequent. It was observed once in the series at 3 years follow-up and once in the 1-year follow-up series (2 of 153 patients). In one case, the infection regressed after debridement and systemic antibiotic treatment; in the other case, an arthrodesis had to be performed after removal of the implant.

The patella is responsible for most of the problems encountered such as subluxation, luxation, or fracture. Since we chose the lateral approach to the knee joint, we have noted a significant reduction in this problem, as the insertion of the vastus internus muscle is no longer weakened. Patellar fracture should become a rarity since the new noncemented prosthesis does not require anchorage deep in the patella. Without doubt the number of re-operations is too high at 7.83%; 4.5% concern only the patella.

### Global Results

Looking at the global results, we can observe that in 114 (75.49%) of 151 cases there is an overall improvement (for pain, range of motion, and functional gain) and that in 21.85% two factors improved. Comparing the clinical data obtained by the physician with the information given by the patients, we note similar results: In 72.55% (physician) and 73.86% (patient), the result is excellent; in 26.99% (physician) and 15.09% (patient) the result is rated good. With a total of 89% good and excellent results, we obtain a figure of almost 90% good results, which approaches the figure obtained with total hip arthroplasty.

## Indications and Contraindications

The present indications and contraindications of the GSB prosthesis are based on the experience we have gained over the years. Principally, all injuries to the knee which are disabling to the walking capacity and cannot be treated successfully through conservative therapy or an osteotomy may be an indication for total arthroplasty of the GSB type. With the exception of septic arthritis of the knee, the indications for GSB arthroplasty are similar to these for an arthrodesis. The GSB prosthesis can be used to correct any kind of axial deformity and ligamentous instability.

The GSB prosthesis is generally recommended to less-trained surgeons, who operate only on a small number of knees every year. For them, implanting a condylar prosthesis requires greater technical skill and may result in a greater risk of failure.

## Recent Type of GSB Knee Arthroplasty

The experience with the second type of GSB knee arthroplasty (1980) was positive compared with the first prototype (1973). Some problems were still unsolved with the new design and led to some modifications in 1987 (Fig. 10). The technique of the lateral approach to the knee joint decreased significantly the frequency of patellar subluxation, which was quite often managed via a medial incision. Nevertheless, there were still a number of patients

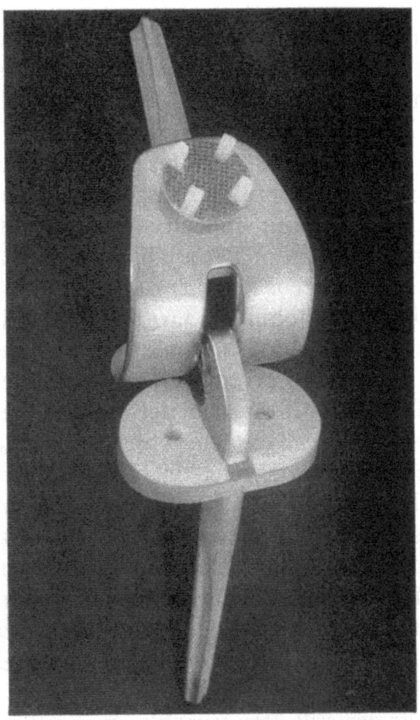

**Fig. 10.** The current type of GSB total knee with a new metal-backed patellar component and enlarged polyethylene contact surface. It has been in use since 1987

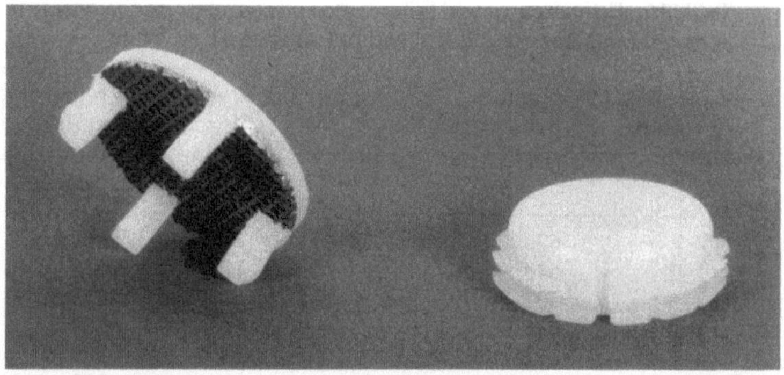

**Fig. 11.** The patellar component of the GSB II, designed in 1987

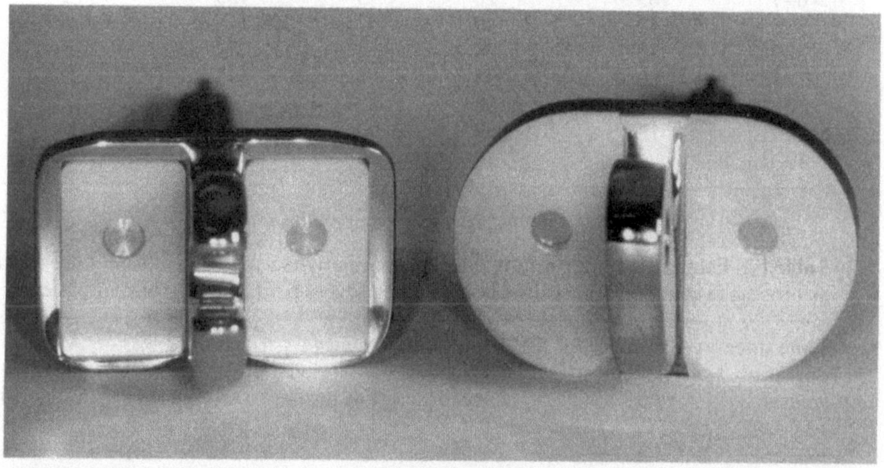

**Fig. 12.** The plateau of the tibial component was improved to this shape and design

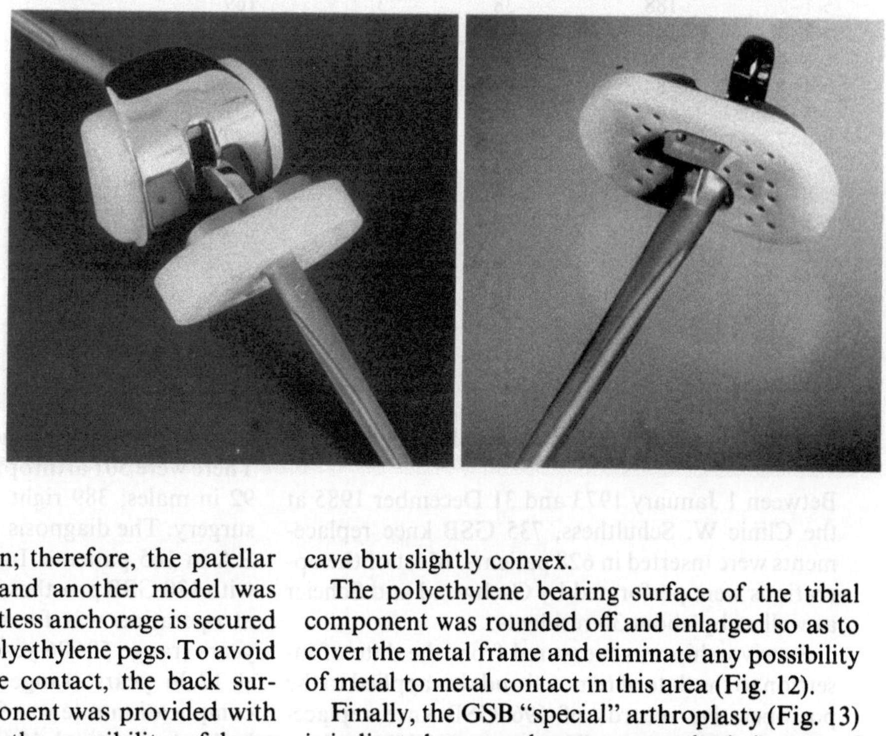

**Fig. 13.** Special type of GSB total knee arthroplasty, designed for revision and exchange operations

with residual patellar pain; therefore, the patellar component was revised and another model was built (Fig. 11). The cementless anchorage is secured by four slightly tapered polyethylene pegs. To avoid a large polyethylene-bone contact, the back surface of the patellar component was provided with a titanium net, allowing the possibility of bony ingrowth. The articulating surface is no longer concave but slightly convex.

The polyethylene bearing surface of the tibial component was rounded off and enlarged so as to cover the metal frame and eliminate any possibility of metal to metal contact in this area (Fig. 12).

Finally, the GSB "special" arthroplasty (Fig. 13) is indicated as a replacement prosthesis in case of failure of a nonconstrained prosthesis.

**Table 16.** Estimated annual failure rate and cumulative success rate of GSB knee replacement, where success is defined as prosthesis remaining in situ without causing severe pain

| Time since operation (years) | Number of patients at start | Result of last review | | Number at risk throughout period | Annual failure rate (%) | Annual success rate (%) | Cumulative success rate (%) |
|---|---|---|---|---|---|---|---|
| | | Success | Failure | | | | |
| 0.5–1 | 696 | 53 | 3 | 669.5 | 0.5 | 99.5 | 99.5 |
| >1–2 | 640 | 122 | 11 | 579 | 2 | 98 | 97.5 |
| >2–3 | 507 | 59 | 12 | 477.5 | 2.5 | 97.5 | 95 |
| >3–4 | 436 | 133 | 11 | 369.5 | 3 | 97 | 92 |
| >4–5 | 292 | 46 | 3 | 269 | 1 | 99 | 91 |
| >5–6 | 243 | 70 | 8 | 208 | 4 | 96 | 87 |
| >6–7 | 165 | 20 | 3 | 155 | 2 | 98 | 85 |
| >7–8 | 142 | 49 | 7 | 117.5 | 6 | 94 | 80 |
| >8–9 | 86 | 24 | 2 | 74 | 3 | 97 | 78 |
| >9–10 | 60 | 33 | 4 | 43.5 | 9 | 91 | 70 |
| >10–11 | 23 | 8 | 2 | 15 | 13 | 87 | 61 |
| >11–12 | 13 | 7 | 2 | 9.5 | 21 | 79 | 48 |
| >12–13 | 4 | 4 | 0 | 2 | 0 | 100 | 48 |

**Table 17.** Estimated annual failure rate and cumulative success rate of GSB knee replacement, where success is defined as prosthesis remaining in situ without causing severe pain in RA group of patients

| Time since operation (years) | Number of patients at start | Result of last review | | Number at risk throughout period | Annual failure rate (%) | Annual success rate (%) | Cumulative success rate (%) |
|---|---|---|---|---|---|---|---|
| | | Success | Failure | | | | |
| 0.5–1 | 206 | 18 | 0 | 197 | 0 | 100 | 100 |
| >1–2 | 188 | 38 | 3 | 169 | 2 | 98 | 98 |
| >2–3 | 147 | 15 | 2 | 139.5 | 1.4 | 98.6 | 97 |
| >3–4 | 130 | 43 | 3 | 108.5 | 3 | 97 | 94 |
| >4–5 | 84 | 21 | 0 | 73.5 | 0 | 100 | 94 |
| >5–6 | 63 | 24 | 0 | 51 | 0 | 100 | 94 |
| >6–7 | 39 | 6 | 0 | 36 | 0 | 100 | 94 |
| >7–8 | 33 | 13 | 3 | 28 | 11 | 89 | 84 |
| >8–9 | 17 | 5 | 0 | 14.5 | 0 | 100 | 84 |
| >9–10 | 12 | 4 | 1 | 10 | 10 | 90 | 76 |
| >10–11 | | | | | | | |
| >11–12 | 8 | 3 | 1 | 6.5 | 15 | 75 | 57 |
| >12–13 | 4 | 4 | 0 | 2 | 0 | 100 | 57 |

## Survival Time of GSB Knee Replacement

Between 1 January 1973 and 31 December 1985 at the Clinic W. Schulthess, 735 GSB knee replacements were inserted in 628 patients. Most of the operations were performed by Gschwend and Scheier as well as by about 30 residents.

Survivorship was measured from the date of insertion to the date of removal and was applied to the postoperative records of 696 GSB knee replacements in 593 patients. There were 103 bilateral arthroplasties; these made up 95% of the total GSB knee implants performed between 1973 and 1985. There were 501 arthroplasties in female patients and 92 in males; 389 right and 307 left knees received surgery. The diagnosis was OA in 428 patients and RA in 165 patients. In the meantime, 102 patients with 120 GSB prostheses have died. The average age at operation was for the OA group 70.67 ± 7.81 years (range 50–86 years), for the RA group 57.90 ± 12.36 years (range 25–76 years). The overall complication rate was 9.77% (68 knees); 41 (5.9%) had to be removed, 10 (1.4%) were reinserted, and a further 17 (2.4%) experienced severe pain.

**Table 18.** Estimated annual failure rate and cumulative success rate of GSB knee replacement, where success is defined as prosthesis remaining in situ without causing severe pain in OA group of patients

| Time since operation (years) | Number of patients at start | Result of last review | | Number at risk throughout period | Annual failure rate (%) | Annual success rate (%) | Cumulative success rate (%) |
|---|---|---|---|---|---|---|---|
| | | Success | Failure | | | | |
| 0.5–1 | 490 | 35 | 3 | 472.5 | 0.6 | 99.4 | 99.4 |
| >1–2 | 452 | 84 | 8 | 410 | 2 | 98 | 97 |
| >2–3 | 360 | 44 | 10 | 338 | 3 | 97 | 94 |
| >3–4 | 306 | 90 | 8 | 261 | 3 | 97 | 91 |
| >4–5 | 208 | 25 | 3 | 195.5 | 1.5 | 98.5 | 90 |
| >5–6 | 180 | 46 | 8 | 157 | 5 | 95 | 86 |
| >6–7 | 126 | 14 | 3 | 119 | 2.5 | 97.5 | 84 |
| >7–8 | 109 | 36 | 4 | 91 | 4.4 | 95.6 | 80 |
| >8–9 | 69 | 19 | 2 | 59.5 | 3.4 | 96.6 | 77 |
| >9–10 | 48 | 29 | 3 | 33.5 | 9 | 91 | 70 |
| >10–11 | 16 | 8 | 2 | 12 | 17 | 83 | 58 |
| >11–12 | 6 | 4 | 1 | 4 | 25 | 75 | 44 |
| >12–13 | 1 | 1 | 0 | — | 0 | 100 | 44 |

Most of the patients have since been reviewed annually. Records up to June 1986 were used in this analysis, so that there is a minimum of 6 months follow-up up to over 12 years.

The statistical method described by Armitage [1] and adapted by Tew and Waugh [10] to estimate survival time was applied. Each patient is thus included once in the table as either a success or a failure at the time of the last follow-up, the time of death, or the time of removal of the prosthesis.

A prosthesis was considered to have failed if it was removed for any reason, or if it frequently caused severe pain but remained in situ either because no defect could be detected in the prosthesis or the patient was too ill or too old to face another operation, or declined such removal. The significance between the sum of the annual expected failures and the total of actual failures was determined by the $X^2$-test.

Tables 16–18 show the survivorship tables for GSB knee replacement for all patients, for the OA group, and for the RA group. Continuous deterioration was observed in all groups and there is a steady decrease of approximately 2%–3%/year over 7 years with a cumulative success rate of 85% at 7 years, 78% at 9 years, 70% at 10 years, and only 48% at 13 years (Table 16). From Tables 17 and 18, it is clear that the annual rate of failure in all years was much lower in the group of RA patients than in the OA group. This difference is highly significant after 5 years ($P < 0.005$).

The predominant reason for failure was deep infection (37 knees, 5.3%), severe pain (17, 2.4%), and fracture of the prosthesis in six patients; loosening was, however, found only in eight cases (1.2%).

## References


1. Armitage P (1971) Statistical methods in medical research. *Blackwell*, Oxford, pp 408–414
2. Gschwend N, Scheier HG, Bähler A (1973) The knee joint. Exerpta Medica, Amsterdam (1982)
3. Gschwend N (1975) Die GSB-Kniearthroplastik. Z Orthop 113: 537–539
4. Gschwend N (1976) Design criteria, present indication and implantation techniques for artificial knee joints. In: Schaldach M (ed) Engineering in medicine, vol. 2. Springer Berlin-Heidel-berg-New York
5. Gschwend N, Scheier HG, Bähler A (1980) Die GSB-Knieprothese. Med Orthop Techn, 100: 128–134
6. Gschwend N, Scheier HJG, Bähler A., Meyer RP (1980) The GSB knee arthroplasty. Int Orthop 3(4): 281–284
7. Gschwend N Kniegelenksendoprothetikbei chronischer polyarthrtis. In: Aktuelle Probleme in Chirurgie und Orthopädie: 15. Huber, Bern
8. Gschwend N, Loehr J (1981) The Gschwend-Scheier-Bähler replacement of the rheumatoid knee joint. Reconstr Surg Traumatol 18: 174–194
9. Scheier HJG, Gschwend N (1978) Zur kniearthroplastik. Therap Umschau 5: 35
10. Tew M, Waugh W Estimating the survival time of knee replacements. J Bone Jt Surg (Br) 64-B: 579–582

## *Discussion*

*Miller* (Montreal General Hospital): Could you repeat your data on survival? I did not quite understand?

*Drobny* (Klinik Wilhelm Schulthess): In terms of success of the prosthesis in situ, the survival rate at 12 years was 60%; but a few of those patients had pain. If you subtract these patients, the survival rate is 48%.

*Miller*: So if you had 60%, then 40% did not survive.?

*Drobny*: I think that the main reason for this is that GSB is usually indicated in older patients. The mean age of implantation was about 70 years.

*Bontemps* (Fabricius-Klinik): You said that metal contact was eliminated by your later modifications, but still the fin that goes up inside the femoral component has the possibility of metal contact.

*Drobny*: Yes, there it has still not been fully eliminated. On the tibial plateau in some knees, there is the tendency toward hyperextension, and there was the possibility that the femur could hit the anterior border of the frame of the tibia. This possibility now no longer exists.

# Experience with a Surface and Total Knee Replacement: Further Development of the Model St. Georg

E. ENGELBRECHT and K. HEINERT[1]

**Summary.** Since 1969, we have had experience with 2373 surface replacements, the so-called sledge prosthesis, and since 1970 with the St. Georg total knee prosthesis in 3190 operations. Both systems present extremes regarding degrees of freedom and stability. Although little was known about knee arthroplasty at the beginning of this type of surgery, our early results were regarded as satisfactory and, therefore, the use and further development of both systems seemed justified.

With the proper indication, considerable relief or freedom of pain was achieved in 95% of cases. Deformities and flexion contractures were corrected and joint function was improved. The durability of a prosthesis system depends on the type of complication, and proper judgement can only be made after medium and long-term follow-up. Careful analysis of the reasons for failure revealed different types of complication for both systems. In the sledge prosthesis, insufficiency of the ligamentous apparatus was the commonest cause of failure followed by mechanical loosening, especially of the tibial component, operative technical errors, contracondylar arthrosis and Sudeck's disease. In the hinge, mechanical loosening and fracture at the tip of the prosthetic stem were the commonest causes of failure.

For both systems, the rate of infection was between 1% and 1.5% after a 10-year follow-up period.

A primary patellofemoral replacement was not performed and long-term results have confirmed our view in this respect. Residual pain was observed in 16%–18% of cases and ranged from minor to moderate, not requiring further revision. In cases of severe residual pain, observed in 1%–4% of cases, we still regard patellectomy as the method of choice.

Analysis of results had a considerable influence on the indication and further development of both prosthetic systems. For the sledge, improvements were made in design stability, operative technique, and in the reduction of bone resection. A further development of the St. Georg total hinge prosthesis led to a stabilizing hinge with axial rotation. The incorporation of a further degree of freedom and changes in design resulted in a reduction of forces at the bone-cement interface, improved operative techniques, and more favorable patellofemoral joint conditions. It is hoped that concurrently with the good short and medium-term results which have been obtained, biomechanical complications will decrease significantly in the future.

[1] Department of Clinical Decision Analysis, Endo-Klinik, Hamburg, Federal Republic of Germany

**Keywords:** Total knee replacement—Sledge prosthesis—Design—Hinge prosthesis—Clinical results

## Introduction

The restoration of normal joint function presents a greater problem in the artificial knee than in the hip. Imitation of the complex physiological knee motion produced over relatively small areas under high compressive load still remains a problem. Attenuation of stresses and a physiological force flow as provided by the cartilage, menisci, and ligaments in a normal joint cannot be reproduced by the implant materials now available. The major stabilizing structures of the joint, namely the ligaments and muscles, are utilized for proper joint function and the stability of the joint is provided by the prosthesis construction. The design of mechanical linkage determines the number of degrees of freedom allowed. The stresses on the prosthesis and its cement fixation are inversely related to the number of degrees of freedom. Therefore, knee prosthesis systems may be classified according to the number of degrees of freedom and the type of joint stabilization (Fig. 1) [13, 14].

Encouraged by our early good results with total hip arthroplasty since 1964, we began in 1968 with the development of knee arthroplasty. Between 1966 and 1969, we gained some experience with the stabilizing all-metal prostheses of the Shiers and Young type [36, 41, 42]. Even in a small series, the main problems of these units, which are also described in the literature, became apparent, namely metallosis, an increased infection rate, extensive bone resection, and an unfavorable shape of the prosthesis with regard to the patellofemoral joint.

In the development of our knee systems, we aimed at the concept of low-friction arthroplasty, cement fixation, and close adjustment of the prosthesis to the joint kinematics. From the very beginning, two knee replacement systems were conceived: a surface replacement relying for proper joint function on the presence of competent ligaments and

| | | Type I | | Type II | | Type III | | | |
|---|---|---|---|---|---|---|---|---|---|
| | | Hinge Joints | | Ball Joints | | Surface Replacement<br>Frequent shape and combination of contact areas (spherical, polycentric) | | | |
| | | a | b | a | b | a | b | c | d |
| degrees of freedom | rotation | 1 | 2 | 3 | 3 | 2<br>1 | 1<br>1+ (1) | 3<br>1+ (1) | 3 |
| | displacement | – | (1) | – | (1) | (1)<br>(1) | 1+ (1)<br>1+ (2) | (3)<br>(3) | 2+ (1) |
| Type of joint stabilization | implant | + | – | + | – | – | – | – | – |
| | Implant + capsule + ligaments + muscles | – | + | – | + | + | + | + | – |
| | ligamentous structures + muscles | – | – | – | – | – | – | – | + |

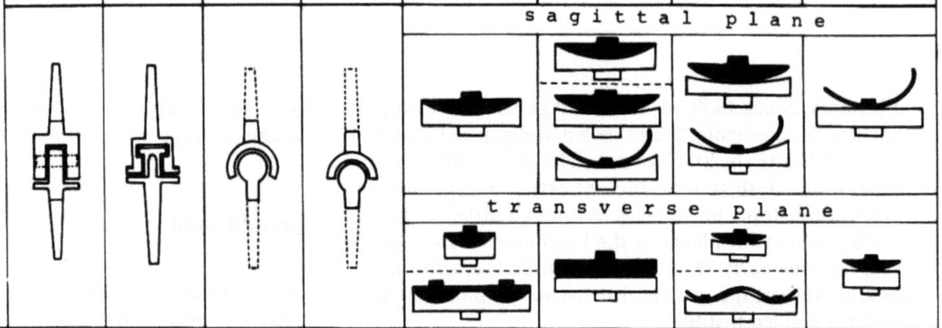


(n) = number of degrees of freedom which are restricted with increase in axial load.

**Fig. 1.** Classification of knee systems [13]

muscles, and a stabilizing total hinge system. According to the main criteria, i.e., degree of freedom and joint stability, the two systems present extremes. The sledge prosthesis, model St. Georg, incorporates the highest number of degrees of freedom, while the stability of the joint is provided by the patient's ligaments and muscles. The total hinge prosthesis, model St. Georg, has only one degree of freedom, but immediate joint stability is afforded by the prosthesis construction (Figs. 2, 3). The effectiveness of both systems, which was noted very early, justified the start of a large series. Surgical practice, medium-term follow-up results, and biomechanical testing were the requisites for gradual improvements of both systems. These were made successively in small steps, but all the improvements made on our knee replacements in the course of years did not affect the basic constructional principles of the two systems.

## Development of Sledge Prosthesis Model St. Georg

The St. Georg sledge prosthesis was developed in 1968 and first implanted in September 1969 [8, 9]. Our concept was greatly inspired by the ideas and initial experiments of Gunston [22]. The principle of prosthetic design incorporating point loading was specifically intended to allow almost normal knee motion. All degrees of freedom and movement including the "screw home" mechanism are preserved. Uni- and bicondylar implantation are possible. The original block-shaped plateau was to prevent severe deformity of the polyethylene. Technical difficulties, such as fracture of the lateral circumference of the tibia, led via several steps to the so-called anatomical plateau in 1976, constructed according to intra-operatively resected medial and lateral tibial surfaces. Metal backing of the tibial plateau in

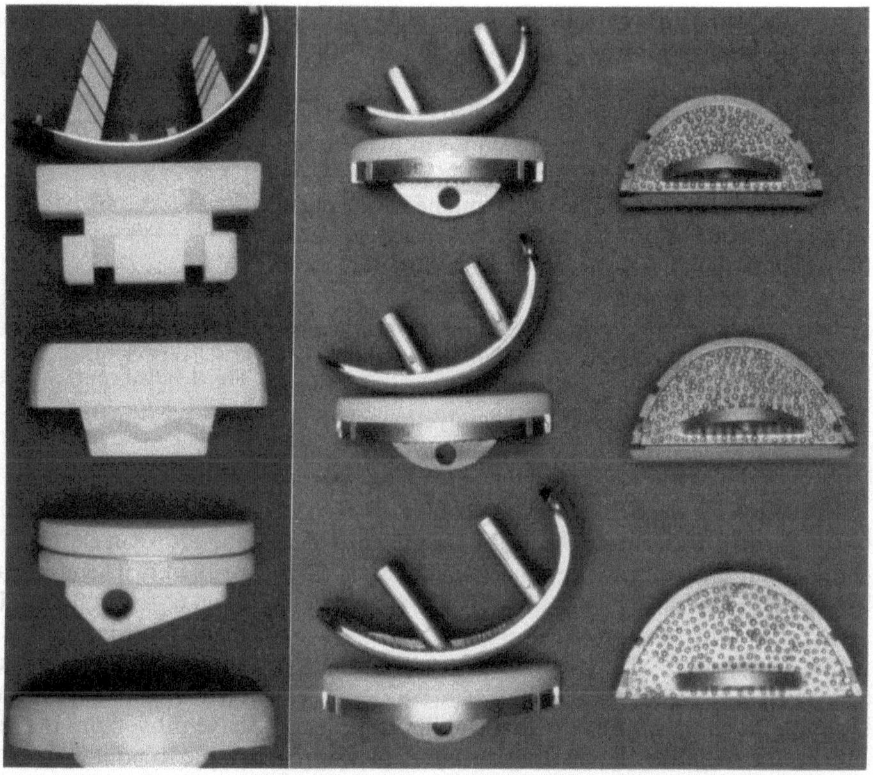

a b

Fig. 2a, b. Development of the sledge. a St. Georg model. b Endo model

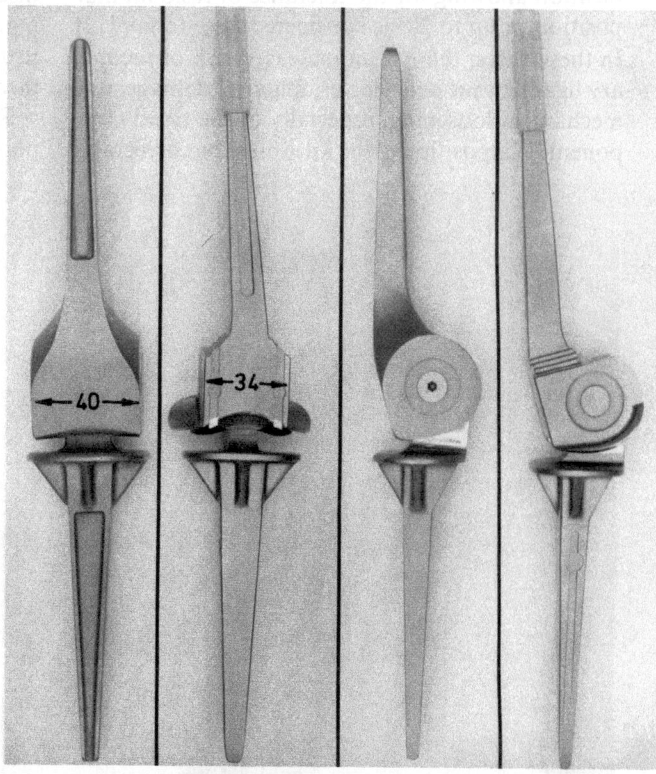


Fig. 3. Total intracondylar hinge St. Georg model—first and second generations

1981 was the answer to the significantly higher rate of mechanical loosening observed (Fig. 2) [10, 17, 38–40].

The polycentric curve of the sledge was derived from different sagittal cross sections of the femoral condyles. Experience has shown the sledge to have an acceptable shape and it has remained unchanged since 1969. The transverse curve resembles an arch, which originally had an 18-mm radius. We now have three sizes measuring 18, 22, and 24 mm. This change was necessary because under certain conditions, such as increased varus deformity, high loads can lead to excessive pressure on the material with an increased rate of wear of the polyethylene. Normally after 60 000 walking cycles, an overall contact zone forms (Fig. 4). This confirms the wear rate predicted for the St. Georg sledge of 0.15 mm–0.25 mm yearly. By enlarging the radius of the transverse arch of the runner, we calculate about a 20% decrease in wear.

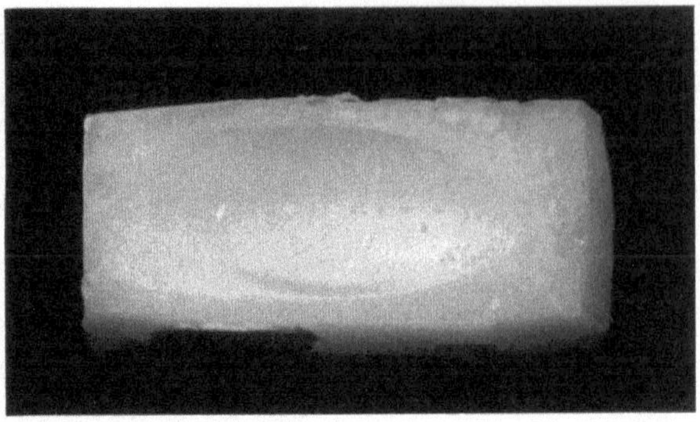

**Fig. 4.** Oval contact zone; wear after 12 years

## Indication

With the construction principle, stabilization is possible through the ligamentous and muscular apparatus alone. Thus, the indication for the system is limited to minor or moderate, mostly unicondylar joint destructions. The original quite generous indication allowing for the tolerance of residual malposition of up to 20° is considered false today [12]. In these cases, there is an increased risk of secondary ligamentous deficiencies, material damage, and mechanical loosening, especially of the tibial component. Malposition in the knee must be correctable without transposition of the ligaments. The maximal angle of correction is 10°–12°. This corresponds to an elevation of the joint surface of about 8–10 mm. Therefore, a varus correction may range from 6° to 8° and a valgus correction may approximate a maximum of 15° (Fig. 5). Additional measures, such as transposing the medial or lateral collateral ligaments in cases of more serious deformity, have proved unsatisfactory in our experience. This is due to poor connective tissue in elderly patients, rheumatoid arthritis, and post-traumatic changes.

The most frequent indication is osteoarthrosis followed by rheumatoid arthritis and post-traumatic disease. A special indication is the fresh predominantly lateral comminuted tibial head fracture, usually calling for simultaneous osteosynthetic measures (Fig. 6).

Rare indications are postinfective cases, dysplasia, and hemophilia.

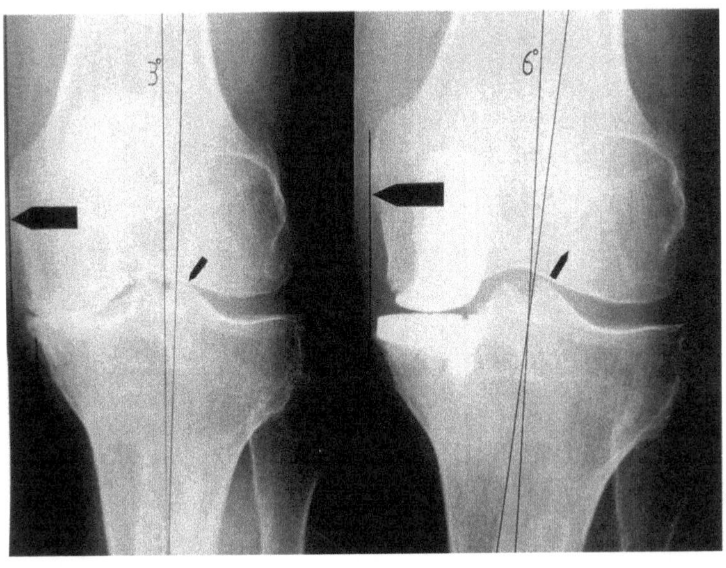


**Fig. 5.** Female, 73 years old with osteoarthrosis. Medial sledge (1986), correction of varus and medial subluxation

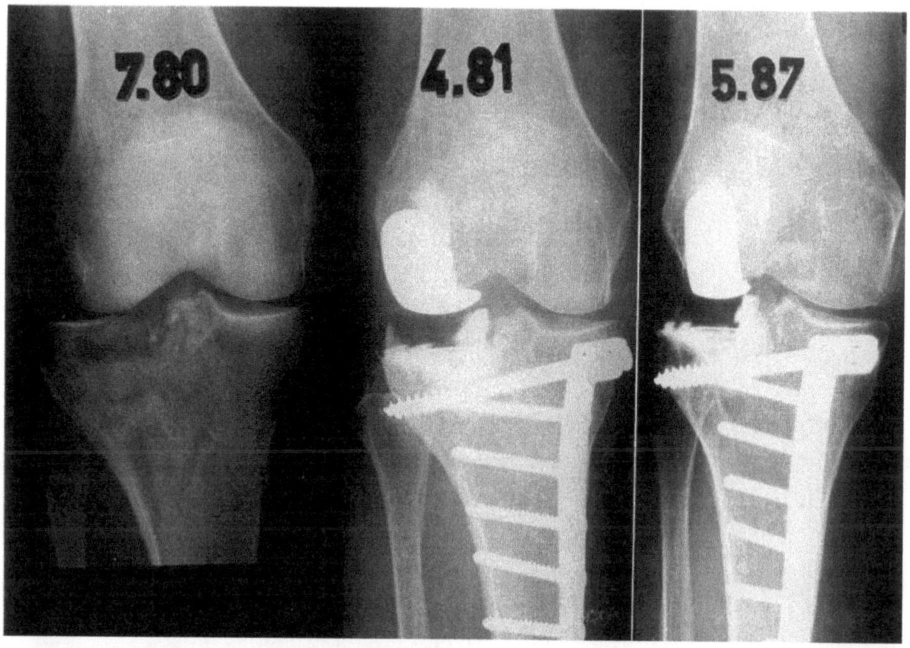


**Fig. 6.** Female, 65 years old. Fresh tibial comminuted fracture (1980), primary lateral sledge and AO technique. Patient had no pain in 1987—0°/0°/100°

## Development of Total Hinge Prosthesis Model St. Georg

The St. Georg total hinge prosthesis was designed for advanced arthritis and first implanted in 1970 [3]. Our early experience with the all-metal hinge was marked by high failure rates from metallosis and infection. Due to extensive resection of bone, only a thin layer of soft tissue remained to cover the hinged part of the prosthesis [1, 19, 35]. We found that the concept of low-friction arthroplasty should be included in our design. With the so-called intracondylar hinge prosthesis, optimal embedding of the implant was achieved, widely preserving the patellofemoral joint. The intracondylar and almost physiological location of the axis of rotation allowed for good joint flexion.

Surgical practice and the complications observed urged us to change the unfavorable design features of the first generation model. The prosthesis construction, especially the femoral component, was inadequate to meet the stresses from high axial load. We regarded deficiency in design and an absent valgus to be responsible for the higher rate of biomechanical complications. This led to the development of the second generation type in 1975. A 6° valgus was incorporated to reduce the varus moment arm. In order to minimize bone resection the width of the intracondylar part of the hinge was reduced to 34 mm for our standard model and to 28 mm for our mini-model. The transition to the patellofemoral articulation was wider adjusted to anatomy. The long stems of the prosthesis remained unchanged to ensure proper positioning on insertion and sound fixation. A polyethylene cap was attached to the tip of the prosthesis stem, easing centering of the stem within the medullary canal and at the same time preventing contact between the stem end and the inner cortex. A marked reduction of mechanical failures after long-term follow-ups and a diminution of residual patellofemoral joint pain have proved the effectiveness of these measures.

### Indication

Almost all, even the most severe damage in the knee, may be treated with the intercondylar total hinge prosthesis due to immediate joint stability and correction of deformities. Special prostheses are used for gross defects after tumor resection and repeated revision for failed total knee arthroplasty (Fig. 7).

The requisite for proper joint function is a competent resilient extensor apparatus. This is particularly true when an attempt is made to remobilize ankylosed or arthrodesed joints. Because of unfavorable clinical results, in particular with respect to postoperative joint function, the indication for

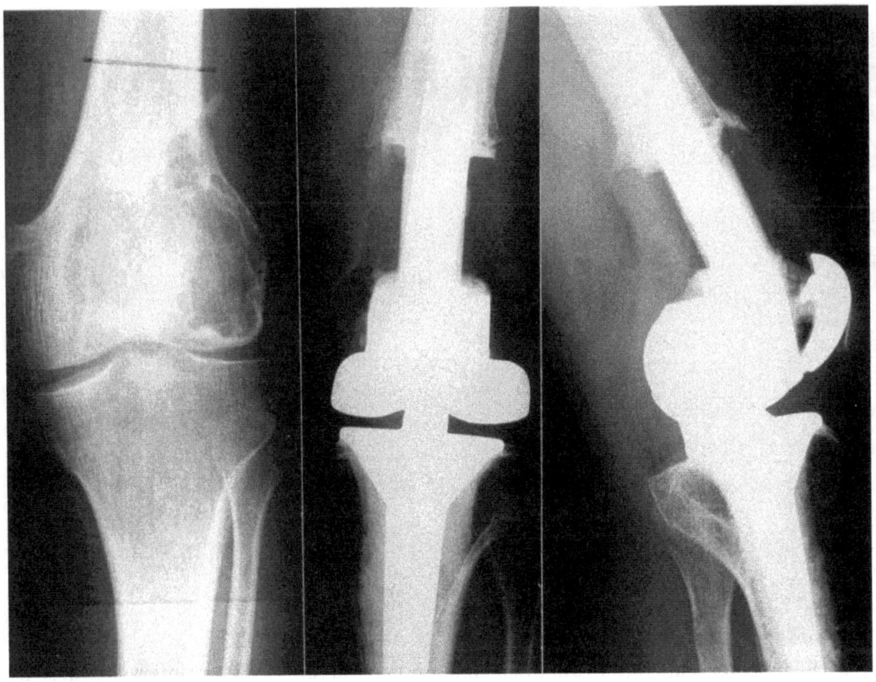

**Fig. 7.** Male, 36 years old with giant-cell tumor. Special long-stem hinge (1977). Patient was painfree in 1986—0°/0°/120°

remobilization must be stringent [12]. This should also be borne in mind when the indication is made for knee arthrodesis. A similar situation occurs when the coupling function of the ipsilateral hip is disturbed due to ankylosis or arthrodesis. In these cases there, is an increased risk for biomechanical complications, such as aseptic loosening and fracture of the femur, especially when osteoporosis is present. After more than 15 years of experience, we still think that total knee replacement for the younger patient is indicated only in special cases as in rheumatoid arthritis, hemophilia, and tumors.

**Patellofemoral Joint**

Replacement of the patellofemoral joint is not routinely provided in any of our systems. We aim at smooth coaptation of the femoral component to the individual anatomical conditions of the articulating surfaces of the condyles. Osteophytes on the patella are routinely removed and retropatellar incongruencies are smoothed out. After correction of a severe valgus, a lateral release may be required at the same time. The vastus medialis insertion is always preserved for muscular balance. Long-term results have shown that we should continue to follow our chosen concept.

Although more or less severe patellofemoral changes were seen in all cases, the medium-term results showed a 16%–25% rate for residual pain, depending on the type of the implant [17]. In about 80% of the cases retropatellar pain did not affect the clinical results. Residual pain was tolerated by the majority of patients and noted only when higher load was applied (stair climbing). In cases of severe residual pain, we either perform hemipatellectomy (10%) or, more frequently, a complete subperiosteal patellectomy, for example with elevation of the patellar tendon according to Kaufer [26] (Table 1).

A comparison of medium and long-term results has shown that the rate of residual pain requiring revision has not increased. Revisions were most frequently performed within the first 3 postoperative years; from then on, we have only seen very few cases even at 10 years and more after surgery. Significant differences in the frequency of revisions were recorded for each model (Table 1). In the rotating knee, the rate of secondary interventions was below 1% at 6 years and tolerable residual pain was below 10%. We think that these favorable results may be attributed to the improved design features preventing postoperative malposition between the femur and the tibia and the ensuing unfavorable ventralization of condyles, resulting in increased stresses in the patellofemoral joint. A prosthetic design adjusted to anatomy and skilled operative techniques will prevent nonphysiological ventralization, which was predominantly seen in our hinged knee (Table 2).

Other arguments against routine replacement of the patellofemoral joint are high compressive load, unknown shear forces, and unfavorable anatomical

**Table 1.** Patellofemoral joint revisions with different designs. Observation time for the sledge/hinge was 10 years, and that for the rotational knee up to 6 years

| Design | Hemi-patellectomy | Patellectomy | Percent |
|---|---|---|---|
| Hinge 1st generation ($n = 237$) | 1 | 12 | 5.0 |
| Hinge 2nd generation ($n = 917$) | 3 | 17 | 2.0 |
| Sledge ($n = 1293$) | 1 | 17 | 1.3 |
| Rotational knee ($n = 1074$) | 1 | 3 | 0.4 |

**Table 2.** The difference between the ventral margins of the condyles and the tibial tubercle

| Design | Measured values (mm) | | |
|---|---|---|---|
| | Average | Minimum | Maximum |
| Normal joint ($n = 40$) | +2 | −6 | +6 |
| Sledge St. Georg ($n = 147$) | +1.9 | −3 | +11 |
| Hinge St. Georg ($n = 155$) | +4.7 | −3 | +15 |
| Rotational knee ($n = 130$) | ±0 | −6 | +5 |

conditions for a secure fixation of the implant. In addition, degenerative bone changes may enhance the problem of proper fixation [28]. Mechanical loosening, fracture of the patella, and an increased wear of polyethylene represent higher risks. In the literature, we found failure rates of up to 5% with a short to medium-term follow-up for these complications [6, 7, 21, 23–25, 27, 29, 30, 34]. For the total hinge of the second generation and the sledge prosthesis, a 15% rate of tolerable patellofemoral pain was recorded and revision was required in 1%–2% of the cases after a postoperative interval of more than 10 years. Therefore, we do not regard routine replacement of the patellofemoral joint to be justified, especially as it is hoped that the incidence of patellofemoral pain will be minimized by our new rotating knee prosthesis, the ENDO model.

In future, these relatively low revision rates must be compared with the complication rates after patellar replacement.

## Clinical Results

Although pain is the main indication for arthroplasty, this phenomenon is highly subjective and can hardly be objectified. All other criteria of evaluation, such as function, stability, walking distance, and walking aids, are strongly based on a subjective assessment of surgeon and patient. Another uncertain factor is proper assessment of results. Clinical results are used to assess the effectiveness of a method but are less meaningful with respect to the durability of a prosthesis system. Therefore, when judging prosthesis systems, we must differentiate the clinical results from the durability of the implant [33]. Evidence of clinical results after knee prosthesis can be given as early as 1 year after operation. In a knee with proper joint function no significant changes must be expected from then on. Should deterioration become obvious years after the operation failure of the implant is very likely. These knees must be separated from the overall assessment and used for the estimation of the implant duration.

**Table 3.** Results from a questionnaire on long-term follow-up examination on knee pain in patients receiving different designs of implant

| Design | No pain (%) | Tolerable residual pain (%) | Severe pain (%) |
|---|---|---|---|
| Sledge ($n = 473$) | 76 | 20 | 4 |
| Hinge 1st generation ($n = 81$) | 66 | 30 | 4 |
| Hinge 2nd generation ($n = 446$) | 78 | 18 | 4 |
| Rotational knee ($n = 364$) | 74 | 23 | 3 |
| Total ($n = 1364$) | 75 | 21 | 4 |

### Pain

Table 3 shows the long-term results derived from the patient questionnaires. The efficacy of this type of information was proved on clinical control examinations because the information given by each patient was free from direct influence of the examiner. With our prosthesis systems, more than 95% of the patients achieved substantial relief from pain or were completely pain-free. Tolerable residual pain was most frequently due to patellofemoral pain, neuroma of the infrapatellar branches of the sap-

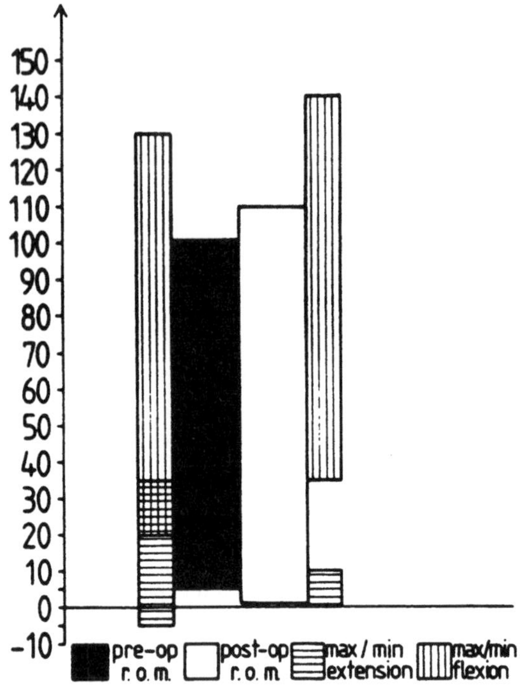


**Fig. 8.** Pre- and postoperative range of motion (*r.o.m.*) in tibial rotating knee ($n$ = 150), including all diagnoses. Follow-up time 1–4 years

**Table 4.** Patient opinion of results of different designs (long-term follow-up examination by questionnaire)

| Design | Content (%) | Discontent, deterioration (%) | No answer (%) |
|---|---|---|---|
| Sledge ($n$ = 473) | 92 | 5 | 3 |
| Hinge 1st generation ($n$ = 81) | 94 | 6 | — |
| Hinge 2nd generation ($n$ = 446) | 92 | 6 | 2 |
| Rotational knee ($n$ = 364) | 96 | 4 | — |
| Total ($n$ = 1364) | 93 | 5 | 2 |

henous nerve, and minor remaining or newly grown instability after surface replacements. In both systems, residual pain was due to mechanical loosening and severe instability was observed after sledge prosthesis.

## Malposition, Joint Stability

Today, we attribute minor (19%) and severe (5%) instability and mild (8%) and severe (8%) deformity to false indication and operative-technical errors in the early years of sledge prosthesis. Now, with a proper indication complete correction of deformity and instability should be demanded with the sledge prosthesis.

With a total hinge, immediate joint stability and correction of deformity are always achieved. False implantation may cause failure of axial rotation. Varus and valgus deformities are widely prevented by the use of long stems and alignment jigs at operation.

## Range of Motion

On average, the preoperative range of motion is regained. Improvements in joint function are related to the possibility of correcting flexion contractures. With the total hinge, the most severe flexion contractures may be successfully treated (Fig. 8) [12].

## Patient Opinion

Depending on the implant model, 92%–96% of patients were satisfied with their results. The opinion of the patient is an important parameter for the assessment of an operation. The results obtained from the questionnaire correspond essentially to the data on pain and show relatively accurately the rates of failure (Table 4).

## Complications

The complications of a system which are based on its principles of construction must be carefully analyzed with respect to implant duration. Only in this way can the need for modifications be noted, for example, change of indication, design, and operative techniques.

Because of the principles of construction, the type and frequency of complications of the sledge prosthesis differ from those of the total hinge prosthesis.

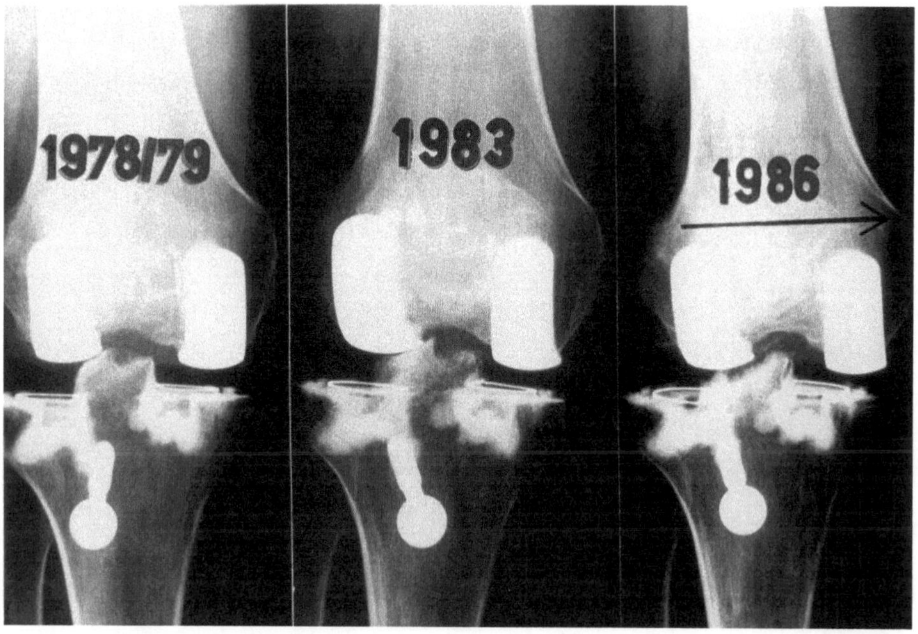


**Fig. 9.** Female, 41 years old with rheumatoid arthritis. Bicondylar sledge (1978). Increasing dislocation and instability (1983–1986). Conversion to a rotating knee was undertaken

### Aseptic Complications after Sledge Prosthesis

The analysis of complications has shown that a number of factors may be responsible for implant failure and retrospectively it may be difficult to trace the original cause of failure. Mechanical loosening, technical errors, false indication, or material defects are considered.

### Ligamentous Deficiency

The most frequent complication was deficiency of the ligamentous apparatus. Postoperative instability and secondary subluxation may occur without loosening the implant. In early presentations, this may be attributed to false indication for the operation, but presentation may be as late as 5 years and more after the operation and then require revision. The reason for this must be seen in newly developing ligamentous deficiency due to progression of rheumatoid arthritis, ageing, and overstress of ligaments due to insufficient damping properties of the implant material now available (Fig. 9).

### Mechanical Loosening

Predominantly, the tibial component became loose while the rate of loosening for the femoral component was significantly inferior. This experience was the cause for subsequent modifications of the component.

### Persistent Residual Pain

This group summarizes the various causes of pain which clinically and intra-operatively are not clearly differentiated in all cases. Hidden failures with respect to indication and technical errors must be considered, because in all cases the results were improved after exchange of the implant against a fully constrained hinge.

*Operative technical* failure will continue to occur in the future because of the complexity of the operative technique. Failure on insertion increases the risk of mechanical loosening and damage of the implanted material.

*Fracture of sledges* was rarely seen and can almost exclusively be attributed to technical failure at the time of operation. So, for example, in the late 1970s, a temporary poor implantation technique led to insufficient underlining with cement. After more than 4 years, we observed an increased fracture rate (Fig. 10).

In the sledge, no revision was required for increased wear of polyethylene. In all cases with increased wear and material flow, this was attributed to ligamentous deficiency, operative-technical errors or fracture of the runners.

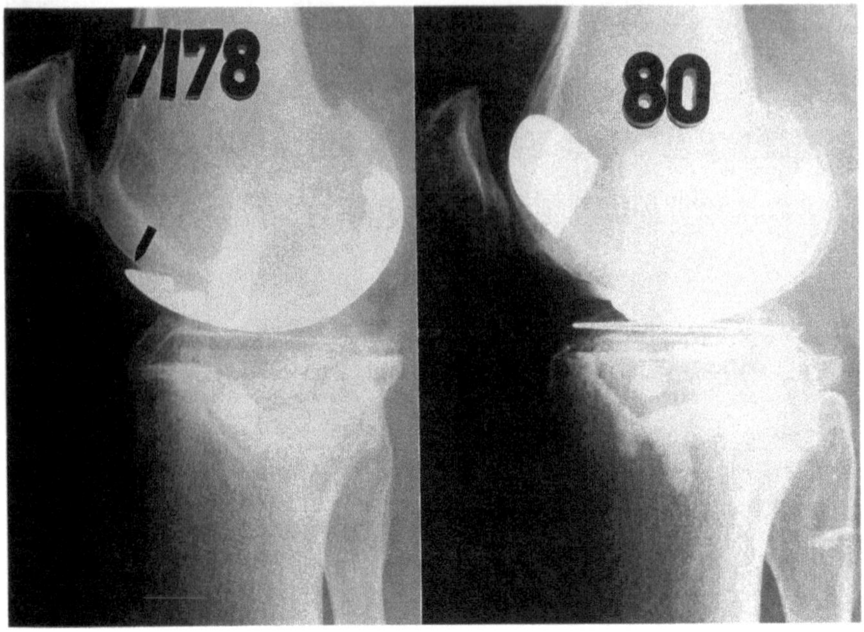


**Fig. 10.** Female, 56 years old with osteoarthrosis. Medial sledge (1978) poor cementing technique. Fracture of runner (1980)

Although Sudeck's disease was seen only in two cases, we think that dystrophic disorders should be considered when patients complain about indefinite residual pain.

### Contracondylar Arthrosis

A specific late complication following unicondylar replacement is the possible development of contracondylar arthrosis. This type of complication is more frequently seen in the rheumatoid patient. Therefore, in cases of unicondylar arthrosis with minor involvement of the contralateral side, we now prefer performing a primary bicondylar arthroplasty.

### Infection

In the long-term follow-up, the rate of infection after surface replacement was noticeably lower when compared with the failure of the hinge. As we expected, the highest rate observed was for rheumatoid arthritis (2.1%) followed by posttraumatic cases (1.8%). The overall infection rate was 0.7% (Table 5).

**Table 5.** Deep infection after knee arthroplasty

| Type of prosthesis | Number of cases | Infections | Percent |
|---|---|---|---|
| Sledge | 1287 | 0 | 0.7 |
| Idiopathic arthrosis | 879 | 0 | 0.0 |
| Rheumatoid arthritis | 239 | 5 | 2.1 |
| Posttraumatic arthrosis | 169 | 3 | 1.8 |
| Total hinge | 1122 | 33 | 2.9 |
| Idiopathic arthrosis | 712 | 16 | 2.2 |
| Rheumatoid arthritis | 347 | 12 | 3.5 |
| Posttraumatic arthrosis | 73 | 5 | 6.8 |

## Complications after Total Hinge Prosthesis

The durability of the total hinge is determined by mechanical loosening and fracture at the stem end. Material defects and operative technical errors were rarely seen (two fractures of the intracondylar part, seven cases of material flow of the impact bearing due to false implantation in hyperextension, and four displacements of the axis). In none of the three systems did patellar dislocation occur [29, 37]. Revisions due to wear of the polyethylene bearing have not yet been observed. This corresponds to the predicted annual wear rate of 0.12 mm on average measured by Strickle in 1974. Material flow of the impact bearing was only observed in four cases following technical failure from the blocking mechanism of the rotation axis.

### Mechanical Loosening

The significantly lower rate of mechanical loosenings seen in our second generation hinge may be attributed to the further development described

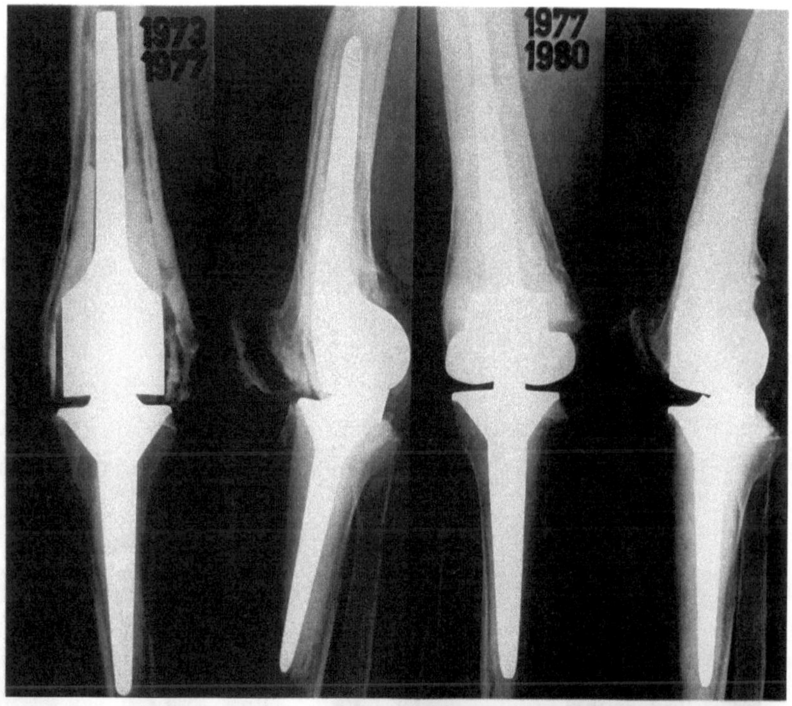


**Fig. 11.** Female, 68 years old with osteoarthrosis. Hinge first generation (1973). Conversion to hinge second generation (1977). Patient pain free in 1980; 0°/0°/95°

above. The mechanical loosenings still observed with this model were predominantly attributed to surgical technical errors, such as excessive reaming of the medullary cavity and poor cementing technique, and restricted hip function and osteoporosis (Fig. 11).

**Femur Fracture**

In cases of severe osteoporosis and restricted or absent rotation of the ipsilateral hip joint, there is increased risk of fracture of the femur at the stem end. This type of complication was also significantly lowered with our improved hinge of the second generation (Fig. 12).

**Infections**

The total rate of early and late deep infection was significantly higher at 2.9%. The high number of rheumatoid patients (31%) with an infection rate of 3.5% may be responsible for this. Noticeably high was the rate of posttraumatic arthrosis at 6.8% (Table 5).

**Treatment of Aseptic Complications**

The complications after sledge prosthesis are successfully treated by direct replacement of loose components or by the conversion to a total stabilizing

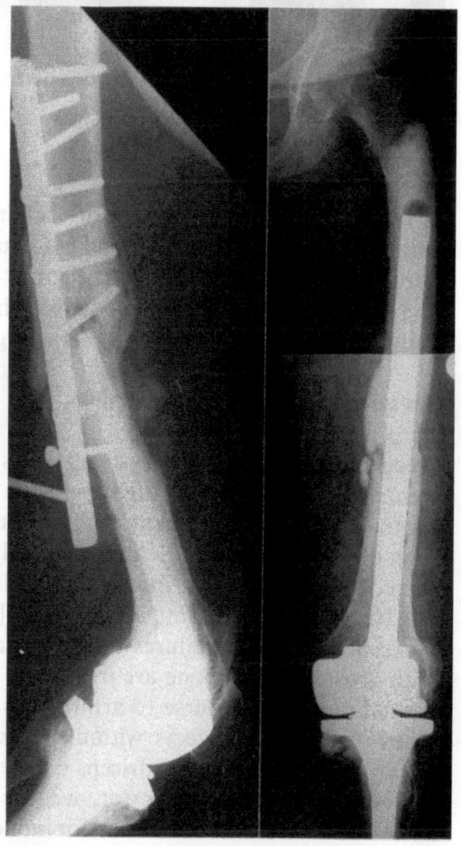

**Fig. 12.** Female, 66 years old with osteoarthrosis. Rotating knee (1985). Accident occurred with femur fracture, note osteosynthesis, and pseudarthrosis. Treated with long-stem femoral component (1986)

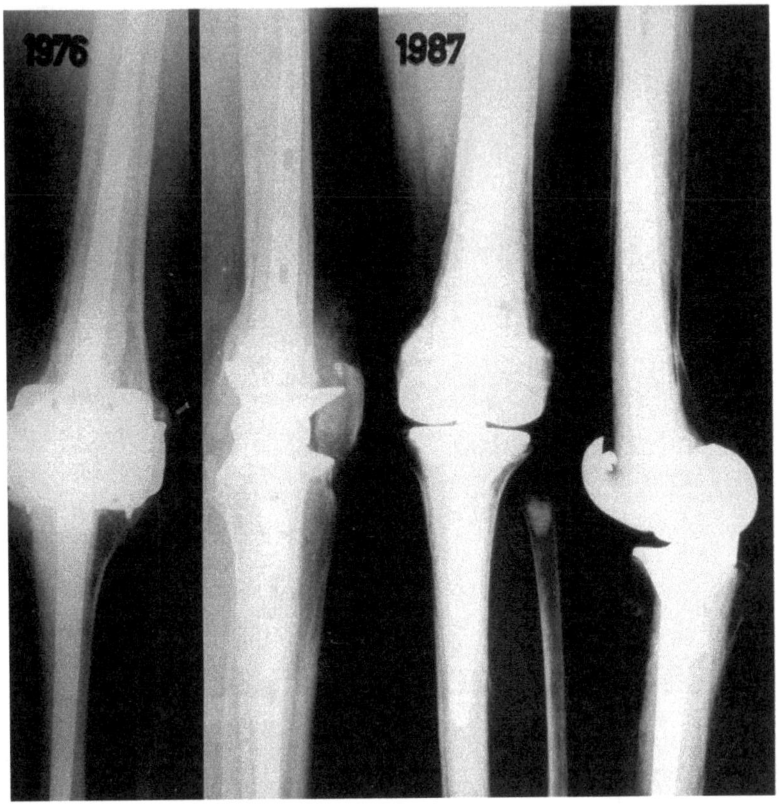


**Fig. 13.** Female, 69 years old with osteoarthrosis. Young knee (1969); late infection with *Klebsiella* (1976); one-stage exchange. No signs of infection or loosening. Patient was pain free in 1987 0°/0°/60

knee.

In the hinge, loose stems are exchanged for a model with long stems and broad plateaux for bony support (Fig. 11). Fractures of the femur at the stem end can be treated by plate osteosynthesis or by using a model with a very long stem (Fig. 12).

### Treatment of Septic Complications

Deep infections of both systems are successfully treated by a primary exchange operation using antibiotic-loaded acrylic cement. The success rate after first exchange at 68% is approximately that obtained in revisions for infected total hip arthroplasty, which is 77% (Fig. 13) [4, 16, 20].

Aseptic and septic failures after knee arthroplasty with gross losses of bone are treated by employing special models. Recourse to arthrodesis is made in cases of extensive defects within the extensor apparatus and/or severe quadriceps deficiencies.

Besides the external fixator, we use in special cases a so-called arthrodesis nail for immediate joint stability and avoidance of leg shortening. In the aseptic case, defects are closed with homografts, while in septic complications antibiotic-loaded acrylic cement is used [18].

### Further Development of Total Hinge

At present, there are no reliable criteria allowing proper assessment of the long-term behavior of ligaments in joint stability after surface replacement. This applies particularly to elderly and rheumatoid patients and frequently to patients with traumatic dysfunction, a group in which joint stability from muscle function is usually limited. However, in all surface replacements the long-term clinical success is directly dependent upon proper function of the ligaments and muscles. At present, it is noted that particularly within the Anglo-American orthopedic community there is an obvious trend to condylar knee prostheses [25, 38]. With this type of prosthesis, attempts are made to compensate for the lack of joint stability by a "built-in" restraint. The stabilizing effects provided by the resilience of the cartilage and menisci in a normal joint may not be compensated by any of the prostheses widely adjusted to anatomy and the unfavorable deformation of materials now available. All these prostheses cause constraints in the joint to a greater or lesser extent since they can scarcely be adapted individually to the ligamentous system. This puts higher stresses on the ligaments, the implanted material, and the fixation

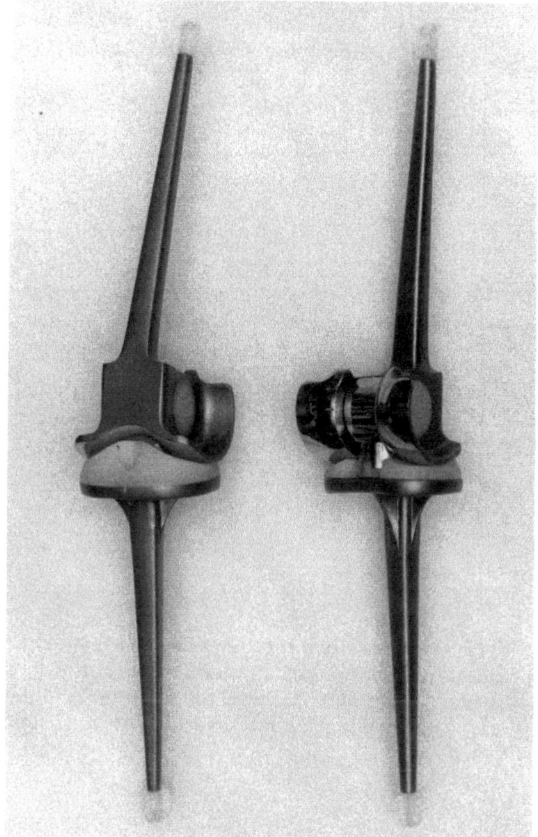

**Fig. 14.** Endo model—tibial rotating total intracondylar hinge

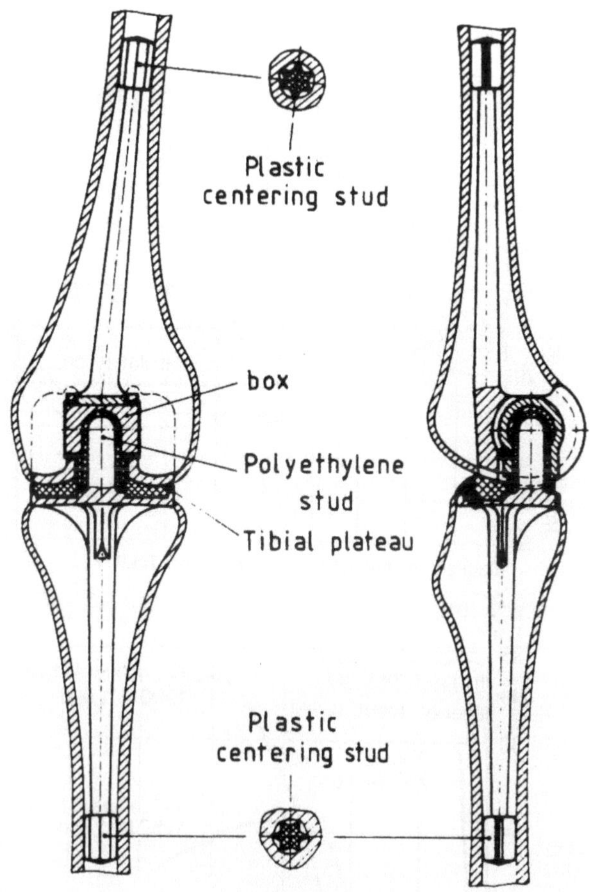


**Fig. 15.** Tibial rotating knee [17]

so that in the long run an increase in the failure rate is suspected due to material fatigue, material wear, mechanical loosenings, and residual and progressing ligamentous deficiencies [2, 5].

In all cases the ligamentous apparatus is more or less involved in the degenerative process and the severity of the damage can hardly be estimated preoperatively.

## Development of Intracondylar Rotating Knee Prosthesis ENDO Model

Where there is doubt that proper function of the ligaments can be maintained for a sufficiently long time, we believed that the stability of the joint must be guaranteed by the constructional principles. This was the main reason for our decision to develop the constrained hinge further.

The tibial rotating knee prosthesis is a hinge construction whose range of motion is almost physiological due to the incorporation of axial rotation. (Figs. 13–15).

Further improvements were made regarding the intracondylar location of the flexion axis and its relation to the long axes of the femur and tibia, which is essential to attenuate stresses in the patellofemoral joint. According to Nietert [32], the so-called compromise axis can be located at 64% of the sagittal diameter of the medial condyle. Using our own anatomical measurements, these relations were improved. The rotation possible at different knee angles is shown in Fig. 16. Mechanical tests were performed under shock loading to prove the damping properties of our rotating knee. In comparison with our total hinge system, the same torsional strain occurred in the rotating knee only, when 15 times the shock load was applied under otherwise equal conditions (Fig. 17).

In a stabilizing system with a fixed hinge and axial rotation, the contact surfaces between both components are determined by the construction. Thereby, the surface pressure allowed on the polyethylene and the frictional wear rate can be calculated (the

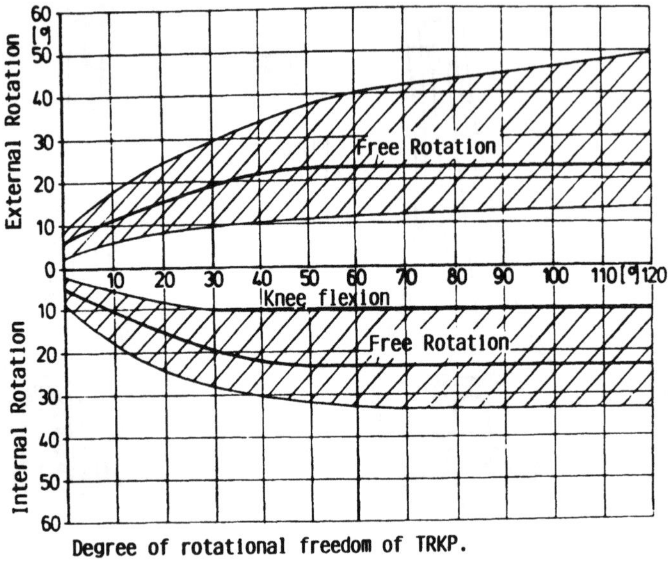


**Fig. 16.** Axial rotation of the tibial rotating knee at different angles of knee flexion [17]

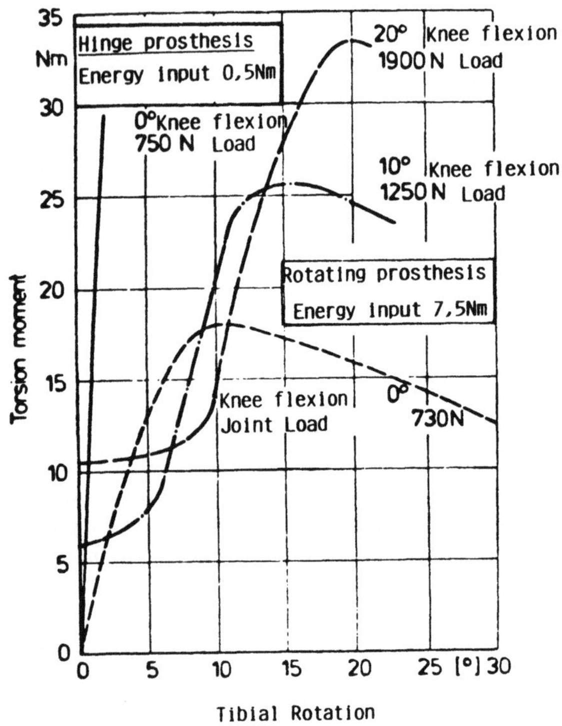


**Fig. 17.** Types of tibial rotation and corresponding torque at different angles of knee flexion for the hinge prosthesis (*continuous line*) and the rotating prosthesis (*broken lines*) while the joint is carrying the load stated [17]

median surface pressure is 5 $N/mm^2$, the wear rate for the tibial plateau 0.03–0.05 mm/year). Improvements in design resulted in a further reduction of bone and a simplified and standardized technique of insertion and removal. Corresponding saw guides for three prosthesis sizes help to ease individual adjustment to anatomy and the preservation and reconstruction of physiological joint axes [14, 15, 17, 32].

## Early Clinical Results

The clinical results correspond mainly with those of the other two systems. Since 1981, more than 1000 primary insertions have been performed. With increasing experience, the rotational knee has widely replaced the total hinge in cases where special prostheses are required (Tables 3, 4; Fig. 8) [11, 31].

### Complications

Up to now, we have seen four luxations. In all four cases, a too extensive resection of bone in the plane of the joint, a too generously performed capsulotomy, and individual ligament laxity and deficiency of the upper thigh muscles were responsible for the failures. Treatment was performed using a fully constrained hinge (Table 6).

### Mechanical Loosening

Mechanical loosening was observed in six cases and was mainly related to the femoral component. It occurred early, which means within the first 3 postoperative years. In all cases, the cause of failure was clearly seen in a false cementing technique.

### Infection

Early and late deep infection was the most frequent complication at 1.3% in the follow-up investigations.

**Table 6.** Complications with the rotational knee ENDO model from 1979 to 1986 ($n$ = 1075)

| Complication | Location | Number |
|---|---|---|
| Aseptic loosening | Femur | 5 |
| | Tibia | 1 |
| Bone fracture | Femur | 3 |
| | Tibia | — |
| Dislocation of comp. | | 4 |
| Material fracture | | 2 |
| Infection | | 14 (1.3%) |

## Discussion

Since 1970, we have had experience with two different knee systems—a surface replacement and a fully constrained hinge model St. Georg. With the surface replacement, the stabilizing joint structures, i.e., ligaments and muscles, are utilized for joint stability without a significant change in the joint kinematics. The fully constrained hinge was intended for severe damage and correction of deformities. Although we had very little experience at the beginning, the effectiveness of both systems soon became apparent. Pain was completely or substantially relieved in more than 95% of cases and deformities and instabilities could be corrected, preserving proper joint function. The operation series was started in 1970 and with the increase in surgical practice we became familiar with the indications for the two systems. The medium-term results justified our continued use of both systems, suggesting a lower failure rate in the late 1970s when compared with the results of total hip arthroplasty. This was demonstrated in our recent long-term follow-up investigation. The specific complications observed for both systems urged us to further stepwise developments.

The higher proportion of failures after sledge prosthesis due to ligamentous deficiency indicated that the percentage of cases requiring stabilization of the joint by prosthetic construction was higher than initially assumed. Nevertheless, we saw no reason to dispense with a system that changed physiological conditions so insignificantly. The consequence was a more stringent indication, which is predominantly restricted to unilateral arthrosis with mild deformity and moderate instability. Changes in design did not affect the original principle of point contact. Metal backing of the tibial plateau was the answer to the significantly higher rate of mechanical loosening. Further modifications led to simplified surgical techniques and improved stability of the model.

The essential system-specific biomechanical complications after hinge prosthesis were mechanical loosening and fracture of the femur. Although the total failure rate is acceptably low in long-term investigations, the severity of these complications must not be underestimated. Due to lack of objective criteria for the assessment of proper function of the capsular ligamentous structures, priority was given to further development of the stabilizing hinge system. Our aim was to reduce the risk of biomechanical complications by changes in the design features. By the incorporation of a second degree of freedom, we expected to obtain a closer adjustment to physiological joint function and a reduction of forces acting on the anchorage of the implant. Nonphysiological ventralization of the condyles frequently observed in the total hinge prosthesis was mainly attributed to false relation of the anatomical axes to each other. In the rotating knee, the location of the flexion axis and its relation to the long axes of the tibia and femur was approximated to anatomical conditions. It has been confirmed that the physiological conditions in the retained patellofemoral joint remained widely unchanged after implantation. Our observation of further reduction of residual patellar pain was attributed to the aforementioned design changes. Therefore, we do not regard replacement of the patellofemoral joint as a routine indication. In addition, the unfavorable loading conditions must be considered.

Further design improvements, the use of saw

guides, and three different model sizes have led to a more simplified surgical technique and a better adaptation of the implant to the individual situation.

After more than 5 years of clinical experience, the complication rate of 2.7% is relatively low and resulted mainly from operative technical failures.

The answer to the question regarding the durability of this type of prosthesis can only be given by biomechanical testing, i.e., long-term observations after more than 10 years of surveillance within the human body.

## References


1. Bagar WL, Cracchiolo A, Amstutz HG (1980) Results with constrained total knee prosthesis in treating severely disabled patients and patients with failed total knee replacement. J Bone Joint Surg 62-A: 504
2. Bartel DL, Bicknell VL, Wright TM (1986) The effect of conformity, thickness, and material on stresses in ultra-high molecular weight components for total joint replacement. J Bone Joint Surg 68-A: 1041
3. Buchholz HW, Engelbrecht E (1973) Die intracondyläre totale Kniege lenksendoprothese "Modell St. Georg". Chirurg 44: 373
4. Buchholz HW, Foerster von G, Heinert K (1984) Management of infected prostheses. Orthopedics 7: 1620
5. Buechel FF, Pappas MJ (1986) The New Jersey low-contact-stress knee replacement system: biomechanical rationale and review of the first 123 cemented cases. Arch Orthop Traumat Surg 105: 197
6. Cameron HU, Fedorkow DM (1982) The patella in total knee arthroplasty. Clin Orthop 165: 197
7. Clayton ML, Thirupathi R (1982) Patellar complications after total condylar arthroplasty. Clin Orthop 170: 152
8. Engelbrecht E (1971) Die Schlittenprothese, eine Teilprothese bei Zerstörung im Kniegelenk. Chirurg 42: 510
9. Engelbrecht E (1972) Die operativen Behandlungsmöglichkeiten bei der Kniegelenksarthrose. Hamburger Ärztebl 26: 346
10. Engelbrecht E, Buchholz HW, Siegel A (1974) Characteristics of the knee-joint prosthesis model "St. Georg" and clinical experiences. Conference on total knee replacement, London 16-18 September 1974. Institution of Mechanical Engineers, London, pp 68–73
11. Engelbrecht E, Engelbrecht H (1974) Totalersatz des Femurs unter Verwendung der Hüft- und Kniegelenkstotalendoprothesen Modell "St. Georg". Chirurg 45: 231
12. Engelbrecht E, Siegel A, Röttger J, Buchholz HW (1976) Statistics of total knee replacement: partial and total knee replacement, design St. Georg. A review of a 4-year observation. Clin Orthop 120: 54
13. Engelbrecht E (1981) Ersatz der groβen Körpergelenke (auβer Hüfte). Chirurg 52: 681
14. Engelbrecht E, Nieder E, Strickle E, Keller A (1981) Intracondyläre Kniegelenksendoprothese mit Rotationsmöglichkeit—Endo-Modell. Chirurg 52: 368
15. Engelbrecht E, Nieder E (1984) Tibial rotating knee prosthesis (TRKP)-"Endo" model: development and early clinical experience. First International Conference on Engineering and Clinical Aspects of Endoprosthetic Fixation. London, 13–15 June 1984. Institution of Mechanical Engineers London, p 23
16. Engelbrecht E (1984) Treatment of infected implants by direct exchange operation. Sixty-second Central Japan Congress of Orthopaedic and Traumatic Surgery 27–28 April 1984, Osaka. Cent Jap J Orthop Traumat 27: 1288–1304
17. Engelbrecht E (1984) Die Rotationsendoprothese des Kniegelenks. Springer, Berlin-Heidelberg-New York-Tokyo
18. Engelbrecht E, Heinert K, Keller A (1985) Interpositionsnagel bei diaphysären Knochendefekten und Arthrodesenagel bei gescheitertem Kniegelenksersatz. Chirurg 56: 712
19. Evans EM, Freeman MAR, Miller AJ, Vernon-Roberts B (1974) Metal sensitivity as a cause of bone necrosis and loosening of the prosthesis in total joint replacement. J Bone Joint Surg 56-B: 626
20. Foerster von G, Wessendorf C (1987) Behandlung und mittelfristige Ergebnisse von infizierten Kniegelenksendoprothesen. In: Buchholz HW (ed) Primär- und Revisionsalloarthroplastik. Springer, Berlin-Heidelberg-New York
21. Freeman MAR, Hammer A (1978) Patellar fracture after replacement of the tibio-femoral joint with the ICLH prosthesis. Arch Orthop Traumat Surg 92: 63
22. Gunston FH (1971) Polycentric knee arthroplasty. J Bone Joint Surg 53-B: 272
23. Hassenpflug J, Holland C, Heupel R, Koebke J (1984) Patellaveränderungen bei Langzeitbeobachtungen der Kniegelenksendoprothese nach Blauth. Z Orthop 122: 185
24. Insall JN, Tria AJ, Aglietti P (1980) Resurfacing of the patella. J Bone Joint Surg 62-A: 933
25. Insall JN, Hood RW, Flawn LB, Sullivan DJ (1983) The total condylar knee prosthesis in gonarthrosis. J Bone Joint Surg 65-A: 619
26. Kaufer H (1971) Mechanical function of the patella. J Bone Joint Surg 53-A: 1551
27. Leval JP, McLeod HC, Freeman MAR (1983) Why not resurface the patella? J Bone Joint Surg 65-B: 448
28. Matthews LS, Sonstegard DA, Henke JA (1977) Loadbearing characteristics of the patello-femoral joint. Acta Orthopaed Scand Supp 48: 511
29. Merkow RL, Soudry M, Insall JN (1985) Patellar dislocation following total knee replacement. J Bone Joint Surg 67-A: 1321
30. Mochizuki RM, Schurman DJ (1979) Patellar complications following total knee arthroplasty. J Bone Joint Surg 61-A: 879
31. Nieder E, Engelbrecht E, Steinbrink K, Keller A (1983) Modulares System für den Femurtotalersatz-Endo-Modell. Entwicklung, Modellbeschreibung, operatives Vorgehen. Chirurg 54: 91

32. Nietert M (1975) Untersuchungen zur Kinematik des menschlichen Kniegelenkes im Hinblick auf ihre Approximation in der Endoprothetik. Dissertation, Berlin University
33. Röttger J, Heinert K (1984) Die Knieendoprothesensysteme St. Georg (Schlitten- und Scharnierprinzip). Beobachtungen und Ergebnisse nach 10 Jahren Erfahrung mit über 3700 Operationen. Z Orthop 122: 818
34. Roffmann M, Hirsh DM, Mendes DG (1980) Fracture of the resurfaced patella in total knee replacement. Clin Orthop 148: 112
35. Roles NC (1971) The complications of total prosthetic replacement of the hip and knee joint. Spring meeting, British Orthop Assoc, Belfast 1–3 April 1971
36. Shiers LGP (1960) Arthroplasty of the knee. J Bone Joint Surg 42-B: 31
37. Sneppen O, Fredensborg N, Karle A, Klaumann U (1978) Lateral dislocation of the patella following Marmor and Guepar arthroplasty of the knee. Acta Orthop Scand Suppl 49: 291
38. Walker PS, Wang CHJ, Masse Y (1974) Joint laxity as a criterion for the design of condylar knee prostheses. Conference on total knee replacement, London 16–18 September 1974. Institution of Mechanical Engineers, London, pp 22–29
39. Walker PS, Ranawat CH, Insall JN (1976) Fixation of the tibial components of condylar replacement knee prostheses. J Biomech 9: 269
40. Walker PS, Greene D, Reilly D, Thatcher J, Ben-Dov M, Ewald FC (1981) Fixation of tibial components of knee prostheses. J Bone Joint Surg 63-A: 258
41. Walldius B (1960) Arthroplasty of the knee using an endoprosthesis. 8 years' experience. Acta Orthop Scand Suppl 30: 137
42. Young HH (1971) Reconstruction of knee joint with Young-type hinged vitallium prosthesis. Reconstr Surg Traum 12: 176

## *Discussion*

*Tateishi* (Hyogo Medical College): I think that the body weight is a crucial factor in the success of an arthroplasty. I take a maximum body weight of 60–65 kg in the indication for unicompartmental arthroplasty. Do you have any such limitations for unicompartmental arthroplasty?

*Engelbrecht* (Endo-Klinik): No we have no such limitations. I think that the patient's ability to move is a much more important factor than the body weight.

*Walker* (Harvard Medical School): On the upper tibia, you have what looks like a plastic bearing surface. What is the purpose of that? It does not seem to articulate except in extension and the extremes of internal-external rotation.

*Engelbrecht*: In extension, this system is stable in weight bearing. We separate free axial rotation from restricted axial rotation. The system is not a constrained one, the two components can be combined. When there is more than 20° of axial rotation, the system separates like a screw.

*Walker*: Is the main bearing carried on the axle still?

*Engelbrecht*: No, the main bearing is on the tibial plateau.

*Walker*: So, instead of bearing on the axle, you bear on the plastic surface, and the axle is just there to hold it all together?

*Engelbrecht*: Yes.

*Walker*: Do you not wish to add a patellofemoral joint?

*Engelbrecht*: I showed one design with a patellar shield; we only use this in special cases—mainly revision cases where we have to change from a design where the patella was primarily replaced. We perform a very low rate of primary replacement of the patellofemoral joint.

*Walker*: With all the attention that has been paid over the last 10 or 15 years to prostheses without patellofemoral replacement, it seems hard to believe that today you can come up with a design which routinely does not use patellofemoral replacement and claim that it is an up-to-date design. I thought that all surgeons over the past 10 years have demonstrated that a prosthesis without a patellofemoral replacement, especially in severe cases, suffers from a high percentage of intolerable pain and loss of function. I cannot see the justification in not having a patellar flange.

*Engelbrecht*: Not all our patients have pain. In recent years, we have been confronted with an increasing number of complications of replacement of the patellofemoral joint. Some of these complications are severe, for example, fracture and loosening with loss of bone stock in the patella. We believe in performing secondary revision when there is residual severe pain.

# The Patella in Total Knee Replacement: A Problem or Not?

I. Goldie, L.-Å. Broström, A. Josefsson, and V. Söderlund[1]

**Summary.** A two-part Imperial College, London Hospital (ICLH) prosthesis with a high anterior flange was used to replace the knee joint in 42 patients between 1978 and 1982. In 1985, 36 patients, 22 of whom had rheumatoid arthritis and 14 osteoarthrosis, were reexamined clinically and radiographically with a special interest focused on the stability and function of the patella.

Three patients were reoperated with an arthrodesis because of deep infections postoperatively. With a mean follow-up of 4 years, the results of the remaining 33 patients, eight of whom were operated bilaterally, were assessed by using the British Orthopaedic Association (BOA) knee function chart. Radiological examination included measurement of alignment of the knee (hip, knee, angle), the patella, and the prosthesis.

Patelloplasty was performed in 19 knees and lateral release in 14. Seven patients were enthusiastic, 24 satisfied, nine non-committal, and one disappointed with the result. A general improvement in pain, range of motion, and walking ability was observed in all except one patient, who had persistent pain and instability. The mean BOA score was 44 points. Pain remained in ten knee joints, all of which were unstable and with subluxation of the patella. There was instability in 14 knees, 12 of which were in patients with rheumatoid arthritis. Clinical subluxation was observed in 30 knees and radiographically in 35.

Except instability, there was no major difference between patients with rheumatoid arthritis and osteoarthrosis. Resection of the patella did not influence the result but there was an increased risk of patellar subluxation when the prosthesis was positioned in valgus.

A lateral release seemed to prevent patellar dislocation and is considered to be of great importance for the outcome; it is advocated in total knee replacement with an ICLH prosthesis.

**Keywords:** Patella—Total knee replacement—Clinical trial—Subluxation—Patelloplasty

## Introduction

Although the main indication for knee arthroplasty is severe pain, improvement of knee function, to which the patellofemoral joint contributes significantly, is important. In recent reports, very good results have been reported after total knee replacement but mostly results are given as scores, sometimes supplemented with a satisfactory registration of range of motion, muscular strength, and walking ability. Seldom, however is there a satisfactory and detailed description of the patella (retropatellar pain, position, and mediolateral dislocation during flexion) and not until postoperative problems can be assigned to the patella does this become a focus of interest [4, 8].

In discussing replacement surgery of the knee joint, the patellofemoral joint attains keynote value and should be included [2, 3, 6, 8, 10, 11]. The patella is entrapped in a funnel-like tendinous extension of the quadriceps muscles and malalignment may occur in aberrations of this extensor mechanism acquired by surgical procedures.

The dynamics of the patella must be kept in mind in total knee replacement with special attention paid to surgical technique, prosthetic design, and implantation of the components to attain proper alignment with optimal force vectors over the knee joint to achieve a good knee function [9].

Surgical treatment of the bone itself has varied over the years. Prior to replacement of the patella with a cemented or noncemented button, which is advocated nowadays [4], a patellaplasty (resection of posterior surface of the patella) or no surgical intervention at all was performed.

To study the problems related to the patella after total knee replacement, we collected patients who had been operated on between 1978 and 1982 with a two-part ICLH prosthesis with a high anterior flange for clinical and radiological reexamination.

## Patients

Between 1978 and 1982, 42 patients received a two-part ICLH prosthesis at Karolinska hospital, Stockholm. Fourteen patients had osteoarthrosis and 28 had rheumatoid arthritis. A reexamination was performed in 1985. Six patients had died, none

[1] Departments of Orthopedic Surgery and Radiology, Karolinska Hospital, Stockholm, Sweden

of whom was registered in the records as having had knee prosthetic complications. Of the remaining 36 patients, three had had a deep infection with the prosthesis extracted and an arthrodesis performed, thus leaving 33 patients for reexamination. Eight patients were operated bilaterally, giving 41 knee joints to be examined. The mean age was 68 years and 25 patients were females. The mean follow-up was 4 years, with a minimum of 2.5 years.

## Surgical Treatment

In all patients, parapatellar skin and a retinacular incision were used. A lateral retinacular release was done in 14 patients, and resection of the patella, e.g., patellaplasty, in 19 patients. In 15 patients, no lateral release or patellar resection was performed. In no patient was a patellar prosthesis used. The tibial and femoral components were both fixed with CMW cement (CMW laboratories Ltd. Blackpool) in a two-step procedure. Drainage was applied for 2 days. Weight bearing was allowed on the 1st postoperative day as well as flexion and extension exercises.

## Methods

Clinical results were assessed by using the BOA knee function chart with a maximum of 55 points [1]. Radiological examination included determination of the position and fixation of the prosthetic components from lateral and frontal films. Development of a radiolucent zone of 2 mm was regarded as an indication of prosthetic loosening. Varus or valgus position of the prosthesis was calculated and tabulated using a 5° interval scale. With the prosthesis in a position of less than 2.5° of either varus or valgus, the alignment was accepted as straight.

Long X-ray films of the whole leg (hip, knee, and ankle joints included) under full weight bearing were used for determination of the mechanical axis and the HKA angle.

Axial projections of the patella at 30°, 60°, and 90° of flexion were used for determination of the position and measurement of any mediolateral subluxation. Dislocation of the patella was measured in millimeters and expressed as a percentage of the width of the patella and divided into four groups: none, less than one-third, one-third to two-thirds, and more than two-thirds of the patellar width. Complete radiographic examination was performed in 37 knee joints.

## Results

### Pain

Preoperatively, all patients had moderate or severe pain. Pain was the main indication for surgery. At reexamination, 23 patients were free of pain, nine had slight pain, and one patient had moderate pain and this patient was disappointed with the result.

### Range Of Motion

At follow-up, the mean range of motion was 95°. In 14 knees the maximun flexion exceeded 100°. Preoperatively all patients had an extension defect. This was corrected in 27 knees and improved in 14 knees, 11 of which had a defect of less than 5°. In two knees, there were still postoperative extension defects of 5° and 10° respectively.

The valgus angle when the tibia was stressed laterally was less than 10° in all knees. The varus angle when the tibia was stressed medially was almost zero for 29 knees and less than 10° for ten knees. In two knee joints, there was a varus instability.

### Walking Ability

Preoperatively, no patient could walk a distance of 1 km. At reexamination, 14 patients could walk 1 km or more and nine of these patients had rheumatoid arthritis but not in an advanced stage. Three patients could only walk indoors. There was an overall improvement of walking ability in all patients but only four patients walked with a free swing. Three patients walked with minmal movement of the knee and the others with a slight limitation of the swing.

Three patients walked without any walking aids, 27 patients used sticks outside, and three patients were in permanent need of walking aids. Preoperatively, all patients used the bannister if they could climb stairs at all. At follow-up, 16 patients were still not able to climb stairs even with the help of a bannister. Twelve patients walked one step at a time and only one patient could climb stairs in a normal way. In general, the walking ability was less good in the rheumatoid patients.

### Patient Opinion

Seven patients were enthusiastic about the results of operation, 24 were satisfied, and nine patients were non committal. One patient was disappointed with the outcome mainly because of instability problems and pain. Reoperation with a lateral release did

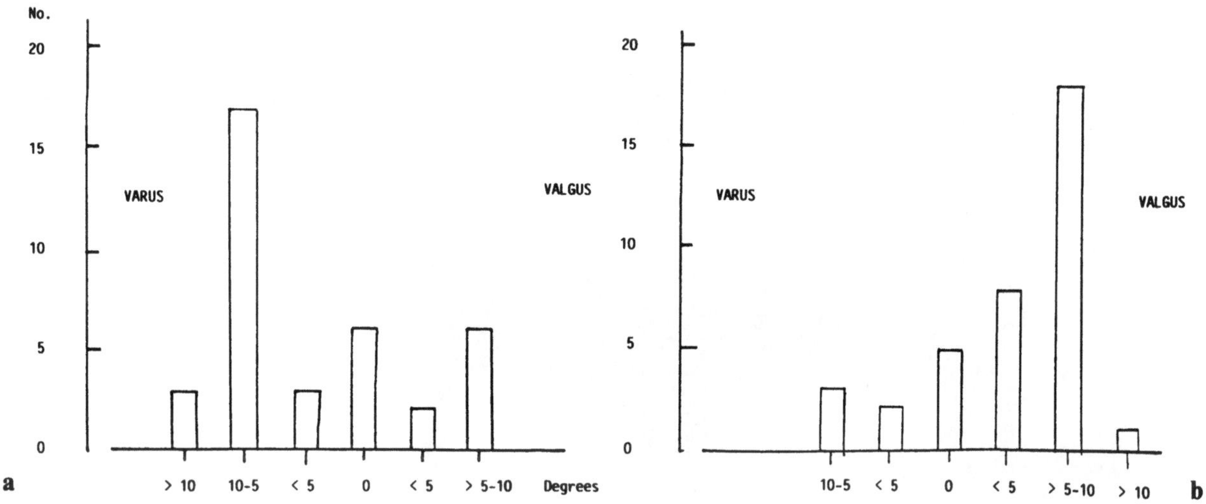


**Fig. 1.** **a** Histogram of numbers of patients with indicated measured values of HKA angle. **b** Histogram of numbers of patients with indicated measured varus/valgus angle

not significantly alter this patient's symptoms and opinion of the result.

**BOA Scoring**

The mean BOA score was 44 points (range 17–50 points).

**Radiographic Examination**

Prosthetic loosening was not registered in any knee nor was there any difference in positioning of the components registered on weight bearing films in comparasion to non-weight-bearing films for 36 knee joints of the 37 examined knees. In one knee joint, instability was evident both clinically and radiographically. The femur component was straight in 15 knees, in a varus position in three knees, and in valgus in 19 knees (Fig. 1).

**Patellar subluxation.** Radiographic subluxation of the patella was observed in 35 of 37 knee joints during flexion. In 13 joints, subluxation was more than two-thirds of the width of the patella (Table 1). In all 35 knee joints with subluxation of the patella, there was a marked deformation of the patella—wear with an angulation over the corner of the femur component (Fig. 2). There was a strong correlation between the degree of subluxation and amount of deformation. Patellar resection was performed in 16 and lateral release in only 12 of these 35 knee joints. The prostheses was positioned in valgus in eight knees wheras a HKA angle of at least 5° was seen in 19 knees. This overrepresentation of patellar subluxation in knees where lateral release had not been performed and the femur component positioned in valgus was even more evident (7 of 12 knees) when subluxation of the patella exceeded two-thirds of its width.

**Table 1.** Dislocation of the patella during flexion measured in relation to the width of the patella and expressed as thirds of the width

| Amount of dislocation | Number of knees |
|---|---|
| None | 2 |
| <1/3 | 9 |
| 1/3–2/3 | 13 |
| >2/3 | 13 |
| Total | 37 |

**HKA angle** After surgery, only 11 knees were considered straight with an HKA angle of less than 2.5° in either varus or valgus. Twenty knees had a varus angle and six knees a valgus angle (Fig. 1).

**Patellar Symptoms**

Clinical examination revealed subluxation of the patella during flexion in 30 patients, ten of whom had pain and 14 instability problems; in 23 of these 30 knees, a lateral release had not been performed. Of the ten patients with patellar pain, seven also had a feeling of instability, but only five had had a resection of the patella and in only four was a lateral release performed. All ten had radiologically a sub-

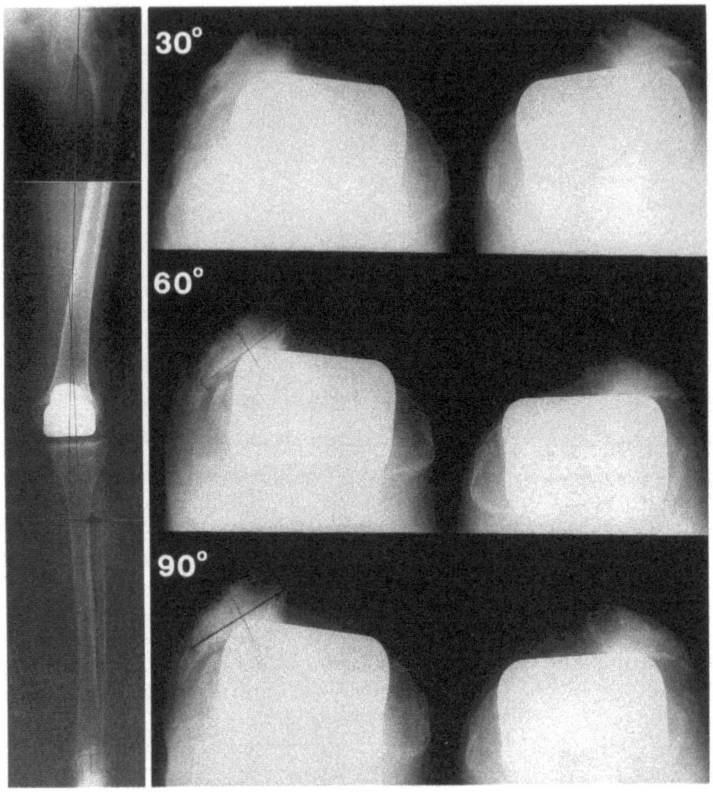


a b

**Fig. 2 a, b.** Radiographs of the knee joint in a patient operated bilaterally with ICLH prosthesis. **a** Demonstration of the knee alignment—the HKA angle. **b** Demonstration of subluxation and wear of the patella at 30°, 60°, and 90° of flexion

luxation of the patella during flexion and in six knees the prosthesis was positioned in more than 5° of valgus. Two patients had an HKA angle exceeding 5° of valgus.

Instability was noted for 14 knees, 12 of these in patients with rheumatoid arthritis. Except for instability, no major difference was observed between patients with rheumatoid arthritis and osteoarthrosis.

## Reoperation

Three reoperations were performed. In all, the indication was pain and patellar instability. Lateral release in two patients gave improvement of function, but patellectomy in one patient only gave this to a limited extent.

## Discussion

This reexamination of patients operated with a two-component cemented ICLH knee prosthesis demonstrated on the whole good results for the majority of the patients: 31 of 41 patients were satisfied or enthusiastic with the outcome and the BOA score attained a mean of 44 points. In our series of patients, there was a general improvement in respect of pain, range of motion, and walking ability in all except one patient who after surgery still had pain and instability problems.

In comparison with other reports on the ICLH prosthesis, many of our patients gained an improved range of motion, with a maximum flexion exceeding 100° in 14 patients.

The results must be evaluated with caution because of the short follow-up period (mean 4 years, minimum 2.5 years), but within the scope of the study may be considered satisfactory. During this period, there were no signs of prosthetic loosening.

The main purpose was to examine knee function after replacement surgery, with special interest focused on the patello-femoral joint, in particular the alignment (mechanical, prosthetic, patellar), the surgical technique, and the implantation of the prosthetic components. A very high incidence of radiographic and clinical lateral dislocation as well as wear and deformation of the patella was observed, but the knee function was not significantly impaired. The wear or grooving of the patella as it passes over the lateral corner of the prosthesis might give a stabilizing effect, as has been proposed by one of the innovators [5] of the prosthesis and may explain why only one-third of the patients experienced instability.

The acquisition of satisfactory results in any type

of replacement surgery of the knee is absolutely dependent on the surgeon's understanding of the technique, the principles upon which a procedure is based, the significance of design, and correct use of the instruments fabricated to facilitate implantation. Lack of this understanding in knee replacement can lead to the insertion of a prosthesis in such a way as to leave the tibio femoral or patello femoral joints misaligned, unstable, and probably in a few years providing an unacceptable function. The manual dexterity required is not exceptional, but it is necessary for the surgeon to be experienced.

Correct alignment is the proper position or state of adjustment of parts in relation to each other. As for the knee joint, it has been suggested that specification of alignment, in particular of the tibio femoral joint, lies in the field of morbid anatomy and surgical technique and not prosthetic design. The opposite opinion exists, however, and most newly designed knee prostheses have a groove in the femoral component for patellar tracking. Interest and practical performance have been focused on the mechanical alignment, implying a restoration of any deformity by special instrumentation to an axis from the center of the femoral head through the center of the knee joint to the center of the ankle joint, the HKA angle. This alignment is static. It certainly has some importance. It cannot, however, be applied to the patellofemoral joint without special prerequisites since the extensor apparatus of the knee makes patellar alignment more dynamic than static. The dynamics of the patella must be kept in mind in total knee replacement since patellar malalignment may occur in aberrations of the extensor mechanism acquired by surgical procedures. The sulcus angle, congruence, and Q angle may become compromised, which will facilitate postoperative patellar dysfunction.

Prior to replacement surgery, a tendency for abnormal patellar function may be present. This information is of utmost importance and should be given due consideration in the preoperative planning of the replacement procedure. A common approach to the knee joint is by a medial parapatellar incision and the injury thus caused to the medial supporting structures may, despite meticulous suturing, provoke a laxity permitting lateral dislocation of the patella. A lateral dislocation of the patella may give a lateral subluxation and external rotation of the tibia, which could with time increase the risk for prosthetic loosening. Post-operative patellar abnormalities, whether the patella is resurfaced with a button or a so-called patelloplasty is performed, like subluxation, dislocation or pain are most often the result of inadequate soft-tissue balance or rotational malalignment of prosthetic components.

Based on the experience of 116 knee prostheses, Figgie and co-workers [7] proposed the following surgical variables of importance to the functional results of knee replacement: joint line of the construction being as normal as possible, prosthetic fitting to the antero-posterior dimension of the natural femur as near normal as possible, positioning of the tibial component posterior to the center line of the tibial condylar plateau, but still covering it and maintaining the patellar height of 10–30 mm. This of course demands meticulous pre-operative planning, which was carried out in a series of 41 knees and in none of these was there any post-operative patellar dysfunction.

Consequently, preoperative planning is essential, in particular estimating the length of the patellar tendon and thus the position of the inferior pole of the patella in relation to the reconstructed articulating prosthetic surface of the tibia.

Defects of prosthetic replacement of the knee have been encountered throughout the period of implant development. This also applies to the technique of insertion. Appropriate modifications have been introduced but progress to a full solution has been slow and is still being awaited. The surgical technique of realignment by soft tissue procedures and balancing the collateral ligaments is generally agreed upon [1].

Nowadays, resurfacing of the patella with a button is advocated but the evidence for the benefit is still not convincing. In patients operated bilaterally with knee prostheses—a patelloplasty performed on one side and a resurfacing on the other—there was no difference in the results [2].

In our own series, we encountered problems like patellar dislocation, wear, and patellar malalignment in a high percentage of cases. Instability was, however, only stated for 14 of 41 knees, 12 of which occurred in patients with rheumatoid arthritis. There was no correlation between dislocation and a moderate valgus angle of the prosthesis, nor did performance of the patelloplasty correlate with valgus angle. There was, on the other hand, an overrepresentation of patellar subluxation among the knee joints in which the HKA angle exceeded 5° of valgus, a finding rationally explained by an increased lateral force vector. Lateral release prevented the patellar dislocation and also contributed to an improved knee function in two of the three re-operations performed. Performance of a lateral release is thus considered of importance for the outcome and is advocated in ICLH total knee replacement surgery.

## References

1. Aichroth P, Freeman M, Smillie I, Souter W (1978) A knee function assessment chart. J Bone Joint Surg 60-B: 308–309
2. Cameron H, Fedorkow D (1982) The patella in total knee arthroplasty. Clin Orthop 165: 197–199
3. Clayton M, Thirupathi R (1982) Patellar complications after total condylar arthroplasty. Clin Orthop 170: 152–155
4. Controversy on total knee arthroplasty (1985) Multian thor symposium. Clin Orthop 192 [section 1]: 2–112
5. Freeman M, Samuelson K, Bertin K (1985) Freeman-Samuelson total arthroplasty of the knee. Clin Orthop 192: 46–58
6. Freeman M, Levak B (1986) British contribution to knee arthroplasty. Clin Orthop 210: 69–79
7. Figgie H E, 3rd Goldberg VM, Heiple KG, Moller HS 3rd, Gordon NH (1986). The influence of tibial-patellofemoral location on function of the knee in patients with a posterior stabilized condylar knee prosthesis. J Bone Joint Surg 68-A: 1035–1040
8. Goldberg V, Henderson B (1980) The Freeman-Swanson ICLH total knee arthroplasty. J Bone Joint Surg 62-A: 1338–1344
9. Kettelkamp D (1981) The management of patellar malalignment. J Bone Joint Surg 63-A: 1344–1348
10. Mochizuki R, Schurman D (1979) Patellar complications following total knee arthroplasty. J Bone Joint Surg 61-A: 879–883
11. Ritter M, Campbell E (1987) Postoperative patellar complications with or without lateral release during total knee arthroplasty. Clin Orthop 219: 163–168

# Panel Discussion

*Miller* (Montreal General Hospital): Dr. Engelbrecht, how would you deal with knees with 20° of fixed varus deformity in terms of realignment with your linked prosthesis?

*Engelbrecht* (Endo-Klinik): We perform the operation by releasing the lateral ligaments tangentially from the point of origin of the condyles. We do not resect them. When we have a severe flexion contracture, we perform posterior release of the capsule and resect the bone on the tibial side as much as necessary. At the end of the operation, we try to achieve in extension a light tension in the medial and the posterior part.

*Miller*: So if you have a valgus deformity you do a lateral release from the femur?

*Engelbrecht*: No, we always perform medial and lateral release of both ligaments.

*Miller*: Irrespective of which way the deformity is?

*Engelbrecht*: Yes.

*Miller*: And additional tibial bone to help correct flexion of contracture?

*Engelbrecht*: Yes. The correction of deformities is performed immediately by the system. The stem has a valgus of 6° and in addition we have three templates. I believe that in particular the long thin stems help the surgeon enormously in daily practice.

*Miller*: Dr. Drobny, suppose there is a varus deformity of 20° which is not correctable, but there is otherwise quite a good range of motion. How do you correct this when you plan to use your linked prosthesis?

*Drobny* (Klinik Wilhelm Schulthess): As Dr. Engelbrecht has already said, we use the lateral approach to the knee in all GSP prostheses. We carry out a lateral skin incision, a lateral arthrotomy. We excise the cruciates, cut the lateral ligament, and the medial ligament posteriorly and obliquely until the gastrocnemius head. In this way, no problems with balancing develop.

*Miller*: You retain the skin, vessels, and nerves?

*Drobny*: Yes. The problem with this procedure is the high rate of infection, which is probably caused by the rigorous approach, with opening of the bone and debridement of bone from the outside and inside.

*Miller*: If, for example, my left knee is rather painful. I had an arthroscopy in November and am now a little better. My knee is perfectly aligned and has quite a good range of motion—125°. I remain perfectly aligned, perfectly stable, and continue to have full extension and flexion to 125°, but I need a knee replacement. Could I induce you to do a Total Condylar, a PCA, or some similar kind of knee replacement? Dr. Engelbrecht, do you ever do anything other than the sledge or St. Georg?

*Engelbrecht*: No. I do not have the right answer for the quality of the ligaments. I am uncertain because of our experience with surface replacement. This is a very unconstrained system; in this system, the stresses on the ligaments are the highest. But in a large number of our cases, there is good stability in the long term.

*Miller*: Dr. Drobny, you are developing a condylar knee. If I came to you with my knee, would I get the GSB hinge or a condylar knee?

*Drobny*: You would not get a GSB from me. At our clinic, we use a variety of criteria according to the stage and age of the patients. We carry out ostotomy; we do unicondylars and condylars.

*Miller*: Do you do Total Condylar?

*Drobny*: No, we do PCA in addition to our own system. We do GSB in severe cases.

*Miller*: Mr. Goodfellow, your indications with respect to varus deformity which is not correctable are very clear. You do your operation on knees that do not require ligament release or need very little ligament release.

*Goodfellow* (Oxford University): I believe there is currently an oversimplified view I often hear expressed, which is that the alignment of the human leg in the anteroposterior plane is the responsibility of the medial and lateral collateral ligaments only. This is not the case; it is the responsibility of all the ligaments, including the cruciates. The proof of this is to take a natural knee, divide the two cruciate ligaments, and then insert a distractor as used in Total Condylar replacement. The knee will be seen to go into varus. This is because the ligaments of the medial compartment of the knee are the medial collateral and posterior cruciate. The ligaments of the lateral compartment of the knee are the anterior cruciate and the lateral collateral. If you simply divide the anterior cruciate you release the lateral compartment of the knee and the knee goes into varus. And so it is the case, at least when I perform Total Condylar replacement, that I find myself performing medial release and this is not because the medial collateral ligament is too short, but because the anterior cruciate ligament has been ruptured and the lateral compartment of the knee is now too long.

*Miller*: If I came to you with my knee, which is very painful, there is a 15° or 20° fixed varus, but otherwise a reasonable range of motion, what would you do?

*Goodfellow:* What do you have—tibia vara or genu varum?

*Miller*: I have a little of each.

*Goodfellow*: There is a difference. Tibia vara is a state common in certain races, e.g., the Japanese, and cannot be corrected at the level of the knee. It is a common precursor of medial compartment arthritis. Genu varum is a deformity occasioned by loss of bone height from the medial compartment of the knee; it is usually acquired and can be corrected by intra-articular replacement. Tibia vara is a perfectly acceptable state of affairs, affects large numbers of the population, and is not universally associated with degenerative change; its presence does not preclude the use of a unicompartmental replacement. If genu varum, i.e., the deformity at the level of the knee, has become uncorrectable due to shortening of the medial collateral ligament, which is much less frequent than is generally believed, a medial soft tissue release has to be performed; a surface replacement arthroplasty is not applicable.

*Miller*: What do you do?

*Goodfellow*: A Total Condylar replacement.

*Miller*: Are you satisfied with the ligament stability that you have a year later, having done a medial release?

*Goodfellow*: If the medial collateral ligament is detached, the knee becomes unstable. The stability obtained after Total Condylar replacement owes very little to ligamentous tension; it is a consequence of the scar tissue that forms around and the fact that the components themselves are inherently stable.

*Miller*: Prof. Yoshino, I would like to ask you the same question. We have a patient with 15° of fixed varus, tricompartmental disease, and quite a good range of motion. The patient is a candidate for a replacement. What is your attitude with regard to the deformity?

*Yoshino* (Nippon Medical School, Tokyo): As I said in my presentation, I would use my system to correct the varus deformity.

*Miller*: How do you form the release?

*Yoshino*: We try to reconstruct the soft tissue that is appropriate for the knee joint. As I showed in my slide, we use Tensor for the alignment as well as for the tension, both medially and lateral. We measure the medial and lateral tension. Until we find a suitable position, we continue to release the ligament and soft tissue as much as possible.

*Miller*: I presume the medial soft tissues from the tissue are in continuity?

*Yoshino*: Yes.

*Engelbrecht*: I would like to stress that I do not sacrifice all the ligaments. I make a complete release; with the Total Condylar, there is a partial release. We are only able to combine the rest of the knee after resection of bone together with the implant. In this system, the point of rotation, the instant center, is predicted. The complete ligamentous apparatus adapts to the new system.

*Miller*: You release and it then reestablishes itself in harmony with the rotary mechanics that you impose on the knee?

*Engelbrecht*: Yes.

*Miller*: Dr. Goldie, how would you deal with a 10° or 15° fixed varus? You use one of Mr. Freeman's many knee designs?

*Goldie* (Karolinska Institutet): Yes, I use the mark II. Part of the surgical procedure is to resect tibial bone and to detach the deep portion of the medial collateral ligament; this puts the knee into alignment without difficulty if there is only 15° of varus. Healing of the soft tissue structures helps the knee to regain stability.

*Miller*: Do you think there is a danger of overreleasing? If you take the medial complex of the tibia can you release excessively, assuming that you release in continuity subperiosteally?

*Goldie*: No, I do not think so. My experience in rheumatoid arthritis has shown that there is good healing and transferring that to osteoarthritic patients I find it is almost the same.

*Miller*: Mr. Goodfellow has presented a knee which in principle is the most attractive in the world. The main case for it aside from the physiological movement is that it diminishes polyethylene wear and debris. What is the effect of polythylene wear and debris in the total artificial knee? And what are also the effects of metallosis? Mr. Goldie, do you think as knees improve and last for 10 or 15 years that polyethylene debris is going to become a problem?

*Goldie*: No, I do not think so.

*Miller*: There is a feeling that this is going to be a problem with the hip.

*Goldie*: This has not really been substantiated; there is a great difference between fact and feeling. In experimental work with rats, the animals were subjected to very large amounts of polyethylene flakes and subsequently developed sarcoma. This situation is not comparable with the human reaction to polyethylene debris. With regard to metallosis, this has also been reported to cause damage to the tissues. The question is, however, whether this has any symptomatic or pathological importance, because we see many patients with metallosis but with no symptoms whatsoever from the inserted foreign material. In patients who have symptoms and we remove the foreign material and observe metallosis, we ascribe the symptoms to metallosis without really knowing if that is in fact the case. So, there again, I do not think there is any great danger in metallosis.

*Miller*: Dr. Engelbrecht, what do you think of debris in the knee joint? We saw some X-rays today with the synovium filled with debris. What are the practical implications of this?

*Engelbrecht*: In the knee arthroplasty that we have used up to now, this has not been a problem. I would imagine also that in the future it will not be a problem.

*Miller*: Willert has made the point that the reticuloendothelial system very quickly becomes saturated in removing debris, and granulomas begin to form. Dr. Drobny, have you observed osteolysis surrounding any of your knees?

*Drobny*: Yes, I have.

*Miller*: Do you think that this is polyethylene debris, metallosis, or something else?

*Drobny*: I do not know.

*Miller*: Mr. Goodfellow, how much polyethylene debris is deposited with your knee design?

*Goodfellow*: With regard to debris, it may not matter a great deal in Total Condylar replacement. In unicompartmental arthroplasty, it is difficult to believe that it is not important—having within the same synovial cavity components that are shedding quantities of HDP. This would clearly seem to be bad for the rest of the joint. There is evidence published by Dr. Larsson some years ago in failed unicompartmental arthroplasties in which he found the articular cartilage on the retained side was peppered all over with pieces of HDP. The amount of debris is I believe related to the load and to the area of contact: The heavier the load, the greater the wear. You cannot do anything about the load, but you can do something about the area of contact. The rate of wear for the Oxford knee is 1 mm in 27 years, based on about 18 collected components. This is because the area of contact is 7 $cm^2$, which is twice as big as a Charnley hip. So the amount of debris should be very much smaller than with the sledge components we saw today.

*Miller*: Prof. Yoshino, what is the feeling of yourself and the Japanese orthopedic community generally about wear debris in the knee? Obviously, this is a matter of some concern.

*Yoshino*: In geometric total knee replacements that had been inserted for over 10 years, we carried out autopsies on some of the patients. We rarely observed HDP wear. The alignment was very good in these patients. Several years ago, Prof. Fukubayashi and I recovered tibial components and studied the geometry of the joint surface. In some of the cases, alignment was poor and loosening occurred. In these cases, the HDP wear seemed to be worse. We have never used alumina prostheses.

*Miller*: I think Prof. Yoshino has raised a good point here. With a well-aligned knee that it is not loose, we do not know what is happening with respect to polyethylene unless we study postmortem speciments.

*Goldie*: Yesterday, as the PCA was being discussed we heard about the beads coming loose. This caused some alarm initially. But I think that the report from Dr. Hastings yesterday proved that so far it does not seem to have caused the patients any harm and there have been so signs of pathological changes. It would be interesting to hear if Dr. Krackow has any information on this.

*Miller*: I think he talked about this yesterday. He counted every bead on the tibial plateau and pointed out that very few of them had come loose. I believe it is quite clear that there are no reports of knees which have been damaged by loose beads. Perhaps in 5 years, we will have definitive evidence.

I would now like to raise the issue of pain in a knee that is not loose and is well aligned. I was rather surprised to see in I believe it was Dr. Engelbrecht's paper that a fair number of patients even with your most modern design have some pain; sometimes, this occurred in cases in which you dealt with the patella well. There were also some cases in your series Mr. Goodfellow, and there were some in mine. What is the explanation of pain in the well-fixed, well-aligned, well-designed prosthesis with a good range of motion and good muscle strength?

*Engelbrecht*: Stability is an important factor. We found in many cases that even slight instability with our surface replacement can cause pain. In addition to this, there may be residual pain in the patellofemoral joint. Most of our patients can tolerate this residual pain. Other pain arises from the intrapatellar branches of the nervus saphenus because our approach is from the medial side. To prevent this, we try to resect all visible branches in the subcutaneous area.

*Drobny*: Pain is a subjective assessment and is the only factor in the evaluation method that we cannot measure. There are many possible sources of pain, e.g., from the soft tissue, dystrophy of the bone. If there is no objectively detectable cause we can only speculate.

*Miller*: Dr. Yoshino, do you have any comments on the perfect knee arthroplasty that still has pain?

*Yoshino*: After artificial surface replacement, we have encountered cases of popliteal pain. We investigated the cause of this pain. Where the popliteal tendon was stretched, we cut the tendon and reduced the pain.

*Goodfellow*: It seems to be a common assumption, particularly I think among North American surgeons, that all patients who complain of pain after total knee replacement have the pain in the patellofemoral joint. But we heard today about a group of patients in whom the patellofemoral joint was not replaced the relief of pain was just as good as in those series in which the patellofemoral joint was always replaced. I was surprised at Peter Walker being astonished at a surgeon wanting to keep a normal patellofemoral joint since he apparently is convinced that the joint should be replaced under every circumstance.

*Miller*: Members of the audience, how many feel that in doing a total knee arthroplasty the patellofemoral joint should be resurfaced in every case? How many feel that total knee arthroplasty can be done frequently without resurfacing the patellofemoral joint? The numbers in the audience are about equal.

I would like to discuss three categories of pain. There is a population of patients who have cementless knees and who have some vague pain; this pain can be compared with the pain around the cementless total hip. I believe that as we improve our surgical techniques, this problem will diminish. I am rather surprised to find another category of pain, which includes patients who have pain around the origin of the lateral ligament of the knee. I have treated these patients with cortisone injections and ultrasound and there has been improvement. The third category I first discovered in an article in the Journal of Arthroplasty: "Sympathetic neurovascular dystrophy following total knee arthroplasty"; one of the authors was Hungerford. The authors made the point that this type of causalgia may not in any way resemble classic causalgia and therefore may be missed. I have been aware of this diagnosis thoughout my career; I have seen a few patients with causalgia and treated them accordingly. However, having read this paper, three of my problem patients came to mind: They had pain to a greater or lesser degree and were discontent; none of them were typical of sympathetic neurovascular dystrophy. But on the basis of the recommendations of Dr. Hungerford and co-workers I sent them all to our anesthetist for epidural sympathetic block. All had dramatic though not necessarily permanent improvement.

*Drobny*: Prof. Yoshino, what was the preoperative range of motion of your patients? Was there any evidence among those patients of hyperlaxity?

*Yoshino*: The patients who were able to adopt the full squatting position did not necessarily have a good preoperative range of motion (ROM). The range of our postoperative ROM takes the form of a bell curve, the minimum being 90°, and the mean 120°. Thus, some patients would have an ROM of more than 140°. With respect to laxity, the ability to adopt the full squatting position is only possible with stability and good muscle strength.

*Miller*: I noticed that one of your patients at least was an older lady of about 60 years age. I would think that among Westerners there are very few 60-year-old women who are able to sit in that way. The population as a whole seems to have greater flexibility than a similar Western population.

# Keyword Index

# Author Index

MIX
Papier aus verantwortungsvollen Quellen
Paper from responsible sources
FSC® C105338

If you have any concerns about our products,
you can contact us on
**ProductSafety@springernature.com**

In case Publisher is established outside the EU,
the EU authorized representative is:
**Springer Nature Customer Service Center GmbH**
**Europaplatz 3, 69115 Heidelberg, Germany**

Printed by Libri Plureos GmbH
in Hamburg, Germany